Spinal Asymmetry and Scoliosis

Movement and Function Solutions for the Spine, Ribcage and Pelvis

HANDSPRING PUBLISHING

EDINBURGH

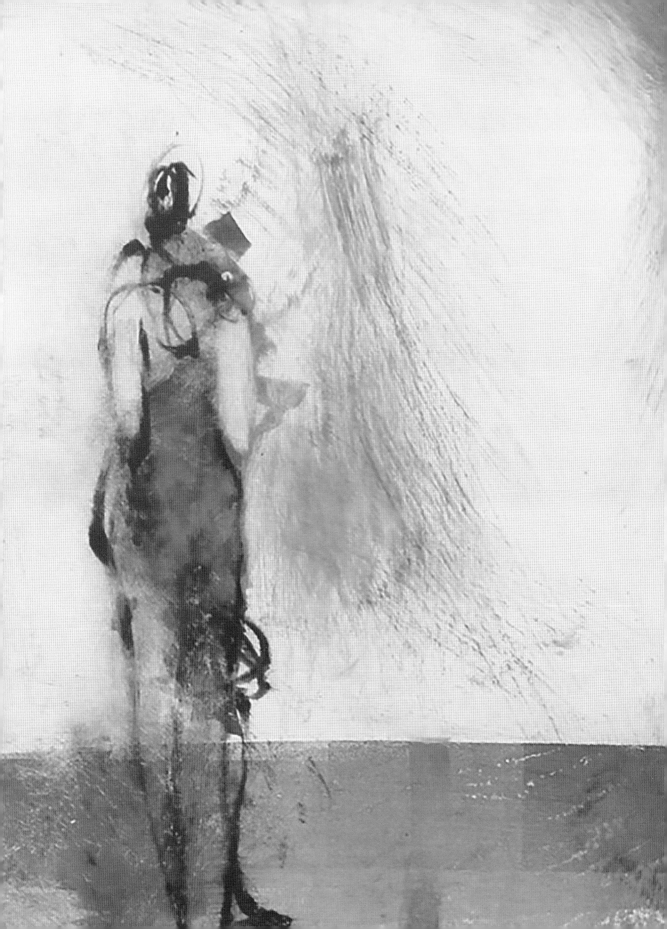

Spinal Asymmetry and Scoliosis

Movement and Function Solutions for the Spine, Ribcage and Pelvis

Forewords
Madeline Black
Lorna Roza
Richard Rosen

Suzanne Clements Martin
DPT, PMA®-CPT, CLT

Sole practitioner, Total Body Development

Founder, Pilates Therapeutics

Lead Physical Therapist, Smuin Ballet

HANDSPRING PUBLISHING LIMITED
The Old Manse, Fountainhall,
Pencaitland, East Lothian
EH34 5EY, Scotland
Tel: +44 1875 341 859
Website: www.handspringpublishing.com

First published 2018 in the United Kingdom by Handspring Publishing

Reprinted 2019

ISBN 978-1-909141-72-8
ISBN (Kindle eBook) 978-1-909141-73-5

British Library Cataloguing in Publication Data

A catalogue record for this book is available from the British Library

Library of Congress Cataloguing in Publication Data

A catalog record for this book is available from the Library of Congress

Notice
Neither the Publisher nor the Authors assume any responsibility for any loss or injury and/or damage to persons or property arising out of or relating to any use of the material contained in this book. It is the responsibility of the treating practitioner, relying on independent expertise and knowledge of the patient, to determine the best treatment and method of application for the patient.

Commissioning Editor Sarena Wolfaard
Project Manager Morven Dean
Copy-editor Lynn Watt
Designer Kirsteen Wright
Cover design Bruce Hogarth
Cover painting Brigitte McReynolds 'Windy Day' www.brigittemcreynolds.com
Indexer Aptara, India
Typesetter DiTech Process Solutions, India
Printer Melita, Malta

CONTENTS

How to access the online videos

Within this book you will find QR codes that will take you to Instructional Videos that accompany the text. These QR codes can be scanned with a smart phone using an app, and many free apps are available to download. If you are using an iPad or iPhone running the latest software (iOS 11 or higher) then no additional app is required. Simply open your camera and point it at the code (no need to take a picture). A notification should pop down from the top and then tap that and you will be taken to the video.

Dedication

AMDG

DISCLAIMER

The information provided in this book and its related resources is intended for educational purposes. The author and publisher are not responsible for:

Inappropriate interpretation and application of the knowledge, principles, and exercises provided.

Injury caused or related to use of this material to the user, the user's clients, or any other affiliated party.

The instructions and exercises presented herein are not intended to be a substitute for medical consultation. The author and producer disclaim any liabilities or loss of any third party, including the end user, in connection with the exercises and advice herein.

If you, as the end user, are a professional using this book and its related materials within the scope of your professional practice, you should follow all screening, assessment, and exercise guidelines as set forth by regulatory authorities governing your professional practice, including relevant certification and instructor competence. If you are not qualified to properly execute any of these guidelines appropriate to your scope of practice, it may be your responsibility to defer to a trained and qualified professional.

Please note that although the author has made every effort to provide current information, updates are continual and you, as end user, should be aware that practices and recommendations may change.

FOREWORD BY MADELINE BLACK

Life is the gift our body bestows upon us to be who we are and how we move through our lifetime. Living in modern times, we are maneuvering ourselves through the complexities and challenges of daily living from birth through death. Along the journey, our bodies are adapting, developing and embodying all that we experience. These experiences shape our physical body in the way we move, our emotional tendencies and the relationship of oneself to the external world. Health and wellbeing requires that we pay attention to our body and do the work necessary to maintain our body as best we can. Even when we are taking care of ourselves, the body brings us unavoidable issues to figure out how to heal. Physical issues arise for everyone. We rely on other human beings to provide us with guidance and methods for directing us toward a healthier body. These people are the professionals, who are passionate, educated and experienced in treatments and methods that bring us to wellbeing. Dr Suzanne Martin is one of these passionate professionals, sharing her expertise and personal history, restoring the spine towards health and function. *Spinal Asymmetry and Scoliosis* is an important source and guide for the movement educators who work with scoliosis and the clients living with scoliosis.

Scoliosis is a mystery to many, unless a direct known cause changes the spine. For most people, scoliosis is idiopathic – meaning there is no known cause. It may begin very early in childhood or adolescence, and it may manifest from our long-term habitual poor posture. Dr Suzanne Martin describes in detail all the possibilities through defining scoliosis, the evolution of scoliosis, the history of treatment as far back as 300 BCE to present, and the modern-day pioneers in scoliosis care. There are rich and important discoveries from our ancestors that provide us with their knowledge and skills to build upon. Recognizing the long history and energy given to scoliosis care is remarkable and useful today.

The growth of care for scoliosis has increased with so many choices and approaches for treatment. In this book, Dr Martin covers all the available medical and non-medical ways to shape a scoliosis plan for wellness. This source, both for the client and the movement educator, is valuable for referencing, empowering oneself with information, and choosing the appropriate path for the individual. She also defines the Pilates Method teacher's role as part of a team that includes practitioners ranging from the medical doctor, osteopath/chiropractor, physical therapist, and bodyworker specializing in fascia.

Asymmetry is nature and all our bodies move and function in an asymmetrical way. Scoliosis greatly emphasizes this fact and can become painful, degenerative and potentially life-threatening. Dr Martin describes the nature of asymmetry, how our preference for right- and left-hand dominance and redirecting it play a role in the development of our asymmetries. And most importantly, how we can use this to our advantage in training the body. Her foundation of the core link is key to addressing the optimal breathing, postural, spinal and pelvic health.

The Pilates Method Movement Educator holds a special place for the care of scoliosis. It is time for us to expand the knowledge base from the initial special population segment of the Pilates comprehensive training programs to fully learn the uniqueness of each person with scoliosis, the medical treatments such as bracing and surgeries, and how to create the individual movement programming for the scoliosis client. There is no one protocol. It requires education, participation and continued searching for the best design and approach to the client.

This book moves us beyond the treatment of scoliosis into learning spinal mechanics, the current functional movement concepts, and assessments specific to scoliosis. There are movement solutions for ergonomics, addressing the nervous system for change, and movement training with the Pilates Method. Dr Martin brings together the recent scientific studies of movement patterns, fascial relationships with the structures of the trunk that have both positive and negative biomechanical effects on the core, breath and spinal support. People with scoliosis are unique in their needs and physical being. She gives us a complete framework for reference and real movement tools to help us make the best and most effective choices for training.

Dr Martin offers a sensitive and gentle side too, bringing our awareness to the emotions of people with scoliosis. One emotion that may be present is grief from their not choosing an irregular body shape or from not having done anything wrong to cause the scoliosis, along with the limitations that come with it. She reminds us to have compassion and empathy.

Dr Martin asks us to "look past the typical curve patterns to discover the interplay of lateralization, preferences and biases along with their neurological aspects of perception shaping personality as a gift." I agree with her that there is never a dull moment and it requires the movement educator to be present, continually researching and learning in the quest to best serve the person relying on you to help them. *Spinal Asymmetry and Scoliosis* by Dr Suzanne Martin does just that.

Madeline Black
Movement Specialist and Author of Centered
January 2018

FOREWORD BY LORNA ROZA

We go about our daily lives observing people. How they walk. How they move. We observe sizes and shapes with wonderment. Why one person stands as tall as a skyscraper, defying gravity while another slouches, barely able to look up. Why one person stands with their head cocked to one side as if listening to the ground beneath them. While another stands with their trunk mysteriously rotated as if about to spin off into space. Expanding and contracting as we move through life. Filling our lungs, expanding our ribs. We wonder why nature is the way it is. What individual differences make us pose like a Rodin sculpture or drape voluptuously like Picasso? What shape is our spine upon whose stability we fundamentally depend? Dr Suzanne Martin offers us this magnificent book in which she takes us on a journey to explore the spine – that inner foundation at the center of our universe.

In 2014 I had the opportunity to meet Dr Suzanne Martin in The Pilates Therapeutics Scoliosis Specialization Program. I was taking her class for my Physical Therapy continuing education and my personal interest in scoliosis. I discovered that Suzanne started her career in the Dance Medicine Pilates program at Saint Francis Hospital in San Francisco and later went on to complete her doctorate in Physical Therapy. This was exciting news since my Pilates teacher, Elizabeth Larkham, also worked in the same program which was started by James Garrick, MD to provide Pilates-based rehabilitation in a clinical hospital setting on the West Coast. Suzanne fuses her experience and expression of dance with knowledge of Physical Therapy and Pilates, creating a visceral sensation of the inner workings of our body. She broadens our understanding of the effects of scoliosis, how to evaluate a client and recommend a plan of care. She cites research that gives us an in-depth view of anatomical changes in the ribs, spine and pelvis that can occur due to a lateral curvature in the spine. Suzanne demonstrates the effects of working on spinal alignment through movement, positioning and corrective exercises to target specific muscles.

My personal interest in scoliosis stems from my own history of developing scoliosis after a traumatic injury when I was 13. I fractured my thigh bone at the age when long bones are still developing. After being in traction for three months I had a leg length difference which caused scoliosis years later. I have always been very active and have a love of exercise and ballroom dancing. Scoliosis has influenced rotational changes in my pelvis and ribs. Listening to lectures and exploring movement with Dr Suzanne Martin, has given me the tools to work on spinal alignment and continue to keep myself strong.

Dr Martin's method of practice addresses the whole body as she describes how to evaluate functional mobility. She describes how one's preferential mobility in the trunk and pelvis may determine which muscles may be dominating to create or inhibit movement. These may be some of the deep core muscles that we target in the Pilates Method of strengthening. Suzanne has a keen eye for observation and vast knowledge to explain how the effects of scoliosis take shape in our bones, muscles and fascia of the spine and pelvis. She discusses how these effects can alter the surrounding tissues.

As a Physical Therapist working with the Pilates Method, I am always looking for new knowledge to add to my toolbox. Suzanne's wisdom and approach conveyed in this book and the Scoliosis Specialization Program has given me insight, direction and the confidence to work with patients that have scoliosis. This book is an amazing contribution to the practice of physical therapy and I am grateful to Suzanne for pursuing her depth of knowledge and interests in the topic of scoliosis.

Lorna Roza PT, CPT
Director, Physical Therapy and Pilates Services,
RehabPilates Physical Therapy and Pilates Inc.
Member, American Physical Therapy Association,
Orthopaedic Section
December 2017

FOREWORD BY RICHARD ROSEN

Welcome to the Scoliosis Team (hereafter ST). You likely didn't imagine you'd be joining a team when you picked up Suzanne's book, but now that you have, you're definitely on board. The idea behind the ST is to bring together a host of 'players,' not only professionals in the ancillary medical and fitness fields, but their clients as well, each with a 'significant role' to play in the treatment of scoliosis. While the ST includes a diversity of skills and experience, like every good team this one has a 'captain,' the Pilates Method Movement Educator (PMME), to whom the material in the book is primarily directed.

I should be clear before going any further that I'm neither a trained PMME nor medical professional. I suppose, as a yoga teacher, I'm considered to be a fitness pro, but I must confess that scoliosis has always been something of a mystery to me. My style of teaching, heavily influenced by the Iyengar method, puts a premium on proper alignment in the practice of the postures and when sitting for breathing and meditation. As you're no doubt aware, scoliosis inevitably creates a greater or lesser degree of imbalance, depending on the severity of the condition. My training at the Iyengar Institute in the early 1980s sought to correct these imbalances through the use of props, various blocks and wedges and straps and so on.

This approach works fairly well as a short term, stopgap measure, but it's effectiveness over the long haul has mixed results, depending again on the extent and history of the scoliosis and other factors, such as the student's willingness to work with the props and the given corrections regularly and attentively. Suzanne's book then, for someone like me, who after over 30 years of teaching is still an ST rookie sitting way down at the end of the bench, is akin to finding an expert 'coach' willing to help me improve all facets of my 'game.' I'm not familiar with any of the literature in this field, but I'd be very surprised if there's a book out there that surpasses Suzanne's grasp of the condition, its background, assessment, and curative approaches.

As an author myself, what also impresses me about Spinal Asymmetry and Scoliosis is the accessibility of its writing. As I'm not well versed in the more technical aspects of the causes of the condition and its treatment, I fully expected as I read the book to at times be in over my head. That really never happened. Suzanne's writing carried me along effortlessly as she generously provided me with a whole new set of scoliosis tools, which I suspect can profitably be applied to the needs of students who aren't necessarily dealing with scoliosis. I'm very pleased and honored that Suzanne gave me the opportunity to make this small contribution to her book, which I've no doubt is destined to become a classic in its field. In closing all that's left to say is, Go Team!

Richard Rosen, E-RYT
Latest publication – *Yoga FAQ* (Shambhala, 2017)
Berkeley, CA
June 2018

PREFACE

Discovering the 'Internal Alien'

I got my first glimpse of the Asymmetrical Internal Alien on an osteopath's treatment table.

As a dance graduate student in the late 1970s at Mills College in Oakland, California, my teachers sent me to the legendary osteopath Dr Muriel Chapman after a hard fall during a performance. Dr Chapman was a diminutive, older-than-yet-as-wise-as God persona who spoke very little yet exuded gravity of authority. My organs swirled under her incredibly gentle skin contacts. How and, most bewildering, why? It was as if I had something otherworldly, living and moving inside me. My journey toward self-discovery really began then, with that first serious dance injury and the work of Dr Muriel Chapman.

Several years later, after teaching at the ballet school that hosts the International USA Ballet Festival, I was driving to a guest artist gig at the University of Southern Mississippi. My pelvis was severely twisted after a four-day car trip. The faculty at USM directed me to the athletic training room where the football coach was a chiropractor. While working with him and his trainers, I had an epiphany moment. I turned to exercise systems I had studied in my Masters Program in Dance at Mills, Feldenkrais training and Bartenieff exercises, for somatic relief. My journey of learning continued.

More years later, while juggling five dance and fitness jobs in the Bay Area, I sought help for my old dance injury at the St Francis Memorial Hospital in San Francisco, where one of my fitness colleagues, Elizabeth Larkham worked. I was invited to join the newly forming Center for Sports Medicine's Pilates division, and thus was introduced to the Pilates Method with the studio founders as my mentors.

I grew up constantly on a swing, loving motion, and my family vacationed every year one block from the Mississippi Gulf Coast beach, where I spent hours somersaulting in the warm Gulf waves. Perhaps the accident in the waves likely set my pre-adolescent spine into its spinal asymmetry. My newly found Pilates practice had it all, spiraling motion with the aesthetics of the dance field I loved. Studying with Elizabeth and with Michelle Larsson, I finally understood that my body was different. Injuries and other factors had caused me to have deep-seated asymmetries, which I have come to think of as 'The Asymmetrical Internal Alien,' because they seem to take on a life of their own beneath the surface of the skin.

Fascinated to learn more, I sought out higher education. Pre-physical therapy study brought neurological concepts into sight with the focus upon balanced and unbalanced motor control. My teaching at home and dance studio became a magnet for those with asymmetrical movement and spines.

In PT school, cadaver dissection revealed the body's incredible infrastructure of connective tissue! It was at once reassuring and distressing! Connective tissue forms unwanted adhesions. Although school faculty encouraged me to give up 'this Pilates thing,' the Method remained my steadfast link between art and science. The more I heard not to not examine the whole body and instead focus upon one area of concern, the more committed my search became for comprehensive bodily order.

Convincing my faculty and co-investigators to approve my dance research of establishing expected functional range of motion was not easy. Surprisingly, as happens with most research, the study showed unexpected results: it was more about the asymmetries of the subjects rather than simply describing what range of motion is to be expected in elite level ballet movers. How satisfying to receive an award and peer publication on the first try!

Undeterred from continuing with dance and 'this Pilates thing,' asymmetry became my obsession. Giving presentations and workshops on high hip, low hip, and feet problems led me into specific scoliosis investigation. Pushing hard to uncover more spurred me to higher education in doctoral studies. I also studied the manual therapy techniques of myofascial release, strain counterstrain, visceral manipulation and cranial-sacral work, and obtained a certificate as a lymphatic therapist. The art of palpation, the art of internal body investigation, became my real-time ongoing anatomy lesson.

In my professional practice as a PT, I was determined to dive deep, and to become an educator as well as a therapist. My studio began to offer months-long programs and I began giving international intensive seminars in scoliosis study that became the backbone for what you read now.

Those of us with different bodies first and foremost want, and deserve, to live life to the fullest. I am convinced that lifestyle and the Pilates Method make this possible. Medicine's obligation is first and foremost to help the individual survive on a fundamental level. Every health field cannot be everything to all people.

Pilates is a piece of the pie that fills the gap that is otherwise impractical or even impossible to fill.

Whether you are an instructor, therapist, clinician or surgeon, my hope is that you will use the information here to instill hope for the myriad age groups who are alarmed, frightened, overwhelmed or lost, when they find out they are different, when they have an 'alien' of their own.

Dr Suzanne Martin DPT, PMA®-CPT, CLT

Pilates Therapeutics, Research and Educational Director; Smuin Ballet, Lead Physical Therapist; Total Body Development, Owner; Continuing Education Provider: Pilates Method Alliance/ California Nurses Association/California Physical Therapy Association; Center for Women's Fitness: Adjunct Faculty; Member: Dance USA, IADMS, PMA, PAMA, CPTA
May 2018

ACKNOWLEDGMENTS

Twenty years ago, my quest for asymmetry solutions began as an internal urge to know more. Ten years ago, I developed my first major scoliosis workshop. Eight years ago, the book pitch started. Five years ago, a formed plan took shape, encouraged by the Pilates community along with several of my faithful clients. Since then, it seems that countless people have contributed time and talent.

With a single conversation, my original Pilates training teacher, Elizabeth Larkham, spurred the evolution of the book that you see here now. Editors Hilary Mandleberg and Laura Daly generously scrutinized the first drafts, along with peer reviewers Lorna Roza, Kris Shevlin and Gail Perry.

Many program specialists and hosts helped to test the framework along with contributors for the detailed work of the last year of writing. Among them are Dr Kevin Vandi for the kinetic analyses, Dr Peter Lewton-Brain for his intention presentation, Dr Ross Pope and Dr Ian Stokes for their scholarly work and generous offers to use their illustrations, Dr Lawrence Lenke for permission to use his diagnostic classifications, and Jill Randal of Shawl-Anderson Modern Dance Center for support of the laterality study.

Technical expertise came from Mitch Silver and Stu Sweetow of Audio Visual Consultants in Oakland, CA; Eliot Kuhner and Ken Mendoza for photography; and the tireless work of Andy Berry for his excellent compilations of all the photographs.

Special thanks to models Autumn Alvarez and Hyun Jung Lee for their generous time and good spirits. Thank you to Lani Fung for her patient support.

Much gratitude for the final push goes to Madeline Black for her helpful insights and my dear husband Tom Martin for his unbelievable patience and excellent editing skills. My tremendous appreciation goes out to Sarena Wolfaard and the Handspring Publishing team for believing in the project, for helping me to see imagination brought into reality.

Imagine. Think. Feel.

REVIEWS

'As a student of Dr Martin's, I can recommend this book without reservation. Suzanne is a rare gem within the Pilates community. She is doing the hard work that we so desperately need in order to develop safe and effective programs for our clients. I, for one, cannot wait to introduce this book to my students.'

Derrick Cope PMA-CPT – Education Director, Synapse Pilates, Shanghai, China

'Suzanne has created a dynamic and comprehensive guide to understanding how to approach the challenges of spinal asymmetry due to scoliosis. It is based on her many years of personal experience in understanding the underlying scoliosis in herself and in others whom she has helped. This book will be valuable to anyone seeking deep insight of how to bring the spine into more balanced and supportive alignment.'

Diego Chia – Director of Core Fitness Physiotherapy Pilates Studio, Singapore

'As an ex-dancer and Pilates Instructor for the past 30 years, I am very thankful to have found Dr Martin. From the first workshop I took with her, I knew she understood to "always infuse art with the science." I had found the person who would take the emotional, mental and spiritual aspect of the body and see how the dysfunction from imbalances of these subtle bodies could impact the physical. Dr Martin has a heart to go with her incredible science and she brings that together impeccably in all her work. Movement instructors lucky enough to work with her will find the missing links – the whole, complete picture that develops over time in the human body. No short cuts, no random promises of miracles. Just well thought out, systematic, layer upon layer of information that makes our bodies, dysfunction or not, what they are. Dr Martin is a gift to our industry.

Carolyne Anthony – Owner/Founder of The Center for Women's Fitness LLC

'As one of the pioneers in combining Pilates with physical therapy for rehabilitation of dance injuries, Suzanne Martin DPT has managed to gift her knowledge to her readers in this book about the rehabilitation techniques she has developed for scoliosis. The book begins with a nice background on understanding the diagnosis of scoliosis and the multidisciplinary approach to managing scoliosis. The remainder of the book details Dr Martin's creative approach which uses aspects of somatization, imagery, Pilates, physical therapy, and breathing techniques to manage scoliosis. This book is beneficial to all who want a better understanding of scoliosis, especially for Pilates instructors and Physical therapists who work with patients with spinal asymmetry.

Dr Martin is well decorated in the field of Pilates and physical therapy as well as dance medicine. She has lectured nationally, internationally and contributed to the field through research. She travels regularly teaching courses to Pilates instructors and physical therapists on the various techniques that she has developed for a variety of conditions.

I have had the privilege to work closely with Dr Martin on several patients. Her ability to combine her knowledge of human movement as a dancer and Pilates instructor and her knowledge as a Doctor of Physical Therapy enable her to treat patients methodically and by using innovative techniques. Her ability to analyze and help correct the biomechanical flaws that underlie injuries enables us to collaborate successfully in caring for patients.'

Selina Shah MD, FACP – Team Physician for USA Synchronized Swimming, USA Figure Skating, USA Weightlifting, San Francisco Ballet School, Diablo Ballet, Oakland Ballet, ODC Healthy Dancers Clinic, Mills College

'Suzanne Martin's masterful book is your guide to spine asymmetry, an increasingly prevalent aspect of the human condition. Whether you live with spine asymmetry, know a family member with this condition, or have a student, client or patient who experiences spine asymmetry, Dr Martin's book is essential. Her clear explanations and superb illustrations illuminate every aspect of this complex condition.'

Elizabeth Larkam – Balanced Body Master Trainer & Mentor

'In the Pilates studio, we have many asymmetric clients, especially with scoliosis. In order to help them, the instructor must be educated. I was very enthusiastic to host Suzanne and learn more because more than half of my clients have Scoliosis since I first started teaching Pilates many years ago. Suzanne Martin's Scoliosis course gives detailed, deep and accurate guidelines. Movement involving science! I love her method. I was also inspired by her enthusiasm at every moment. I am grateful for such a deep study and glad to be with her. I hope that Pilates instructors are encouraged to learn Suzanne Martin's method to ensure that more clients are safe and receive effective training.'

Hyun Jung Lee – CEO and Co-founder of Epilates, Seoul, Korea

In her fascinating book, Dr Suzanne Martin shares the perspective about scoliosis from the fathers of medicine to the pioneers in early scoliosis treatment who gave us the terminology we use today. She skilfully gives us functional and creative exercises and backs up her information with case studies and scientific research. While this book is mainly for Pilates practitioners, all readers would benefit from this treatise on Lifestyle Medicine. *Spinal Asymmetry and Scoliosis* is one of the most comprehensive books about this very 'difficult to treat' condition that affects all ages. Scoliosis is explored with a multidimensional focus on musculoskeletal, visceral and fascial influences and interactions. It is a must read for all practitioners working with asymmetry and scoliosis.

Marika Molnar PT, LAc, FIADMS – President and Founder, Westside Dance Physical Therapy; Director of Physical Therapy for New York City Ballet and School of American Ballet, New York

'Appreciating the complexities of spinal asymmetry and scoliosis can be a daunting journey for experts and those discovering them for the first time alike. This book by Suzanne Clements Martin brings a fresh overview of the subject giving important keys to understand the reasoning and outcomes from a wide perspective of treatment possibilities. As well as offering positive take home advice for movement-based therapists in diverse domains of practice, she empowers the reader to continue their acquisition of knowledge while working within a multidisciplinary approach.'

Peter Lewton-Brain, Doctor of Osteopathy – Director, Pôle Santé de Danse, France

GLOSSARY

Imagery and cue legend

Breathe into – a body area, such as the face, the eyes, the ribs or the vertebrae, to describe direction of the breath toward an area, creating a mild activation or expansion in that area.

Bulldog or Push-up Plus Position – a quadruped position where the sternum is elevated with the scapulae engaged with the serratus anterior, the Adam's apple supported by the neck flexors, and the face plane looking down forward of the line of the hands.

Claw hands – a neutral, firmly held, cupped palm to hold hand grips or the foot barre to avoid wrist or hand injury.

Cones of the lungs – breathing from the bottom of the base of the imaginary cones upwards where the tips of the cones come above the clavicles.

Diamond of the hands – a position with the thumbs together and the index fingers touching, which is placed upon the pelvis to note whether the pelvis is in neutral rotation.

Duck hands – handling or supporting a client with the palm of the hand instead of gripping with the fingers.

Flat plateau of the pelvis – a neutral pelvis in supine.

Finding a back door – indicates that a modification or more deconstructed version of an exercise will help to eventually gain the full acquisition of an exercise.

Gills of a fish – an image to encourage posterior lateral breathing of the ribcage.

Headlights of the hips – using the facing of the anterior superior iliac spine (ASIS) forward to balance pelvic disorientation.

Hollow – the combined action of the lift of the pelvic floor fascial slings with the abdominals to create a small dip in the soft tissue just above the pubic symphysis.

Hollow/lift – the combined action of the activation of the pelvic fascial slings along with abdominals and spinal elongation.

Line of the spine – the imagined line of vertebral stability during the isometric compressions in Chapter 8. Since spinal asymmetry is not in a true line, it must be imagined.

Inner Envelope – a fascial lining inside the abdomen and pelvis, which fascially connects the respiratory diaphragm with the pelvic diaphragm.

Lizard hand – a position of the hand used in sidelying exercise to give support needed due to rotational imbalance or side flexion spinal weakness. The pads of the fingers are used instead of the palm so that the top shoulder does not protract forward.

Motorcycle shoulders – the use of both hands in tactile aid to gently pull client's skin away from the clavicles to facilitate lower trapezius use as if revving up a motorcycle.

Moving the spine like a chain – describes lumbo-pelvic rhythm, a smoothness of the coordination and transitions between the lumbar spine and the pelvis, since the sacrum directly connects to the spine, not the ilia. Optimally there is a smooth transition of flexion to extension, and the reverse when vertebrae when transitioning between a forward bent position and standing.

Navel to spine – a cue for the transverse abdominals to contract, not to be misunderstood with a cue for spinal flexion.

Over the fence – describes spinal flexion where the transverse abdominals are held tightly through the transition between the psoas flexion phase of hip flexion during a roll-down, roll-up or any spinal flexion activity. When performed with the coordination of the posterior pelvic floor musculature, this action supports the spinal motion in the transition between deep spine flexion to hip flexion.

Parachute of the pelvic floor – describes the lift potential of the anterior and posterior pelvic diaphragm coordinating with the internal fascia to elongate from the bottom to the top of the spine.

Pearls into sand – describes the compression of the soft tissue on the spine while the spine remains mostly neutral without resorting to strong spinal flexion or posterior rotation of the pelvis.

Pelvic Slings or Pelvic Parachute floating toward the head – describes the fascial connections from the pelvic diaphragm and pelvic floor musculature to aid internal organization for spinal protection during exercise.

Pelvic Spool – orientation which helps describe the alignment of the pelvis in relation to the trunk.

Protruding ribs – an asymmetry cue involving the shapes of the cartilage of the false ribs 8–10 that attach to the 7th rib cartilage, indicating a non-normal transition from one to another, perhaps due to fascial tightness or twisting, or muscle imbalances between the internal and external oblique abdominals.

Puppy Dog Prep – a preparation used in supine exercise to facilitate segmental head-to-shoulder, girdle-to-spine control when performing upper body spinal flexion.

Rooster hands – a position with the thumbs embracing the top nose bridge, the index fingers on the forehead and the little fingers touching one another. The hand hold is helpful to safely guide cervical rotation.

Semi-circle arc with the knees – imagine the knees are sliding inside an upside-down bowl to express the natural spiral motion of the leg as the legs move from one side to the other.

Smile lines – describe the lines of the gluteal folds between the lower gluteals and the upper thigh.

Solar plexus – a chest region literally in front of the diaphragmatic crurae at T12.

Tailbone heavy, head is heavy – describes the head-to-tail connection for full spinal engagement.

X to align the ZOA – two lines converging from the front to the back, one from the xiphoid to the sacral promontory and the other from the pubic symphysis to the anterior 12th thoracic vertebra.

ZOA – the Zone of Apposition of the respiratory diaphragm, an important zone and concept in connecting the upper body and trunk with the lower trunk and body. If the zone is non-optimal, it encourages the twist of spinal asymmetry by decreasing rib rotation, vertebral action, vertical head position and compromises pressures inside the thorax and abdomen.

1st Parallel – a position of the legs in standing where the second toe of each foot lines up with the mid-knee-cap and the mid-hip to create a pelvic archway of support for the lumbar spine.

4 diaphragms – describes the connective tissue of the level of the eyes (cranial), the ring above the clavicle and shoulder girdle (thoracic outlet), the respiratory diaphragm, and the pelvic diaphragm, which when acknowledged together allows more comprehensive trunk activation.

7 under the foot – where the weight is optimally placed on the sole of the foot, beginning with weight at the lateral heel, moving toward the great toe, then the fifth toe, inscribing the number 7.

9 areas of the visceral torso: Rubik's Cube – describes a useful geography of the lower ribs, waist and anterior pelvic region to break apart the waist into regions for more precise attention.

Introduction

A dancer's story

A young dancer sustained an audible fall on her pelvis during a graduate performance at a local college. Undaunted, and spurred on by the excitement of the mock fight in the choreography, she and her partner completed the piece, bowing appreciatively to the applause. Backstage, the concerned faculty quizzed the young woman as she came offstage, "That was a loud bump. We saw the bounce off of your pelvis. Are you all right?"

Young and healthy, the dancer laughed and shrugged it off as one more bump in the road. Three weeks later, the spasms came. The faculty directed care toward the local osteopath, a retired obstetrician still practicing osteopathy in the pool house of her Berkeley Hills home.

Within the treatment, the old healer laid the young client on her side. With seemingly light, yet obviously targeted touch, the physician created a swirl within the young dancer's internal viscera, providing much relief.

After the dancer resumed training in a few weeks, left hip pain began. This time, obtaining X-rays and an examination from the local orthopedist, the young dancer received a diagnosis of common hip tendinitis.

Weeks later, disabling back spasms during ballet barre alerted desk staff to carry the dancer out of the studio to rest. Once again returning to seek spinal X-rays, nothing seemed to be wrong. She was determined to become non-symptomatic and resumed fitness conditioning.

As she became less symptomatic, her work life brought her in contact with the Pilates Method. Training from Michelle Larsson, a protégé of Pilates Elder Eve Gentry, hit the nail on the head. She had scoliosis.

I was that young dancer. I have scoliosis.

Scoliosis

Scoliosis derives from *skolios*, the Greek word meaning 'bent' (www.dictionary.com/browse/scoliosis). Underneath the skin, an observer can see curving of the spine, indicating that the axial spine twists in a non-expected fashion. Scoliosis is a particular category of *spinal asymmetry*, and throughout this book, we will examine the world of asymmetries through the lens of scoliosis.

Scoliosis: the basic terms

Scoliosis is defined as *non-neutral* in relation to an expected *neutral*, centrally vertical, spinal position. Did you know that although its cause may be congenital, developmental, or degenerative, most cases are *idiopathic*, meaning of no known cause (https://www.spine-health.com/glossary/scoliosis)? That a medical diagnosis occurs at or greater than a 10° measurement (Levine, 2013)? And that most right-handed people experience a right spinal convex asymmetry and left-handed people experience one on the left (Cramer & Derby, 2005)?

Scoliosis is both a medical diagnosis and a basic body type condition, and the term includes both structural and functional asymmetry.

The curve of scoliosis takes time to develop, whether in utero, in the infant or child, in the second growth spurt of puberty or over a lifetime of physical experiences that lead to a spine veering from the normal vertical line (Mitchell Jr, 2002). In my case, as the young dancer described above, it was an injury that began the process. In my practice, I encounter scoliosis cases of all kinds.

As a medical diagnosis, scoliosis is traditionally confined to the *axial skeleton*, the part of the skeleton that consists of the bones of the head and trunk, where a deformity creates an *abnormal lateral curving of the spine* often accompanied by ribcage and pelvic deformities. As a condition, the entire body recognizes the disparity between form and function, striving to create detours weaving about blocked routes for motion.

Despite generally being considered a non-life-threatening medical or body type condition, scoliosis can mean exacerbations of pain, absence from work, diminishment of family roles, and loss of social engagement. How many cases are hidden within the staggering statistics of a general 80% prevalence of low back pain within the United States?

The National Scoliosis Foundation calls scoliosis a 'silent epidemic.' Scoliosis does not discriminate according to any socioeconomic, race or age group, although genetic evidence points to both Caucasian and Asian heritage prevalence. It affects infants, children, adolescents and adults worldwide. The foundation estimates roughly 2 to 3% of the general US population, about seven million people, mostly women, are affected by this condition (National Scoliosis Foundation, 2017).

The Scoliosis Team

In this book I will refer to the Scoliosis Team often. I want you, the reader, to think of yourself as a member of the Scoliosis Team, whether you are the patient, a Pilates Method Movement Educator (PMME), or ancillary medical or fitness professional treating the person with scoliosis. All members of the Scoliosis Team can have a significant role in the treatment of this condition.

I primarily address the PMME in this book, but I am also addressing all of the above. As with myself, one can be a PMME, a patient and a medical professional all at once!

PMMEs include Pilates instructors at every level, but for purposes of this book we assume that a PMME is certified and trained in the Pilates Method by a reputable certifying organization and trainer or trainers.

Some medical and health professionals add Pilates certification to their toolbox, and these would be considered PMMEs as well.

The Pilates Method and scoliosis

The time is perfect for PMMEs to move forward into their place within the Scoliosis Team, since the Pilates Method is a lifestyle resource offering the potential of wellness for all age groups.

The Pilates Method is an excellent movement adjunct for populations such as those with spinal asymmetry seeking specialized movement guidance of either a non-medical nature as well as medically therapeutic purposes involving *pre-habilitation* (before an impending surgery), during *rehabilitation* of a specific injury or surgery, and *post-rehabilitation* of that injury or surgery, usually under the supervision of a higher-level healthcare provider in medically acute situations. The Method stands alone in the forefront of core conditioning, with evidenced effects upon conditions of the spine and many other body parts affected by spinal asymmetry, such as shoulders, hip and legs (Keays et al., 2008; Bialek et al., 2009; Levine et al., 2009; Lin et al., 2010).

Scoliosis is a lifelong condition. Whether or not it is a medical issue, scoliosis and spinal asymmetry often converge with other health issues, conditions and diseases called *comorbidities*.

The Pilates Method in its variety of exercises and applications expands readily beyond general wellbeing exercise into very effective use for the overlap of chronic illnesses and conditions such as aging, cancer survivorship and neurological disorders, including Parkinson's disease, brain injury and even diabetes.

Lifestyle healthcare

A lifestyle approach to healthcare moves chronic non-disease conditions into a preventative model of healthcare, when active attention to lifestyle makes the difference in long-term health, especially when comorbidities come into play. A proactive approach includes judicious choices in nutrition, such as predominantly whole food plant-based meals, stress management, alcohol and tobacco control, sleep hygiene and healthy relationships in addition to exercise (What is Lifestyle Medicine?, 2015).

The Pilates environment is the perfect place for lifestyle exercise. Joseph Pilates advocated this approach in his classic book, *Return to Life*. Using the knowledge that was available at the time, he advocated spinal suppleness, heart control, lung control, hygiene, dry brushing (a lymphatic stimulation technique), sunshine, fresh air, good sleep and proper diet (Pilates, 1945).

Although the complexity involved with lifestyle influence on the special population client with spinal asymmetry appears daunting, every PMME has the ability to make a difference. This book will guide you.

Be the difference maker.

The wheelchair dancer

A young local dancer made an appointment with me for dance physical therapy and Pilates training. Upon opening the door and looking down my office door's four steps to greet her, my face fell, stunned to see a wheelchair. Assertively and a bit apologetically, she humbly requested not to be sent away.

As I welcomed her with trepidation, she assured me she needed no help entering the office. With halting steps, she began on the journey from her wheelchair onto and up the stairs, into the entrance. She then stumbled onto the nearby Trapeze Table. Thankfully it is situated close to the door.

Flipping her head repetitively to the right about every 15 seconds, she told her story. Given the verdict of 'it's as good as it will get,' she wanted more.

The next three years became for me one of the most unimaginable, fascinating journeys into the world of spinal instability, hypermobility and scoliosis.

Starting with an incredible story of vitamin B12 deficiency that left neurological damage, this young woman had already attained a dance career in her wheelchair. During our work together, her stability improved almost beyond recognition after undergoing intense exploration and training on the Reformer.

Very few people will present such a dramatic display. Many of us will see those with common curves under 20° and fewer cases of the neurologically involved

varieties of scoliosis. Helen Keller (1968) said, "Life is an exciting business and most exciting when lived for others." Every PMME can make a difference and have influence.

Everything worthwhile takes time

A recent high-wind storm in my neighborhood sent tree limbs and tree trunks toppling into piles on the back wall of a two-story Victorian house. Debris scattered far and wide damaging the fence, house and surrounding structures. Cleanup and repair had to happen.

Processes are journeys. Before accessing the debris, the workmen had to move a giant truck up an incline. Before the trunk could be removed, a crane had to be positioned. Before the trunk could be moved, a chainsaw had to chop it into pieces. Then the workers could haul it away.

Some journeys are best not rushed. No matter how much talent or resources, a baby cannot be produced in one month by getting nine women pregnant. To create a make-a-difference mindset, a number of *befores* must take place on the journey to equip the PMME.

Before a PMME earns the respect to influence those with spinal asymmetry and scoliosis, certain steps must occur. One must form the intent to grow. An intention of growth is a requirement before taking on any new course of action.

A number of obstacles keep many PMMEs away. Many assume professional growth happens automatically with the passage of time. Some believe the concepts and exercise sequences must be perfect before beginning to accept special population clients, being afraid of making mistakes. Still others expect to understand scientific material on the first time of exposure. Still others believe the time must be right before special population clients are added to the schedule.

The time is now

Learn a philosophy of influence that transforms exercise instruction from skill-focused movement acquisition into preparing the client with a framework for lifelong management. This client-focused process equips the PMME to possess the background, knowledge, technical tools and confidence to lead an effective win-win clientele interaction. The clients are coming. They are there already.

Transforming teaching into coaching allows the client to gradually assume responsibility by trouble-shooting how the lifestyle approach is mixed into daily life.

Begin simply.

The framework

Breaking down the framework philosophy for helping those with spinal asymmetry into several groups of three aspects makes the work memorable, explainable and understandable.

The Rule of Three is an ancient mathematical formula of proportion sometimes referred to as the Golden Rule. Architecture employs this concept of three, building efficient structures of proportion off of this basic rule.

Ergonomics, exercise and emotion comprise the Rule of Three for the client. Somatics, correctives and conditioning comprise the Rule of Three for the PMME. The Rule of Three also extends to the three points and planes that create the all-important unit of human physical function, fascia, discussed in Chapter 6.

Another important set of three, history, anatomy and asymmetry, begin the journey. Before addressing the client's asymmetry, learn from the past. Stand upon the shoulders of the scientists, researchers and PMMEs who came before you.

Scoliosis in history

Attention to spinal asymmetry, and the attempt to control or tame it, are not current phenomena.

Evolution studies to better understand the *Homo erectus* skeleton show evidence of axial skeleton asymmetry as far back as 1.5 million years in the Nariokotome boy skeleton (labeled KNM-T 15000).

The actual term *skoliosis*, meaning 'a bending' in Greek, appears throughout the writings of the Greek physician Hippocrates (460–376 BCE), in his treatise, *On Articulations*. Hippocrates presents many of the concepts, protocols and apparatus to treat spinal deformities like scoliosis that are remarkably similar to those that we use today in manual

therapy, and in the Pilates environment with both our Reformer and Trapeze Table. The Hippocratic ladder, much like a modern CoreAlign® Ladder, was a vertical ladder system used to elongate the spine. Hippocrates invented a horizontal table that also applied corrective pressure at three points (shoulder, ribs and pelvis) by means of straps (Hippocrates, 460–376 BCE).

The Greek philosopher Aristotle (384–322 BCE) gave the West the first written idea about how the human body moves and the organization of the human body. In *Parts of Animals* and *Movements of Animals*, his study of movement of the muscles shows how muscles create a geometric organization in order to create movements. Thus, Aristotle became the father of kinesiology, the study of movement.

Aristotle's *Progression of Animals* analyzes why different animals have different propulsive elements, "why some animals are footless, others bipeds, others quadrupeds, others polypods, and why all have an even number of feet, if they have feet at all." Aristotle concluded that no forward propulsion in the human occurs without the flexion of two limbs, and that symmetry is important to humans for optimal biped walking. His famous statement, "Life requires movement" was echoed by the modern educator, Moshe Feldenkrais, who said "Movement is life."

Claudius Galen (130–200 BCE) is the successor to Hippocrates and Aristotle, becoming the first recognized Western physician. Expanding and further developing spinal theories and practices, his *On the Usefulness of the Parts of the Body* assigned names used today by beginning the classifications for spinal abnormalities. His terms such as lordosis and kyphosis are retained today along with identification of spinal deformities in which the spine veers forwards, backwards or sideways out of a usual position, scoliosis. (Vasiliadis et al., 2009)

Pioneers in modern treatment

Many physicians in the past few centuries, most notably in the European community, researched, experimented and sought to understand better why spinal abnormalities develop and how to treat them. However, it is important to note three figures from the orthopedic medical community in the US who established namesake tests still in use internationally. These individuals along with their international historic predecessors and colleagues are to be commended as ground-breaking heroes.

Dr William Kane, Dr John Cobb and Dr Joseph Risser are perhaps the three most-used names in the history and current field of scoliosis medicine worldwide.

Dr John Cobb

Dr John Cobb codified present medical diagnosis terminology of scoliosis as a spinal line differing from the typical spine in its characteristic veering from the *central vertical spinal line* (CVSL) sideways into the coronal plane by at least 10° (Cobb, 1948). His radiographic measurement procedure remains the gold standard of diagnosis. Dr Cobb trained surgeons at the teaching Hospital for Special Surgery (HSS) in New York in the 1950s.

Dr David Levine, who studied under Dr Cobb, recounts the history of the HSS regarding the lengthy and arduous surgeries done in an effort to correct the spinal effects of polio and tuberculosis.

> *"In the time of Dr Cobb, surgeons used a full-body turnbuckle technique for curve correction. The child was bed-bound for about one year for the whole process. The patient first wore a cast from the head down to one thigh. We then cut the cast in half with a big tree saw and applied a metal screw-type lever called a turnbuckle on one side. Over a period of about five weeks, we turned the turnbuckle.*
>
> *This turning motion corrected the curve. The patient had to lie down in this cast for five to six weeks. After the curve was corrected, surgeons cut a window in the cast, through which they performed surgery. Since anesthesia in the late 1950s and 60s was limited, surgeries could not last longer than two hours, so several surgeries on one patient were staged at two week intervals. Recovery from surgery was often nine months. Finally, the patient needed to learn how to walk again before going home."*
>
> Levine, 2013

Many of the patients at that time were hospitalized in a sanitarium situation due to quarantine conditions for tuberculosis and polio. Dr Levine's article spurred a number of appreciative responses by older adults who were treated at the HSS. Although in contemporary

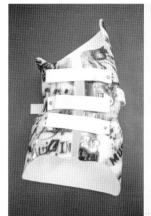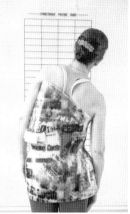

Figure 1.1

terms, these treatments may seem frightening and extreme, it is touching to note the positive experiences many patients reported, expressing gratitude for the care which allowed them to live normal lives. The contemporary 'night brace,' or nBrace, is remarkably similar to the one worn by patients in historic photographs of the HSS. Figure 1.1 shows me modeling the night brace of a recent client, a charming young adolescent woman who is a budding cellist.

Multiple braces exist on the market for the treatment of scoliosis. The nighttime brace creates a mirror image countering the spinal curves in contrast to daytime or around-the-clock braces that promote a more central vertical line (Ortholutions GmbH & Co., 2017).

The Harrington Rod procedure replaced the turnbuckle procedure in 1963 when Dr Wilson, Jr and Dr Konstantin Veliskakis first performed the procedure at HSS. Hooks attached a metal rod to the spine. An inserted wire then pulled the vertebrae together, straightening the curve. Next, bone chips harvested from the pelvis or the spine are inserted to fuse and to heal the abnormal curve into one vertical relatively straight fused bone. The rod serves to keep the vertebrae in place until the bones achieve fusion and healing. Some clients remove their rods later.

Originally the lumbar region was set into flexion to try to lessen the spinal rotation. Contemporary

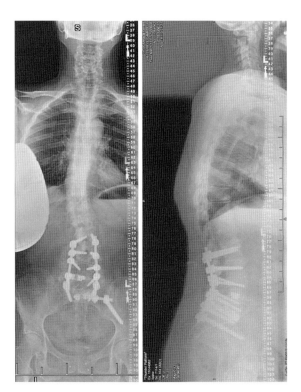

Figure 1.2

surgeries are now more variable in their use of metal as well as attention to preserving the normal lumbar lordosis (Levine, 2013). Figure 1.2 shows X-rays from one of my recent clients. Notice the bolt affixing the ilia to the hardware. The rod or fixation is not enough to keep the torso erect. Clients like these need a special approach for active work. Chapter 12, on individual programming, contains ideas on how to work with this population.

Dr William Kane

Dr William Kane is an orthopedic surgeon who helped establish the Scoliosis Research Society. He began research on establishing the normal expected level of spinal asymmetry as a response to an article published by *Time* magazine in 1975 titled *A dangerous curve*, which produced a heightened public perception of scoliosis.

This article somewhat sensationally focused on several individuals with more extreme conditions. Reportedly, Dr Kane's concern with the article was that

the public would see any spinal asymmetry to be as life-threatening as those described in the article.

Dr Kane found that a marker of 10° or below, as measured on a standard radiograph, should be regarded as an expected physiologic measurement, within the normal limits range of deviation. Ten degrees remains the contemporary standard.

His standard of curves greater than 10° warranting medical surveillance along with implementing bracing and more frequent medical observation at 20° for an immature individual is still in use today (Kane, 1977).

School screening in the US

Controversy continues to exist over the emphatic public health call for school screening caused by the 1975 *Time* magazine article, *A dangerous curve*. In 2004, the US Preventive Services Task Force authorized an end to scoliosis screening in US public schools.

However, international healthcare providers and scoliosis societies differ in their opinions regarding the continuation of implementing school screening. A trend observed in my teaching travels outside the US is that a number of nations no longer carry out screening programs. Some of my clients still report school screening here in California, usually in private school settings.

When the mid-twentieth century discovery of antibiotics and vaccines essentially eradicated polio and tuberculosis, diseases historically associated with scoliosis, surgeries such as those related by Dr Levine at the HSS diminished in frequency due to reduced necessity for spinal correction.

The American government remains conservative in the belief that public health fears associated with spinal curvature as being a sure sign of disease or disability never fully dissipated. The term scoliosis may still be misunderstood by the American public as a 'dangerous curve,' fostering non-useful interventions (Linker, 2012).

The Cobb angle: measuring scoliosis

I refer above to the pioneering physician Dr John Cobb. In this book I make frequent reference to the Cobb angle. The Cobb angle is a measure of the curvature of

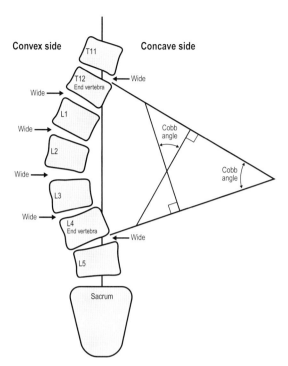

Convex side

Concave side

T11

T12
End vertebra

Wide

Wide

L1

Wide

Cobb
angle

L2

Wide

Cobb
angle

L3

Wide

L4
End vertebra

Wide

L5

Sacrum

Figure 1.3

The Cobb angle is measured from the top vertebra
of the curve to the bottom vertebra. These two lines
meet at a perpendicular point, called the Cobb angle.

the spine in degrees, which helps a physician to determine what type of treatment is necessary. A Cobb angle of 10° is regarded as the minimum angulation to define scoliosis. PMMEs should be aware of the measure of the Cobb angle when planning an exercise regime. A radiologist draws two perpendicular lines, one from the upper end and one from the lower end of the curve. The lines that intersect give the degree of spinal curvature, the Cobb angle (Figure 1.3).

Minimal curvature

Long-term studies of up to 50 years indicate that *adolescent idiopathic* (of unknown cause) scoliosis shows that the medical consequences, involving *morbidity* (severe illness) or *mortality* (death), over a lifetime are minimal for smaller degrees of curvature (0–30°).

Perhaps the main issues at this level of severity are the cosmetic effects of the deformity, along with functional issues and soft tissue compensations. Even at the beginning of the moderate severity level of a 40° Cobb

angle, actual medically significant physiologic consequences are not seen, although the cosmetics and compensations increase.

The greatest impact medically appears upwards of 80° of Cobb angle measurement. Even at this level of potential obstruction of breathing capacity or actual breathing mechanics does not compare with the life-threatening effects of other long-term cardiopulmonary diseases.

Despite his introduction of the 'dangerous curve' idea, Dr Kane's research inadvertently paved the way for management of this condition through exercise, by beginning the conversation that scoliosis in and of itself is not necessarily fatal or always medically severe (Weiss et al., 2013).

Case example

A woman with an energetic voice on the phone explained she had an 80° Cobb angle. Her physician recommended she contact me. She explained she had no pain but wanted some exercises.

A diminutive force of nature of Asian heritage bustled into my studio. The top of her head literally veered toward the side wall. At 71 years of age, she had been a nurse and reared two, now grown, children. With co-conditions of menopause, osteoporosis and intermittent lung infections, she still did many of her chores and attended social events. She had stabilized in youth with a 40° curve. Unable to comfortably lie flat, sitting and standing became the session focus after assessments. Targeting balance and body awareness for beginning goals, we set out in sitting and standing training using the Chair. By the end of the session, she better understood some body skills on which to focus for balance.

Dr Joseph Risser

A third figure in our historical study, Dr Joseph Risser, established the gold standard test in 1958 for determining whether a youth's skeleton is at risk for scoliosis progression, a worsening of the curve.

Until Dr Risser's study, the carpal bones of the wrist were used to determine the full closure of a youth's skeleton. He argued that the last ossification centers of the skeleton are the iliac crests and ischial tuberosities of the pelvis, not the carpals, and are easier images to observe. His study confirmed through rigorous testing that most subjects at risk for curve progression did not continue to progress in severity of curve once the growth plate was fully ossified (Risser, 2010).

Adult scoliosis progression is another matter. Although Dr Risser's score indicates a likelihood of minimal progression upon reaching maturity, it does not address a full life span. Once fully developed, an adult undergoes the physical burdens of life with a spinal abnormality.

Although the condition of scoliosis may not cause further illness or death, the asymmetry may cause more pain and limit physical participation if not checked over time. Once the spinal curve begins to progress, the waist may collapse at a rate of 1° per year. The previous case of the diminutive woman with the 80° Cobb angle illustrates this point.

The progression scale or care of the adult with scoliosis is not as medically well defined as for the adolescent. Progression at any age occurs at a Cobb angle increase upwards of 5°. Stemming this progression in an adult focuses on the avoidance of the collapsing waist causing a severely flexed spine (Kim et al., 2010).

General stretching or tissue softening methods are not advised at this time to limit de-stabilizing the spine. Instead, the recommended exercises focus on increasing neuromotor control to counteract the gravity force of flexure, along with extension posture promotion, in essence, functional control of asymmetry (Silva & Lenke, 2010).

The nature of asymmetry

How is asymmetry an essential part of nature, our material world, our human body? Human asymmetry strives toward symmetric balance within its asymmetry, since as Aristotle noted, symmetry is essential for function and locomotion.

Did you know that the embryonic neural tube with its emerging central spinal system is intact in utero by the fourth week after conception, often before the knowledge of pregnancy awakens within the mother?

How does it happen that vertebrate bodies develop asymmetrically along three axes: superior to inferior (top to bottom), ventral to dorsal (belly to spine), and left to right?

Polarity, the disparity of positives and negatives, are the push and pull of predetermined asymmetric processes, similar to cells, which migrate to unite through a lock and key system as in a jigsaw puzzle, to form shapes, textures and functions of each group of tissue cells, culminating in a unique organ system. The spine and its nervous system, connecting head to limbs, lie at the heart of this overall scheme. Human movement emanates from the spine (Bryant & Mostov, 2008; St Johnston & Ahringer, 2010; Moore & Persaud, 1993).

Normal asymmetries in the body

Look underneath the skin and muscles of the abdomen and chest to see a normal asymmetric arrangement. Each body has one heart lying to the left side of the chest. The liver borders inside the right-most internal ribcage and extends like a large pancake underneath the left breastbone. The lobes of the lungs differ in size, amount and position from one side to another. The complete right lung is slightly larger than the left and has three lobes, whereas the left comprehensive lung has only two lobes to accommodate the girth of the heart. The resulting right lung then has a higher volume and weight, than that of the left lung, affecting the symmetry of the respiratory diaphragm. These disparities can, in fact, be some of the driving factors in spinal asymmetry.

If we are normally asymmetric inside of the ribcage and the abdomen, how is it that what appears externally to be a symmetric body is indeed not?

How is it that despite the visceral asymmetry, the normal spine possesses the appearance of a straight CVSL when observed from behind?

Closer inspection underneath the body surface reveals the enormous variety of the shapes of the vertebrae from one region to the next. Entwined and anchored by interlocking bony shapes, stability and collagenous strength give mother-of-pearl-like sturdiness combined with the mobility of a snake.

Each spinal region possesses unique characteristics, creating function out of form. Yet function can also dictate form, especially in a young undeveloped body (Ritchie et al., 2009).

Form and function

The spine

Every PMME should know that the *axial skeleton* (the part of the skeleton that consists of the bones of the head and trunk) is made of 33 vertebrae of the vertebral column, 12 associated ribs interlocking with three bones in the sternum and summing up with the 22 bones of the skull. The spine is an anchor for the activity and use of the limbs, guided by the gravitational pull of the head.

In referring to the vertebrae, we use initials for the region of the spine where they occur: **C**ervical, **Th**oracic, **L**umbar and **S**acral; and a number for where they occur in the region. For example, T1 therefore refers to the first thoracic vertebra.

What is often overlooked is that each vertebra has common characteristics along with certain variations from region to region that help to dictate the function of the vertebra.

What about the pelvis? Although technically the pelvis is not a part of the scoliosis definition, attention to its form and function definitely has ramifications into the spine as well as the legs.

Of the roughly 206 total bone count in the body, how many figure critically into the issue of spinal asymmetry and its ramifications? Three areas of natural structural asymmetry occur in the head, one in the respiratory diaphragm area and the other in the pelvis. All can have significance in scoliosis.

From the head, with its 22 bones composing the skull, spill arteries, veins, nerves, inner fascial network and lymphatic vessels, all down the stem of the neck, emptying into the thoracic inlet, a ring of soft tissue and bone forming a convergence where the cervical spine meets the torso.

With some exceptions such as the C1, each vertebra generally has a body, lamina, pedicles, transverse processes, spinous processes and facets. The angles and orientations of the interlocking pieces of the vertebrae dictate their basic movement patterns and uses. One vertebra cannot operate without the cooperation of the others on either side, a system called a motion segment.

The cervical region

Each vertebral column region has its purpose, shape and function. Note in Figure 1.4 that the seven cervical vertebrae are more flat in shape and as a whole slope in a 45° angle to the transverse plane. Besides allowing a liberal amount of rotational swiveling one upon the other, a forward telescoping capability occurs due to their sloped orientation in the frontal plane.

This is a reason why the forward-head phenomenon is so prevalent. Cervical vertebra can slide straight forward and are held in check by the soft tissue constraints of fascia, ligaments, tendons and muscles (Agur, 2013).

The thoracic region

The thoracic region is special with its connection to the sternum, creating a full ring-like effect from one side of the ribs to the other. An important connector between the weight of the head and the trunk's center of gravity at S2, the apex of the thorax at T8, is a critical element in finding functional solutions for gravitational spinal curve management.

Each level of the anterior sternum cartilage serves as a connector to the opposing ribs and provides a flexible structure for the ever-changing optimal internal pressures driven by the respiratory diaphragm. The bodies of the vertebrae in this region are smaller than in the lumbar spine since the ribcage provides the perfect suport structure to protect the all-precious heart and lungs. The vertebrae here are unique in their beak-like spinous processes.

See how the lengths of the processes increase in Figure 1.4 beginning at the neck at C7 to the apex of the thoracic region at about T8. Figure 1.5 shows that they function with great rotational ability like rudders in a sail boat, allowing muscle and fascial attachments to create a comprehensive swiveling action, rotating each ring of the ribs. This is a critical element in the development of scoliosis, where a rotating force may be reinforced by the musculature attached to the

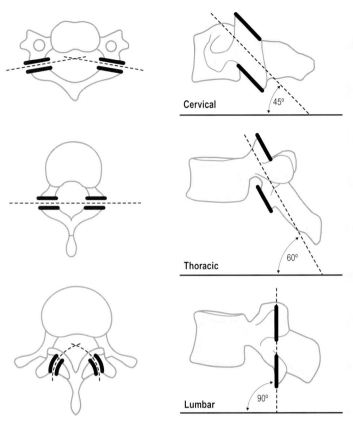

Figure 1.4

Note the differences between the facet orientation angles of the spinal regions.

Cervical 45°

Thoracic 60°

Lumbar 90°

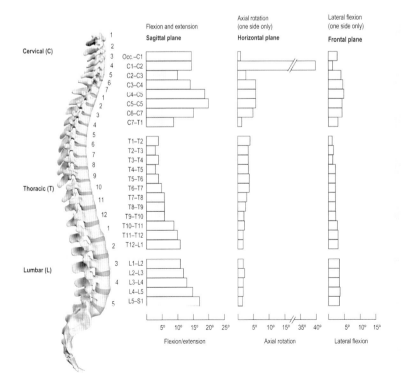

Figure 1.5

Note the degree of average ranges of the different regional areas.

Flexion and extension
Sagittal plane

Axial rotation
(one side only)
Horizontal plane

Lateral flexion
(one side only)
Frontal plane

Cervical (C)

Occ.–C1
C1–C2
C2–C3
C3–C4
C4–C5
C5–C5
C6–C7
C7–T1

Thoracic (T)

T1–T2
T2–T3
T3–T4
T4–T5
T5–T6
T6–T7
T7–T8
T8–T9
T9–T10
T10–T11
T11–T12
T12–L1

Lumbar (L)

L1–L2
L2–L3
L3–L4
L4–L5
L5–S1

5° 10° 15° 20° 25°
Flexion/extension

5° 10° 15° 35° 40°
Axial rotation

5° 10° 15°
Lateral flexion

vertebral segment and level. In addition, alterations in the ribcage affect what is called the *zone of apposition* (ZOA) from T8–L1, the functional area for the respiratory diaphragm.

Is it possible for asymmetric bodies to find side-to-side balance within the ring? Think of the two sides of the moving rings. Ideally both sides of the ring should elevate and lower at the same time. However, it is also possible to form a wave-like effect from one side to the other. Optimizing the ZOA is an essential component for function solutions (McKenzie et al., 1994).

Case example

A woman called about her adolescent son who had just undergone thoracic surgery to re-shape his concave sternum. As a nurse and PMME, she looked for familiar help. Her son had only mild scoliosis, but had insisted on ribcage straightening, a known procedure that other young people had undergone. The goal was to keep a metal bar underneath the sternum for two years to help the sternum achieve a better shape. We began Pilates exercises with mat and apparatus, the mom accompanying me for safety. As we worked together, the bar caused complications that finally meant mandatory removal. After the bar was removed the boy recovered quickly with the resilience of youth. For the next two years, we built him up through Pilates, and he has made excellent progress.

The lumbar region

The lumbar spine region, the waist, is vulnerable. With no bony help between the ribs and the pelvis, this situation creates a susceptibility for collapse, muscle imbalance and fascial distortions in the soft tissue, often disturbing the internal pressures of the abdomen and the all-important thoracic pressure associated with the anterior bowstrings of the respiratory diaphragm (Kleinman & Raptopoulos, 1985).

Figure 1.4 shows the vertebral facet orientation here is a full 90° perpendicular to the transverse plane, blocking most rotation. Figure 1.5 also illustrates that the lumbar region's 45° orientation to the frontal plane freely allows flexion and extension. Thoracic

spine and pelvic/hip stiffness produce more motion in the waist, leading to undesirable effects of lumbar spine motion segment wear and tear. This is why a supple thoracic and hip region helps keep the lumbar spine safe.

The pelvis

The pelvis houses the last two regions of the spine, the fused sacral segments and the coccyx. Because of its large structure, the pelvis is often viewed as an immobile, impermeable block. Yet closer observation reveals domino-like motion around the bones of the pelvic ring among the sacrum, ilia, femurs and lumbar spine.

The relation of the bone shapes here exert a strong effect on whether the spinal curves above the pelvis will achieve the true 'S' shape. A measure used by surgeons to determine balance of proportions in the pelvis and hip joints is called the *pelvic incidence* (PI). It is a relationship between the sacral base and the acetabular hip joints. The PI is the main axis of the sagittal balance of the spine. Looking at this distance helps to understand the importance of the lumbar spine lordosis in those with scoliosis. A low level of PI (smaller distance from sacral base to femoral heads) is associated with less lumbar lordosis (Figure 1.6). Less lumbar lordosis is associated with scoliosis.

Apparently, the PI influence goes both up and down the spine. Less lordosis is associated with vertebral axial rotation. The higher a severity of scoliosis rotation, the more restricted the lordosis is and less able to adjust to other level spinal changes (Legaye et al., 1998).

Did you know that it is possible that one side of the pelvis may possess non-equal measures from side to side versus actual bone shape asymmetry? That each side is not a mirror image?

Three-dimensional imaging reveals that each side of the pelvis, for instance the right iliac bone and the right part of the sacrum, is not necessarily a mirror image of the comparable bone areas on the left. The functional implications of such discrepancies occur in the pelvic-to-leg function. Pelvic asymmetry essentially follows a spiral path where the upper part of the iliac blades move in a clockwise fashion while the lower part with the pubic symphysis rotates

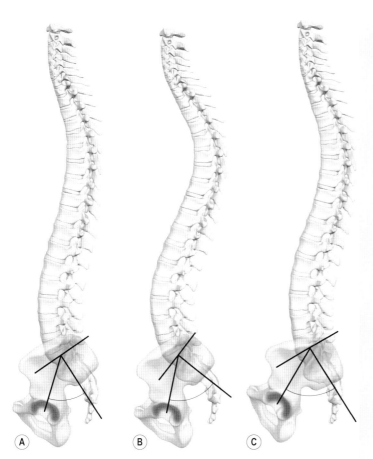

Figure 1.6
Relationship of pelvic incidence to amount of lumbar lordosis. Low angle of pelvic incidence is associated with development of scoliosis. Note the subtle differences in the three models. Generally we are looking at the shapes of the sacrum (how curvy or flat) and their relationship to the sacral promontory (base), the low lumbar (L4–L5) vertebrae, and femoral head distances along with their accompanying gravitational loads. The idea is to see how slight anatomic differences either potentiate or diminish lumbar curvature. Place a pen vertically at the acetabulum toward the cervical spine. See how (A) shows less lumbar extension due to the flattening of the lumbar curve, (B) shows too much lumbar extension and (C) shows the most normal acetabular to lumbar ratio.

oppositionally due to bone shapes. In addition to individual pelvic bone rotation, the entire upper body at T12 counter-rotates in relation to the global lower body, where the spiraling spine is the driver of ambulation.

Czech surgeon Dr Milan Roth researched spinal cord length issues as a cause of scoliosis in the 1980s. He noted how evolutionary influences made possible counterclockwise torques in the torso. Bipedal man is the only animal with a spinal cord ending at the thoracolumbar joint which freed the lower body for independent movement (van Loon, 2012).

Did you know that it is possible to have equilibrium within an asymmetric pelvis and disequilibrium within a symmetric pelvis? Walking in itself is not a symmetric activity even if stride length appears equal. Flexibility in the motion of each limb at hip, knee and ankle joints along with muscle length, and activity, particularly of the soleus, determine similarity of stride length.

Is it possible that handedness affects gait? Right-handed people use the dominant limb for propulsion and the non-dominant side receives more loading in typical stride. Upper limb dominance surely plays into this scenario given that limb dominance varies according to task within Gracovetsky's spinal engine concept of counter-torque of the torso (Boulay et al., 2006).

Defining neutral skeletal form

If the internal body is asymmetrical, how do we interpret the difference between what's expected and not expected when looking at the external body?

In analyzing a person's structure from the outside, a guideline of basic posture helps. Most people possess seemingly symmetrical right and left sides of the body, with two eyes, two arms and two legs. Globally, there are three horizontal postural lines defining the relationship between the two eyes, the two sides of the shoulders and the two sides of the pelvis.

The neutral spine

Determining neutral spine begins by observing someone from behind. Look closely at the center line of the back. The outline of the spine appears. The term 'neutral' is the starting point from which scoliosis, a deviation from the norm or 'neutral,' is analyzed. 'Neutral' refers to the position where the person is standing straight up without an intentional bend or twist to either side.

Next, imagine a plumb line hanging from the middle of the head to the coccyx (the tailbone) to the floor (Figure 1.7). A person's mid-line, plumb line and neutral spine line are all terms for the same central, vertical line of observation. Now find the line of vertebrae protruding from the spine at the central line or close to it.

Any sideways deviation from this plumb is called a *lateral (or sideways) spinal curvature*. Another, kinder, term is *lateral prominence*. As previously mentioned, a lateral or sideways spinal curvature lies within normal limits if the curve is 10° or less Cobb angle as measured on an X-ray.

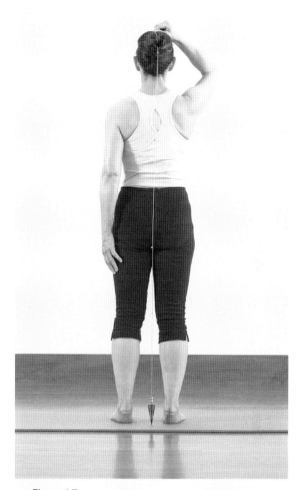

Figure 1.7

Neutral vs normal spine

How is neutral not the same as normal? There is a hair-splitting difference between the terms 'neutral' spine and a 'normal' spine. Both terms refer to the characteristics of the spine. A 'neutral' spine is observed from the rear. The 'normal' spine refers to observation from both the back as well as the side, observing both the central spinal line and the gravitational, sagittal 'S' curves from the side.

A flattened back, where the gravitational curves of alternating lordosis and kyphosis are diminished, is not a normal back although it may look straight from behind. Every spine needs to develop the customary gravitational curves, and this begins as an infant learns to sit, stand and walk. These curves form an 'S' shape when observed from a person's side.

The neck part of the 'S' curve arcs in a concave direction, called extension, or technically, *lordosis*. The thorax, encompassing the ribcage, follows a convex direction, called *kyphosis*, which means the mid- and upper-back is more rounded in shape.

Continuing down the body, the low back, the lumbar spine, alternates with a concave curve (extension/lordosis), and the sacral bone inside the middle of the pelvis follows a convex design (flexion/kyphosis).

Case example

A mother called for help for her daughter, a young equestrienne, for her mild scoliosis, chest concavity and hypermobility. Upon assessment, the spinal gravitational curves appeared absent. Lumbar recoil and rebound is important in riding. For this obviously athletic child, the next two years focused on evening out leg lengths, equalizing shoulder strength, getting schoolwork ergonomic sitting under control, along with fostering development of the curves, which gave her confidence to continue competition. Her spine would always be straighter than normal, yet the motion and strength was now functional.

These sagittal gravitational curves are an ingenious design to allow for a springboard type of effect against the loads of gravity. This springboard concept is an important element in functionality. The mechanical links and the fascial connections participate in the dynamic interplay of body weight going down into the ground, recoiling or rebounding and then coming back up into the body. Structure and function cooperate (Fukashiro et al., 2006).

The context of usage of the terms 'kyphosis' and 'lordosis' is important, determining whether each term indicates a mere anatomical description or a description of a problem.

In common clinical usage, the terms may indicate a severe, more than expected curve, or a diminished, less than expected curve value. Be sure you notice the difference.

The coupling of the neutral spine: Fryette's laws

The osteopath Harrison Fryette devised two laws in 1918 and later a third was added by osteopath Dr Nelson to make three laws, Fryette's laws of spinal mechanics, to help analyze the treatment of painful spine problems (Table 1.1).

Fryette noted that the junctions of the spinal bones link together in a jigsaw puzzle-type arrangement where as one vertebra moves, another must move

Table 1.1

Fryette's laws summarize vertebral mechanics concerning the coupled nature of vertebrae and the occurrence of dysfunctions such as scoliosis

Principle 1	Principle 2	Principle 3
Applies when a spine is in a neutral position, not in another position such as flexion, extension, side bend or rotation	Applies when a spine is in a non-neutral position, intentionally in a flexed or extended position	Applies when the spine is either in a neutral position or a non-neutral position as in both Principles 1 and 2
Describes a coupled nature when a group of vertbrae side-bend out of the neutral position. Side-bending to one side will be accompanied by horizontal rotation to the opposite side, an expected occurrence due to the coupled nature of vertebrae	Describes a coupled nature when one vertebral segment begins to side-bend, the one next to it will rotate toward the other side in mostly the thoracic region, and to the same side in mostly the cervical region. An expected ocurrence due to the coupled nature	Describes the relationship of the whole spine, a total coupled nature, where either a group or one vertebral segment moves out of one plane. Motion is modified, usually reduced in the other planes of motion
Observed in spinal dysfunctions where when a spine is side-bent for a prolonged period of time, the vertebrae adapt into a permanently rotated shape, as in a true structural scoliosis. This dysfunction applies to a group of vertebrae, not just one segment in relation to another	Observed in spinal dysfunctions where when a particular vertebral segment becomes restricted, the side-bending and rotation relationship is altered, causing more pain in flexion or extension. This dysfunction applies mostly to one vertebral segment in relation to an adjoining vertebral segment	Observed in expected spinal mechanics and also dysfunctions where either a group of vertebrae or a particular segment changes from its expected neutral or non-neutral position; motion will probably be reduced. This principle applies to either a group of vertebrae or just one in relation to another

by virtue of their connection, their positioning to one another an interaction called coupled motion. This term applies specifically to the understanding of spinal interlocking motions.

Fryette's three conventionally accepted laws define manual clinical practice. The vertebral pairings fit into interlocking pieces much like facets on a precious beveled jewel. The irregular surfaces occur as a result of tendons and ligaments along with their fascial slings pulling and pressing on bony areas to cause irregularities that create bumps and ridges. Just as a

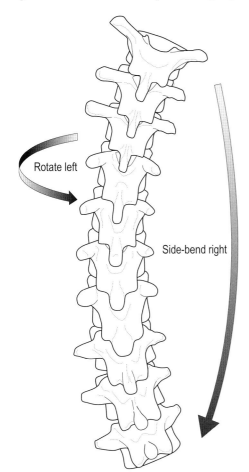

Neutral spine mechanics

Figure 1.8
A group of vertebrae that side-bends alters the Central Vertical Spinal Line creating an adapted curve which then also rotates in formation.

thumbprint is highly individual, so are the nooks and crannies of our individual bone surfaces.

Fryette observed that coupled motion occurs due to the bony architecture of the vertebral column in all motion segments. A motion segment consists of three vertebrae coupled together. With one vertebra interlocked into another, the other two must move in a domino effect. Rotary motion occurs almost simultaneously as the coupled vertebrae are bent to the side, out of a neutral Central Spinal Vertical Line (CSVL).

A side-bending action out of the expected CSVL is the hallmark of a person with scoliosis as observed from the back. With every side-bent lateral curve, the neutral CSVL experiences a rotation due to the locked links of the jigsaw puzzle of the spine (Figure 1.8).

Fryette's third law is the main principle that PMMEs should keep in mind. Moving one part of the spine has ramifications on all the other parts. The spine with asymmetry follows these laws to a large extent, but not always, especially as the vertebrae change shape as a result of the spinal twist. For instance, Cobb angles of less than 25° are thought to follow expected spinal and muscular mechanics where the convex and concave scoliosis is able to coordinate around the central vertical spinal axis. However, theories such as the chaotic dynamical system question this assumption so that measures near this level may change accepted spinal rules. For this reason, PMMEs cannot go it alone as the Cobb angle increases.

To better understand how the spine and body of a person with scoliosis moves differently, follow the link below (Code 1.1) to a pilot observational study illustrating via kinetic analysis a view of some very simple motions. Watch and compare the subjects with varying scoliosis issues.

The skeletal images are not X-rays showing individual spinal shapes yet do show the functionality. Look at the distance between the legs and see where the plumb line falls. Notice the difference in strategy as the subjects move on one leg versus the other.

The first subject has had a Harrington rod for 20 plus years and has difficulty standing erect now. She exercises regularly, has been doing adapted Pilates

Code 1.1 (free code)
Computerized scoliosis analyses: standing

exercises and swimming, and has improved with less discomfort and more function. The second subject has significant thoracic rotation over 45° and is a Pilates and yoga instructor. The third subject had a Harrington rod removed when in her 20s and is just about to start Pilates training. The last subject has minor lumbar scoliosis with multiple level rotations in the pelvis, along with a recent significant left leg injury.

Discovering the adaptive curve

Scoliosis is detected by various ways, through school screening, by family or self-observation, or medical observation. The person is usually diagnosed in a standing upright position, or so the person thinks. Osteopath Fred Mitchell, Jr categorized scoliosis as the abnormality of a spine with a lateral curve observed from the back in a 'Type I dysfunction.'

The reason Mitchell used the Type I dysfunction designation is because the bend is the result of some long-term sort of adaptation to mechanical stress, skeletal pathology, or neurologic abnormality. Type I indicates the veering from a neutral plumb line position, without the intent to move into a twist, side bend, forward flexion, or upward extension.

What this all means is that the lateral curve, often appearing as a 'hump,' is not just ribs out of position but is, in essence, a side bend. Therefore, according to the 'coupled motion law,' the spine must also twist in a type of corkscrew effect not only in the spine but also throughout the rest of the body creating functional along with structural elements of asymmetry.

A twisting DNA-helix is a fitting image to describe the three-dimensional twists of scoliosis. From the outside, the spinal side bend appears flat, yet it is a true corkscrew shape internally. The internal twisting essentially pulls many other structures into its vortex, creating a ricochet sequence of imbalances.

Note that the twisting does not necessarily cause the spine to fall apart. The whole body normally participates in spiraling.

Did you realize that spiraling in the body is what defines normal function? The lower limb bones assume a spiral in their basic geometry. The knee is known for its screw-home mechanism locking the femur into the tibia and fibula. The fascial slings help to wind and unwind the knee, its four joints comprising the hinge, as they function in a recoil effect of stored potential energy to facilitate dynamic, kinetic motion, much like the winding of a clock spring.

The groundbreaking work of physical therapist (PT) Maggie Voss and Dr Kaiser, who devised the renowned PNF (proprioceptive neuromuscular facilitation) therapy patterns, found that 'mature' movement always involves rotation, spiraling (Morad Pour Taleb et al., 2016).

The video above (Code 1.1) shows how non-neutral, yet still intact, spines are still functional, retaining their unique spiraling elements that create the individual's preferred movement patterns.

A delicate balance

The phenomenon of the spine with scoliosis is that it attempts to assume a vertical position in spite of lateral adaptive curves, due to automatic reflexes that help a person maintain erectness. It is as if an elephant wishes to ride a unicycle. It is possible, yet it is a delicate balancing act.

Fascial areas of stiffness creating internal and external buttresses and pulleys also come into play. Imagine an ankle sprain where the ligaments, connective tissue that holds bones together, stretch apart when the ankle joint bends into an unnatural alignment as a result of stepping incorrectly off a curb, rolling over on its side. These ankle bones either transiently or permanently lose their couple, called *congruency*, not fitting together as before the injury.

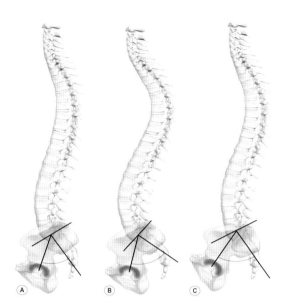

Figure 1.9
Illustration of altered rib and vertebral anatomy due to spinal asymmetry.

A structural scoliosis, adapting over time, goes beyond transient misalignment to become permanent (see Figure 1.9). Eventually it can create a balanced asymmetrical structure through the help of fascial buttresses and muscular reflexes that start out attempting to help the asymmetry remain stable yet if not checked may exacerbate the condition over time.

Although the bones become just slightly differently shaped, they fit into their interlocking facet orientations unless there is a ligamentous or degenerative instability preventing them from holding together. Nature achieves perfection despite imperfect replication or development. It is what makes us individual (Mitchell Jr, 2002).

As Fryette's third law states, one area of misaligned spine affects all other parts. Schaumberger takes the malalignment aspect one more step to explain that a malaligned spinal section involves compensatory curvatures along other areas of the spine, thus affecting the rest of the skeleton. Asymmetrical ranges of motion of the head and neck, trunk, pelvis

and joints of the upper and lower extremities then create asymmetrical tension in the muscles, tendons and ligaments.

This situation in turn causes asymmetrical muscle bulk and strength, an apparent (functional) leg length difference culminating in an asymmetrical weightbearing pattern (Schaumberger, 2012).

PT Marianna Bialek found that those with an asymmetrical spine, scoliosis, exhibit asymmetrical loading patterns of the foot. She found a consistent trend where the right forefoot exhibited less loading in the propulsion phase. The good news is that combining scoliosis training with Janda short foot exercises helped to re-establish right forefoot activity, indicating that functional compensatory patterns have *plasticity*, the ability to change (Bialek et al., 2009).

Asymmetry: nature and nurture

Did you realize that what you do on a daily basis engrains asymmetry? Most people possess some small amount of symmetrical non-perfection, asymmetry, slight changes from average expectations, which form the human thumbprint. When these variations in average expected measure are small they are referred to as 'within normal limits.'

Being right- or left-handed dominant makes a difference in side-to-side development. Is the side-to-side deviation genetically encoded, such as the cowlick shared by my sister, on one side of our forehead hairlines? In terms of habitual or required behavior there are side-to-side differences, directional biases seen in daily driving with the right or left foot on the gas pedal. There are individual habits of preferentially crossing one leg over the other while seated. These habits create a repetitive activity causing muscle pattern preferences. In turn, the repetitive activity becomes our comfort position, our preferential direction, a feeling of ease.

The core link: fetal life, birth and early life

Let's explore why these possibilities of behavior exist. Going back to our early life, prenatal positioning in the womb and perinatal labor and delivery have an impact on anatomic structure. The first possibility of asymmetry in life goes back to cranial asymmetry that establishes what osteopaths term 'the Core Link,' which is the cranial-sacral relationship of the *dura*, which covers the spinal cord, linking the head to the pelvic base.

Did you know that positioning in the womb affects your directional preferences? Prior to birth, a phenomenon called vestibular lateralization begins to occur due to natal positioning. Because of the relationship of maternal-to-child circulation and nutrition, the fetus tends to receive left-sided vestibular input.

With a left-lying fetus, which is typically inverted, the fetus receives a left dominant vestibular input as the mother walks with her right side dominantly forward. This typical scenario sets up a more left-dominant stabilizing side as the infant and child begin to sit upright.

The labyrinthine reflex is the righting reflex, hard-wired into our neurological system to help us maintain verticality. Those who suffer birth delays and complications causing lack of oxygen in the first moments of exit from the birth canal suffer more, causing diminishment or actual loss of this reflex, a condition associated with cerebral palsy. And so lateralization begins (Pope, 2017).

All people with spinal asymmetry benefit from exercises, some included in later chapters, which stimulate this natural reflex. One such movement therapy is hippotherapy, where the riders sit horseback without saddles. The input from the horse's bones up into the rider's bones helps individuals who have brain issues, but not necessarily spinal cord issues. The spinal cord then exerts its own intellect to help the rider sit upright, although the brain vestibular system in the inner ear is having difficulty finding balance.

Case example

The clinical director called a group of PT students into the office to anounce the good news. They were selected for the Woodside internship. The director explained it was a unique environment using therapy horses. At five foot two inches and with no equine background, it was hard for me,

as one of the students, to believe how it could be positive!

After the 1.5-hour drive to a rural spot, the grounds came into view. The program director, an assertive occupational therapist and equestrienne, began her duty. Off the group went to view videos of how the horse's spine and pelvis, with their winding and unwinding in simple equine gait exert influence into the rider's pelvis and spine. An adolescent girl in a back-supporting walker clumsily labored her way to the ring to begin treatment, observed by all us students.

As her head hung forward and to the right side almost past her shoulder, she struggled to move one leg and then almost threw her shoulder weight over to the other side in order to free her opposite leg to swing forward. Obviously, it was impossible for her to be upright without the back-handled walker. After she was assisted onto the horse, she abruptly fell sideways, draping her abdomen over the horse's back. Her head was down along the horse's thighs on one side, and her feet were about the same height from the sandy ring ground on the other side.

After pleading with the director that we should help this girl not to slide off of the side, she explained to just wait and see. As the horse began a plodding, rhythmic stride with the therapists at the horse's muzzle and flank, the girl's body appeared as if it would flop right off. The therapists cautiously guarded the girl and the stride proceeded all around the large ring. As the girl approached about halfway, her posture began to change. Somehow she had swung herself forward to catch the horse's mane and now was in line with the horse's spine. By the time she reached the starting point, she was upright, riding, smiling and in sync with the horse's motion. This stunning display was a valuable lesson in the *righting reflex* of the body. The value of the Pilates balance point is a similar tool helping spinal extension through stimulation of the righting reflex.

Lateralization and separate sides

When does handedness begin in life? Study of early life indicates awareness of separate sides begins soon in the infant's life with the most basic sense of laterality in a child's cognitive and perceptual development.

Detection and correct labeling of the two different sides of the body when parents coax a motion from the little one around age five is a major accomplishment. This awareness of right versus left differs from an actual lateral or directional preference, or bias.

Early life begins with manipulation of objects with both hands by age one yet turns into true preferential treatment of sides such as in handwriting, throwing, hopping and kicking once common activities of play commence. Setting the stage for handedness and leg-gedness, the preferential use of the limbs begins with manipulating space and objects (Loffing et al., 2016).

In addition, a sense of asymmetrical external space develops about the body with the favored side enlarged in comparison to the non-favored side. The majority of us are right-handed. Right-handers show a bias not only with respect to judging external space but also with judging the spatial characteristics of their own body (Hach & Schutz-Bosbach, 2014).

Dominance of sides

The role of dominance of sides is trickier than it seems. When performing tasks with both hands, each hand usually performs a unique role such as stabilizing an object with one hand while manipulating it with the other. Tasks that require coordination of arm and leg motions often switch off role sides as the task changes, especially if added to neurological complexity such as the teaching of multiple cues common within Pilates instruction. For this reason, the PMME should avoid offering only one-sided exercise to those with spinal asymmetry. As a rule of thumb, exercise both sides of the body and always perform the exercise in both directions, deciding which side is the first side.

Biased practice, using each side of the body in a certain role, such as playing the violin, influences learning. The brain adapts to the new specialized skill and learning takes place. Skill is dependent upon neuromuscular control and not just on physical parameters. The ability to learn is also affected by our perceived competence in performing a task or skill to one side or the other. For this reason, allowing the direction of the exercise to be performed first in the direction of ease, the one with more confidence and comfort, and then reversing the exercise to the more challenging direction, is a favored plan (Loffing et al., 2016).

> ### Case example
>
> The parents of an adolescent male called me about their son's new diagnosis of scoliosis. The young man was an avid archer, in good physical health. When the group came to the studio, his developed favoritism was evident. He was similar to another young client of mine, a fencer. Fencing, archery and other sports such as golf, skeet-shooting, along with many others, orient the body in one direction and depend upon perfecting the one-sided eye vision to body coordination system. Both young men showed rotational favoritism along with asymmetrical upper body to lower body dominance. In both cases, we used cross-training to break up the pattern, involving eye use and other techniques to develop more balanced strength. These cases form the foundation of the youth progressions found in the Scoliosis Specific Physical Observational Test Part 2 (SSPOT™-2).

Motor skills and handedness

A basic brain asymmetry promoted in childhood development creates a lateral preference in motor skills. These skills then become biased motor experiences that also converge with a right-biased world.

These influences then lead to asymmetrical proficiency, even if it serves a good function, such as creating the desired choreographic movement, dunking the basketball into the net or hitting the ball with the right angle to foil the opponent. However, asymmetry is also associated with injury potential, a major reason to cross-train especially when developing specialized motor skills for athletics and dance (Kimmerle, 2010).

Boyle and colleagues found an inherent postural tendency in a general athletic population. Right-handed individuals tend to shift their body weight with the center of gravity to the right in conjunction with right rotated lumbar vertebra and thoracic and pubic symphysis rotated to the left.

This tendency to stand on the right leg shifts the center of gravity to the right, potentially creating a tight left posterior hip capsule, poorly approximated left hip (less congruence in the joint), and long, weak left hip adductors, internal obliques, and transverse abdominis. Additionally, strong, overactive and short paraspinals, muscles on the right anterior hip outlet (adductors, levator ani, and obturator internus), a left rib flare (tight internal obliques) and a decreased respiratory diaphragm *zone of apposition* (ZOA) complete the list (Boyle, 2013).

Described as the Left Anterior Interior Chain (Left AIC) Pattern, it is similar to Florence Kendall's Right Handed Pattern, which she ascribes to organ position, asymmetrical growth and development along with neurologic patterned function and not literally tied to hand dominance (Kendall et al., 1993).

Did you know that the majority worldwide is right-handed, and that distinct advantages of left-handed dominant people include creativity, musicianship, mathematical capacities as well as higher socioeconomic status (Loffing et al., 2016)?

In an effort to better understand the impact of lateral preferences, six volunteers participated in a casual laterality exploration. Variables of eye dominance, rotational preference and standing leg preference associated with pelvic sway were explored. After functional interventions altering the variables were implemented, all six volunteers reported greater ease in their everyday walking task (Martin, 2017). Watch the video of the synopsis of the pilot study (Code 1.2). It illustrates some of the functional tests and interventions in this book. This study

Code 1.2 (free code)
Beta study: laterality interventions

was repeated in several conference venues where surprisingly similar results of improvement in symmetrical posture and spinal rotation were achieved through simple laterality correctives.

Neuromotorial laterality

Besides knowing about the lateralization in the womb, early life, childhood milestone and skill acquisition, an additional knowledge tool for PMMEs involves brain plasticity and an understanding of compensatory patterns involving the neuromotorial system.

Lateral favoritism and ensuing compensatory patterns in the neurological system consist of more than muscle imbalances. Take into account visual and perceptive brain integration along with balance, vestibular and hearing patterns that begin in utero, continue through childhood and persist into adulthood.

In a functional model of asymmetry, scoliosis perpetuates in a cascade of systematic neurological interactions. The Herman Theory provides an inspiration for all PMMEs working with spinal asymmetry to understand the complexities of the individual and not just the skeletal curve type (Table 1.2).

Table 1.2
Using Herman's Theory to consider scoliosis as a compensation from neuromotorial alterations

Input into	Processing through	Output gives the outcome
Sensory system (innate and/or environment)	Perception (the reality to the client)	Altered body spatial orientation creating neurological alterations
Rearranged sensory/neurological integration	Oculomotor system (eye control of motor system)	Altered eye control creating altered axial (vertebral) motor control
Adapted motor system	Axial and balance motor systems	Altered motor patterns
Motor pattern alterations	Patterns of habits now favor alterations	Musculoskeletal and neuromuscular asymmetry creating and reinforcing spinal asymmetry

When major spinal adaptations occur in the axial motor system of postural muscles, a sensory re-arrangement occurs giving both an altered body awareness and an altered external orientation in space.

Next, spinal motor control is altered to adjust to the sensori-muscular changes, giving an altered perceptual awareness. Altered perceptions impact the eye reflexes and balancing. The eyes seek out a horizon in order to maintain uprightness and coordinate with feet hitting the ground surface and hands performing fine motor activites at the appropriate time, force and manner.

This altered perceptual awareness operates within a narrow window of functional meeting dysfunction-al border. Sensory disturbances, motor dysfunctions are a matter of meeting a threshold where alterations become true problems. This is why the training of good mechanical and behavioral habits in daily life is an important aspect of lifelong scoliosis management (Romano et al., 2015).

Case example

A young college-aged woman called me to explain that she and her twin both had scoliosis. The caller was more affected by pain and concern than her counterpart. Both were in good health otherwise. When the two women arrived together, their positioning in the womb became apparent. Although twins, one was a structurally larger woman than the other. One stabilized out at a near 50° primary spinal curve and the other had a smaller primary lateral spinal curve at 30°.

Most interesting about the two were the discrepancies between their head shapes and orientations. The larger woman's frontal face plane was clearly rotated so that her right eye, face and head rotated significantly to the left. Her pelvis was also significantly rotated to the right in the transverse plane. Her primary scoliosis curve was a left lumbar curve, causing posterior pelvic rotation on that side, severely restricting her sitting comfort. This twin needed specific female pelvic help due to her pelvic imbalances.

The second had more leg and ankle issues due to her asymmetry. They had had the same activities growing up, yet each body found different strategies around their specific asymmetries. Each case warranted her own focus within the Pilates work. The young women found their way, building on the foundation we started. One went into environmental research and the other works with an agency involving international travel.

Conclusion

Say that a client just came into your studio with a 50° thoracic curve. Are you ready to use your mind's eye to see the body and beyond the personality standing before you? Did you know that it is a skill to read the creases in the clothes, the tilt of the head, the client's stance, the symmetry of the eyes, probing the unexpected curving of the spine?

Talent is born. Skill is hard won. *Skolios* is Greek for bent yet the asymmetric aspects reveal more than a bent spine. Concepts of preference and laterality form a major principle for helping those with asymmetry and scoliosis. Poll your friends. Do the majority of your right-handed friends have some slight spinal convex asymmetry?

If each person with spinal asymmetry deserves individual attention, some large curves and some small, how is this skill accomplished beyond general knowledge of the exercises of the Pilates Method?

PMMEs do benefit from understanding the basic two or three types of generalized scoliosis patterns. Yet look past the typical curve pattern exercises to discover the interplay of delivery of the Method to a young person versus a middle-aged adult, probably with comorbidities. Look at preferences and biases in motion and perception shaping personality to give the work *lagniappe*, as New Orleanians say, the something extra, to bring art into the science of the client's program.

The desire to work with those with spinal asymmetry, whether as part of a medical team or non-medical team, takes forethought, integrity and courage. Did you know that PMMEs who work with scoliosis have many reasons to want to belong to the Scoliosis Team? If the PMME should possess a special skill set for not only effective Pilates instruction but also to work within a Scoliosis Team, how does that happen?

Each person with spinal asymmetry deserves individual skilled attention, which requires more specialized training. Although PMMEs benefit from understanding the basic two or three types of generalized scoliosis patterns, look past the typical curve patterns to discover the interplay of lateralization, preferences and biases along with their neurological aspects of perception shaping personality as a gift. Boredom never comes into this arena. Take the challenge. Use the strategies in this book as the guide to discover the influence of the PMME in the world of spinal asymmetry and scoliosis.

Bibliography

Agur, A. M. (2013). Clinically Oriented Anatomy, 7th edn. Baltimore: Lippincott Williams & Wilkins

Aristotle (367–347 BCE). Aristotle: Parts of Animals. Movement of Animals. Progression of Animals (Loeb Classical Library No. 323) (Vol. 1). (A. L. Peck, Trans.) Athens, Greece: Loeb Classical Library

Bialek, M., Pawlak, P., Kotwicki, T. (2009). Foot loading asymmetry in patients with scoliosis. Scoliosis, 4(Suppl. 019): 1

Boulay, C., Tardieu, C., Bénaim, C. et al. (2006). Three-dimensional study of pelvic asymmetry on anatomical specimens and its clinical perspectives. Journal of Anatomy, 208, 21–33

Boyle, K.L. (2013). Clinical application of the right sidelying respiratory left adductor pull back exercise. International Journal of Sports Physical Therapy, 8(3), 349–358

Bryant, D.M., Mostov, K.E. (2008). From cells to organs. National Review of Molecular Cell Biology, 9(11), 887–901

Cobb, J.R. (1948). Outline for the study of scoliosis. American Academy of Orthopaedic Surgeons Instructional Course Lectures, 5261–5275

Cramer, G., Derby, S. (2005). Basic and clinical anatomy of the spine and spinal cord and ANS. St Louis: Elsevier Mosby

de Mouray, J.-C., Ginoux, J.-M. (2012). Is AIS under 20-30° a chaotic dynamical system? Studies in Health Technology and Informatics, 176, 473

Fukashiro, S., Hay, D.C., Nagano, A. (2006). Biomechanical behavior of muscle-tendon complex during dynamic human movements. Journal of Applied Biomechanics, 22(2), 131–147

Hach, S., Schutz-Bosbach, S. (2014). In (or outside of) your neck of the woods: laterality in spatial body representation. Frontiers in Psychology, 5, 23

Hippocrates. (460–376 BCE). On articulations. Athens: The Perfect Library

Kane, W. J. (1977). Scoliosis prevalence. Clinical Orthopaedics 126, 43–46

Keays, K.S., Harris, S.R., Lucyshyn, J.M., MacIntyre, D.L. (2008) Effects of Pilates exercises on shoulder range of motion, pain, mood, and upper extremity function in women living with breast cancer: a pilot study. Physical Therapy, 88(4), 494–510

Kendall, F.P., McCreary, E.K., Provance, P. G., eds. (1993). Muscles: Testing and Function, 4th edn. Baltimore: Williams and Wilkins

Kim, H., Kim, S.H., Moon, E.S., et al. (2010). Scoliosis imaging: what radiologists should know. Radiographics, 30(7), 1823–1842

Kimmerle, M. (2010). Lateral bias, functional asymmetry, dance training, and dance injuries. Journal of Dance Medicine and Science, 14(2), 58–66

Kleinman, P.K, Raptopoulos, V. (1985). The anterior diaphragmatic attachments: an anatomic and radiologic study with clinical correlates. Radiology, 155(2), 289–293

Legaye, J. Duval-Beaupère, G., Hecquet, J., Marty, C. (1998). Pelvic incidence: a fundamental pelvic parameter. European Spine, 7, 99–103

Levine B., Kaplanek B., Jaffe W.L. (2009). Pilates training for use in rehabilitation after total hip and knee arthroplasty: A preliminary report. Clinical Orthopaedics and Related Research, 467(6), 1468–1475

Levine, D. D. (2013). History of scoliosis surgery at HSS. Retrieved February 25, 2017, from Hospital for Special Surgery: https://www.hss.edu/playbook/history-of-scoliosis-surgery-at-hss/#.WK-XzoWcGMo

Lin, JJ., Chen, WH., Chen, PQ., Tsauo, JY. (2010). Alteration in shoulder kinematics and associated muscle activity in people with idiopathic scoliosis. Spine, 35(11), 1151–1157

Linker, B. (2012). A dangerous curve: the role of history in America's scoliosis screening programs. American Journal of Public Health, 102(4), 606–616

Loffing, F., Hagemann, N., Strauss, B., McMahon, C. (2016). Laterality in Sports. London: Elsevier

Martin, S. (2017). Explorations in Asymmetry and Laterality in Dance Training. Berkeley: Suzanne Martin

McKenzie, D.K., Gandevia, S.C., Gorman, R.B., Southon, F.C.G. (1994). Dynamic changes in the zone of apposition and diaphragm length during maximal respiratory efforts. Thorax, 49(7), 634–638

Mitchell Jr, F.L. (2002). The Muscle Energy Manual, 2nd edn, Vol. 2. East Lansing: MET Press

Moore, K.L., Persaud, T.V.N. (1993). Before We Were Born, 4th edn. Philadelphia: WB Saunders

Morad Pour Taleb, F., Sokhangouyi, Y., Valipouri, V., Faghihi, S. (2016). Effect of one period of PNF receptors on lower-crossed syndrome. International Journal of Biology, Pharmacy and Allied Sciences, 5(1), Special Issue: 507–522. Retrieved August 30, 2017, from http://ijbpas.com/pdf/2016/January/1452607749MS%20IJBPAS%202016%20JAN%20SPCL%201127.pdf

National Scoliosis Foundation. (2017). Retrieved December 21, 2017 from: http://www.scoliosis.org/early-detection/

Negrini, S. (2010). Rehabilitation in adult scoliosis: an introduction. Scoliosis, 5(Suppl. 1), 049

Ortholutions GmbH & Co. (2017). The scoliosis night brace nBrace. Retrieved March 7, 2017, from www.orthosolutions.com: http://www.ortholutions.com/tlso-trunk-orthoses-brace-orthotics/scoliosis-night-brace-rigo-cheneau-ortholutions/

Pilates, J. H. (1945) [2010]. Return to Life Through Contrology. Miami: Pilates Method Alliance

Pope, R. (2017). The common compensatory pattern. Thesis, Oklahoma City. Retrieved August 30, 2017, from ericdalton.com: http://erikdalton.com/article_pdfs/articleCCPThesis.pdf

Risser, J.C. (2010). The classic: the iliac apophysis: an invaluable sign in the management of scoliosis. Clinical Orthopaedics and Related Research, 468(3), 646–653

Ritchie, R.O., Buehler, M. J., Hansma P. (2009). Plasticity and toughness in bone. Physics Today 62(6), 41–47

Romano, M., Negrini, A., Parzini, S. et al. (2015). SEAS (Scientific Exercises Approach to Scoliosis): a modern and effective evidence based approach to physiotherapic specific scoliosis exercises. Scoliosis, 10(3), 1–19

Schaumberger, W. (2012). Malalignment Syndrome, 2nd edn. Edinburgh: Churchill Livingstone Elsevier

Silva, F.E., Lenke, L.G. (2010). Adult degenerative scoliosis: evaluation and management. Neurosurgery Focus, 28(3: E1), 1–10

St Johnston, D., Ahringer, J. (2010) Cell polarity in eggs and epithelia: parallels and diversity. Cell, 141(5), 757–774

Tensegrity – the geometry of thinking. (2017). Retrieved August 30, 2017, from Buckminster Fuller Institute: https://www.bfi.org/about-fuller/big-ideas/synergetics/tensegrity-geometry-thinking

Vasiliadis, E.S., Grivas, T.B., Kaspiris, A. (2009). Historical overview of spinal deformities in ancient Greece. Scoliosis, 4(6)

Weiss, H.R., Moramarco, M., Moramarco, K. (2013). Risks and long term complications of adolescent idiopathic scoliosis surgery versus non-surgical and natural history outcomes. Hard Tissue, 2(3), 1–12. Retrieved August 29, 2017, from http://www.oapublishinglondon.com/article/498

What is Lifestyle Medicine? (2015). Retrieved January 26, 2017 from the American College of Lifestyle Medicine: https://www.lifestylemedicine.org/What-is-Lifestyle-Medicine/

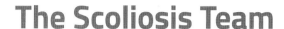

The Scoliosis Team

My first exposure to the treatment of asymmetries and scoliosis was as a Pilates instructor, before becoming a physical therapist (PT), while attending Pilates training with the legendary Jean-Claude West, a motor control expert.

He recommended a book on muscle testing and scoliosis developed by PT Florence Kendall, along with her colleagues, Elizabeth Kendall McCreary and Patricia Provance. They devised muscle testing and posture exercises to treat the musculoskeletal imbalances caused by polio and scoliosis.

The scoliosis chapter opens with a statement made by Dr Risser, the namesake of the pelvic test to determine closing of the skeleton:

> "It is customary at the scoliosis clinic at ... Orthopedic Hospital, as late as 1920–30, to send new patients with scoliosis to the gymnasium for exercises. Invariably the patients who were 12 to 13 years of age showed an increase in the scoliosis ...it was therefore assumed that exercises and spinal motion made the curve increase."

No wonder the 'wait and see' model has persisted for so long. Yet Ms Kendall was ahead of her time, and the time is ripe for the tide to turn. At the end of the same chapter, Ms Kendall questioned whether scoliosis should be a part of the 'wait and see' observation monitoring system, where the only intervention is repeat X-rays to see if the curve worsens over time. She offered, "Instead of waiting to see if a curve gets worse before deciding to do something about it, why not treat the problem to help prevent the curve from getting worse?" (Kendall & McCreary, 1993). Her statement is the inspiration for my personal pursuit to the transition of the Scoliosis Team.

Did you know that there is more than one type of Scoliosis Team? Encompassing a variety of healthcare givers divided into direct medical and non-medical categories, many active players participate in dispensing care for spinal asymmetry.

Medical physicians, along with their staff of radiologists, assistants and nurses, are largely *allopathic*, treating disease symptoms and effects with conventional means such as surgery, medication and injections. Some are multidisciplinary allied healthcare practitioners, such as physiotherapists, who work directly under the orders of supervising medical physicians.

Another medical team, the non-allopathic group, are known as *Complementary Alternative Medicine* (CAM) practitioners and are composed of chiropractors and osteopaths. These groups, allopathic and CAM, sometimes work together for scoliosis patients, depending upon their individual philosophies and ideologies. The types of care delivered by the teams are categorized into conservative and non-conservative care.

Allopathic medicine and scoliosis

Traditional Western Medicine (allopathic) physicians include orthopedists or neurologists who specialize in spinal pathologies. They administer injections and perform structural re-engineering involving surgery and other technologies to treat their patients.

When clients with asymmetries or possible scoliosis are referred into the medical system, these physicians are generally responsible for making a medical determination of the patient's level and severity of spinal abnormality. They deliver both conservative and non-conservative care. These physicians collaborate with other allopathic physicians within their specific team to deliver pain control or other necessary interventions to stabilize the client.

Conservative medical care

Conservative medical care, by definition, is care that is not extreme or drastic. It is the norm of care until certain criteria are met for more aggressive measures.

Conservative care's main goals are to restore or pre-serve function. It is designed to avoid radical thera-peutic measures or operative procedures such as spinal fixation.

Allopathic physicians prescribe conservative care according to their philosophy of care and it is based on the relevant evidence found in the field. Included in this category of care are injections, medications prescribed to lessen pain and inflammation, along with brace prescriptions attempting to stabilize a cli-ent's curve. Conservative care measures are usually the first level of care after the observation and onset of scoliosis.

Bracing

The 'wait and see' method of watchful waiting with periodic monitoring for minor curves for both ado-lescents and adults includes the use of a progression-inhibiting brace, an orthotic that can be likened to the use of braces to straighten teeth. Braces are pre-scribed according to the individual correction and are made in either hard or soft materials.

The goal of each type of brace is to stop the progres-sion of the curve; however, a brace neither removes the actual deformity or straightens it out entirely. It attempts to stabilize the abnormal growth. Adoles-cents typically wear a hard brace for about a two-year period. The use of hard braces is known to help curves at 50° and upwards in prevention of the need for surgical fixation, although typical bracing begins at smaller curve measures (Weistein et al., 2013).

More physicians now recommend a multidisciplinary conservative approach involving other allied health-care providers for exercise, posture and ergonomic advice. These are the physical therapists or physio-therapists (PTs), occupational therapists (OTs), chiro-practors (DCs), along with paraprofessionals such as PMMEs and PT and OT assistants.

Multidisciplinary conservative approach

Chiropractic

Doctors of chiropractic (DCs) treat the asymmetry or scoliosis condition non-surgically. Typically, this group refers patients into the allopathic system if the client worsens. A wide variety of philosophies and treatments exist within the chiropractic field of sco-liosis treatment.

Some prescribe bracing in the form of the Montreal SpineCor® bracing, a soft brace that is custom fit with bands to correct the curves and is meant to be worn especially with exercise activities (SpineCor® Train-ing, 2013).

Others employ lateral pressures against the torso combined with bodywork and corrective exercise. Still others use vibration plates to alter propriocep-tion, exercising afterwards to re-instill new motor control neurology.

Innovation is high in both allopathic and CAM to find non-surgical as well as cutting edge surgical interven-tions. Although well-meaning, it is prudent to advise all persons wishing to pursue either allopathic medical or non-allopathic medical strategies to research the care type that each offers and gain multiple opinions before entering any specific approach. Many clients combine systems. Older adults especially need advocacy since any system will not guarantee success of outcome.

Occupational therapists and physical therapists

Other medical healthcare practitioners in the con-servative medical care approach are OTs or PTs.

Occupational therapists are especially involved with young people affected by scoliosis. These governmentally licensed therapists are primari-ly concerned with activities of daily living such as school attendance and participation, grooming, toilet care, and food preparation and consumption. Their skills extend into knowledge of developmental development and sensory integration techniques for children and adolescents, helping with reading and sensory normalization.

Once the treatment objectives and methods are deter-mined, the treatment plan is implemented. Once the goals have been reached, discharge from the OT's care is planned and the intervention is terminated.

Physical therapists are governmentally licensed allied healthcare providers who also deliver conservative care. An allopathic physician or non-allopathic physician may refer into an allopathic physical therapy system.

Generally, PTs receive referrals to address a specific problem or limitation associated with the scoliosis, such as with the knee or foot, or in specific spinal areas such as the lumbar spine.

Pediatric services similar to the OT, such as sensory-motor exercises, are often a part of the PT's plan. PTs that work with youth tend to work on seating and walking special aid issues. PTs that work with adults with scoliosis and spinal asymmetry usually employ a combination of manual therapy and therapeutic exercise focusing on stability of the lumbar spine. The referral to discharge process is the same format as the OT's.

Scoliosis-specific systems in physical therapy

There are a number of recognized physical therapy systems. They are specifically designed to stem the progression of the adolescent scoliosis spine, yet also address the non-progressing or slowly progressing spine of adulthood. Three are discussed here.

The most well-known and patented system is called the Schroth Method® from Germany. The other two are also European models: the FITS (Functional Integration Therapy for Scoliosis) from Poland, and the SEAS (Scientific Exercise and Approach to Scoliosis) from Italy.

The Schroth Method®

The Schroth Method® was developed in the 1920s by physiotherapist Katerina Schroth, originally in an inpatient hospital setting, and is proven to either partially or fully correct particularly the adolescent onset of scoliosis. Its original principles, becoming more popular today, were revolutionary in their attention to the 'cylindrical muscular core,' as well as the three-dimensional and block analysis of the spinal scoliosis curve. The Schroth Method®'s emphasis is on abnormal curve correction.

Ms Schroth's ideas and principles are probably the basic foundation for all forms of PT that directly address exercise regimens for scoliosis. The Pilates Method's breathing and exercise to address bodily asymmetry has significant overlaps with the Schroth Method® (Weiss, 2011).

The FITS method

The FITS method from Poland, credited to PT Marianna Bialek, is mainly an inpatient hospital administered therapy. It equips the patient with a home follow-up program, similar in philosophy to the Schroth Method®.

A main principle of the FITS method is to educate the patient to see their own curve patterns. After initiating treatment with manual therapy, FITS treatment follows with an individually designed program of exercise using breathing exercises on a wall ladder, much like the Schroth® system, but also includes stretchy therapy bands that bind the patient in specific individualized counter-force patterns. Outcomes show the FITS program improves especially the 20°–30° Cobb angle curves (Bialek & D'Hango, 2008).

The SEAS method

The SEAS is an individualized approach in rehabilitation that is meant to address the three main stages of scoliosis: 1) to aid rehabilitation in youth to stop the need for possible bracing; 2) to aid medium severity to severe curve progression during bracing and prepare the individual for eventual weaning from the brace; and 3) to aid the adult in stabilizing the curve and so prevent disability in later years.

The SEAS is a neurological approach in that the PT teaches the patient to use reflexive self-correcting postures in activities of daily life. Coined as an active self-correction technique, it is an outpatient therapy that initially meets regularly per week and reduces to about once per year for refinements and accuracy (Romano et al., 2015).

Each scoliosis-specific program has a primary aim to educate and rehabilitate the patient for the particulars of the condition.

The Scoliosis Team: non-traditional members

This is where additional elements of the Scoliosis Team, the Movement Educators and body workers, along with complementary licensed providers such as acupuncturists, matter.

Body workers

Body workers, such as Rolfers as well as chiropractors and osteopaths who perform body work, tend to concentrate on altering the soft tissue texture or joint malalignments and subluxations (minor dislocations) with direct hands-on therapy. They often delegate movement education as an adjunct to other parts of the team, such as PMMEs (Blum, 2002; Cottingham, 1988; Managing scoliosis with osteopathy, 2017).

Acupuncturists

Pain may or may not be an indicator for an individual or a parent to seek alternative care but in seeking pain remediation they, especially the older adult population who tyically suffer from the musculoskeletal effects of aging, may wish to try acupuncture. Acupuncture is known for its anti-inflammatory and pain-relieving properties for conditions such as migraine, arthritis, neck pain and low back pain, which are also common symptoms associated with adult scoliosis. Acupuncturists also generally refer their clients to other providers for exercise instruction (Marty-Pourmarat et al., 2007).

The Pilates environment

The Pilates Method approach emphasizes quality and education of movement process as well as the ability to concentrate on and coordinate with many body parts at once. The Pilates environment specifically promotes facilitation of postural muscles to stabilize movement preceding large muscle group use. This is consistent with exercise physiology principles of motion (Henneman et al., 1965).

The Pilates environment encompasses working both within the mat environment as well as within the various forms of Pilates apparatus such as the Reformer, Trapeze Table, Wunda Chair, Spine Corrector and Ped-O-Pull, among other props and adjunct pieces of equipment.

These components environmentally allow the variability required by the principles of the Pilates Method. This diversity of tools gives the educator room to individualize the client's comprehensive human experience. A person with spinal issues requires deep body learning on an elemental level.

The environment itself both assists and challenges the individual. Traditional progress moves from the establishment of a stable skeletal base to a dynamic, moving base of support that withstands external forces from either one's own gravitational weight,

or the resistance of a spring system. These types of resistance ultimately offer functional resistance training.

The specific tools also include imagery, and the use of props, along with the way that the education is delivered, which may or may not include the use of the Pilates devices.

The PMME within the Scoliosis Team

How can the PMME be of help within the Scoliosis Team? In physical therapy, rehabilitative attention by definition is single-issue focused, such as on one level or one region of the spine, usually promoting basic activities of daily life. Physical therapy is defined by its acute rehabilitative nature, and not maintenance follow-through.

Not all clients move swiftly through the therapy pathway. The PMME has more freedom to work past a pre-determined timeline. With the PMME's involvement, the PTs and other members of the allopathic medical team receive the additional support they need to attend to the acute, direct therapeutic procedures involved with any specific degenerative or disease states of the client.

The PMME both takes a burden of supplemental education and adjunct motor learning from the PT, while the PMME can rest assured that the client receives the acute structural care that only medically based personnel can deliver. Most PT treatment includes manual therapy, healing modalities such as sound, light or electrical applications, as well as home exercises directed toward alleviating muscle spasms, spinal segment malalignment and stiffness, or composes a treatment plan for a critical issue such as recent hip replacement or lymphedema from cancer treatment. It is a win-win situation. For this reason, astute PTs include Pilates, which may be undertaken by themselves or by PMMEs.

The self-care model

Did you realize that a number of people will seek out the expertise of a PMME on their own? Whether the patient is inside or outside of the allopathic, traditional medical model, ultimately it is the patient's decision, not the physician's or any member of the Scoliosis

Team, on how and why to seek care. Be a part of the solution. Mother Teresa of Calcutta encourages us, "Never worry about numbers. Help one person at a time, and always start with the person nearest you" (20 Mother Teresa Quotes, 2017).

Become transparent through local, regional, national and even international venues so that clients will find you. However, whether an individual who has scoliosis is looking for self-care, or is a parent seeking care for a child, body–mind movement approaches that clients decide to pursue depend upon individual and family beliefs about the efficacy, safety and value of exercise systems.

For this reason, the PMME must answer the call for specialized training so that clients can identify Movement Educators appropriate to their needs, verifying their qualifications and how to access them (Ajzen, 1991).

A call for advanced training

Due to the complexities of working with those that have non-neutral spines (scoliosis) and bodily asymmetries as well as time-of-life issues, there is a need for advanced qualification training for both licensed allied healthcare providers as well as PMMEs.

In addition to the fitness instructor registries, qualified Movement Educators are identified in other ways.

It is to the advantage of the consumer to seek out verification of the Movement Educator's background. National registries, such as the United States Certified Registry of Exercise Professionals (USCREP), and the National Registry of Registered Personal Trainers (NRPT) in the UK, as well as the International Confederation of Registries for Exercise Professionals (ICREPS), help to identify the level of training of the individual personal trainer or Movement Educator.

Advanced qualification is a higher level recognized by the registry organizations. Generally, when working with scoliosis, PMMEs should maintain a Level 4 qualification as established by the ICREPS, and seek specialized training focused on spinal abnormalities.

Recommended ICREPS qualifications include:

- An in-depth knowledge of the acute and chronic responses, as well as adaptations, of both healthy individuals and individuals with the special condition to the physical activity.

- A clear understanding of the responses of medications used for the conditions during the physical activity.

- An understanding of how various co-morbidities (note: explained in Chapter 12) affect the response to the physical activity.

- A comprehensive knowledge of the design and implementation of safe and effective exercises for those with functional limitations or disabilities.

- Effective skills in educating healthy behavior modification.

- A thorough knowledge of indications and counterindications to physical activity.

- An ability to determine when to terminate exercise activity during a session or suspend sessions until further medical intervention is sought.

- An ability to respond to emergency situations.

- An ability to create and respond to a written emergency plan for the facility or when working within the facility.

- An understanding of the behavioral change model and strategies that need to be considered and applied when working with individuals with a certain condition (Warburton et al., 2013).

Scope of practice vs qualification

Level of movement education qualification is similar but not the same as scopes of practice. A licensed PT allows differing skills than a Movement Educator or personal trainer. This scope of practice varies from country to country and state to state within the US.

For instance, in the US PTs can perform manual therapy for the client, such as specific joint mobilizations and maneuvers, as well as apply physical agent modalities, such as ice, heat, light, sound and vibration.

In the US, the legal ability to administer modalities varies from state to state. For instance, dry needling, a form of musculoskeletal acupuncture, is allowed in some states but not in California. In Canada, PTs are allowed to administer dry needling throughout the country.

In general, the PT is licensed to perform joint measures and tests using specialized equipment in order to arrive at a working PT diagnosis. The PT comes up with a prescriptive treatment plan that directly involves rehabilitation of a specific injury, pain or dysfunction with a finite discharge plan once the patient is deemed at a plateau, allowing periodic monitoring for maintenance of the discharge program. However, PTs are also allowed to provide wellness services such as ongoing asymmetry training when not treating a specific injury, pain or dysfunction. Wellness includes maintaining a level of fitness, strength, and skills such as fall prevention or decline of health (Wellness and cash-based services, 2013).

The certified PMME may not diagnose a physical or mental condition, or measure a client with instrumentation commonly used by PTs unless they are a PT.

In addition, although PMMEs generally provide encouragement and support to the client, referral for individual counseling is important when necessary.

When administering touch in the manner of tactile aid, request the client's permission, being sure to only "facilitate movement, position the client, and to prevent injury or damage." Do avoid inappropriate, even if trained and useful, touch beyond the level of certified training. This scope of practice rule is not to limit the PMME, yet rather to protect the PMME as well as the client. Referring a client for appropriate emotional or physical help demonstrates wisdom and prudence. Actively develop collegial relationships within your community (PMA® Scope of Practice, 2015).

A long-time client came in noticeably upset. At 85 years old, she was a poster girl for lifelong fitness. As a fitness instructor in her local community program, she had started as a member of my dance classes years ago and eventually had become a permanent client. Perspiring a bit, looking pink and a bit winded, she seemed more tense, bloated and symptomatic than was usual when her asthma flared up. After watching her a bit, I took her blood pressure. I always keep a digital device on hand. The reading was exceptionally high. I stopped the session and insisted she go to her doctor, who determined she needed to increase her blood pressure medication. In my heart, I knew a medical incident was avoided by allowing referral to another provider who had other skills than myself. When in doubt, refer out.

Is the PMME moving toward the role of a paraprofessional to the PT?

The PT probably has the most similar role to the PMME in that they both work with special populations. Exercises for the two often overlap. Some countries even require a PMME to also be a licensed PT.

Research and evidence increasingly point to the use of Pilates for a variety of health issues, especially in the case of low back pain (Aladro-Gonzalvo, 2013). For this reason, the public may view PMMEs as skillful providers of spinal care, even when the individual PMME may not possess a higher skill level.

Additionally, PMMEs may or may not be licensed as another type of healthcare provider, such as PTs, chiropractors, athletic and fitness trainers, as well as physicians and nurses.

As part of my research I queried some PMMEs who have participated in my trainings and some who are also educators within the Pilates Method field. They represent a mix of PT, PT-assistant and jurisprudence, and are all certified Pilates teachers either with the Pilates Method Alliance in the US or a similar certifying agency in another country. The majority agreed that a multidisciplinary Scoliosis Team is best, where the PMME has extra training beyond the Pilates Method vocabulary as that training alone does not best address the needs of those with scoliosis.

Most felt the PMME should be a collaborator on the healthcare team, offering insights and suggestions.

Most agreed with the notion of the PMME standing in the role of a paraprofessional where a particular aspect of a professional task is delegated yet is not a fully qualified licensed professional such as PT, podiatry or chiropractic. However, disclosure regarding level of training is important so as not to mistake a PMME for a medical professional.

The tide is beginning to turn as new methods, training and collaboration, sharing conservative care techniques and technology, make certain appoaches to exercise, both within and outside of the PT world, a more viable option.

The conversation is likely to continue for many years as the PMME becomes closer and closer to defining their role beyond CAM to be fully recognized as part of an allopathic medical team. It cannot be denied that PMMEs possess a special opportunity to share their unique talent with the Scoliosis Team.

The job of the medical team is to cure, repair and fix the body. The job of the PMME is to build the body. Chapter 3 explores further how the PMME exerts influence within the Scoliosis Team.

Bibliography

20 Mother Teresa Quotes. (2010). Retrieved December 27, 2017, from: https://www.goalcast.com/2017/04/10/top-20-most-inspiring-mother-teresa-quotes/

ACE Personal Trainer Manual, 4th edn. (2017). Retrieved January 22, 2017, from LinkedIn: http://www.slideshare.net/ravostulp/week-1-scope-of-practice-15923951

Acupuncture: in depth. (2016). Retrieved January 20, 2017, from National Institutes of Health: https://nccih.nih.gov/health/acupuncture/introduction

Aladro-Gonzalvo, A.R., Araya-Vargas, G.A., Machado-Díaz, M., Salazar-Rojas W (2013). Pilates-based exercise for persistent, non-specific low back pain and associated functional disability: a meta-analysis with meta-regression. Journal of Bodywork and Movement Therapies, 17(1), 125–136

Azjen, I. (1991). Theory of planned behavior. Organizational Behavior and Human Processes, 50, 179–211. Retrieved January 20, 2017, from: https://www.scribd.com/document/145805916/Ajzen-Theory-of-Planned-Behaviour-1991

Bialek, M., D'Hango. A. (2011). Conservative treatment of idiopathic scoliosis according to the FITS concept: presentation of the method and preliminary, short-term, radiological and clinical results based on SOSORT and SRS criteria. Scoliosis, 6: 5. doi: 10.1186/1748-7161-6-25

Blum, C.L. (2002). Chiropractic and pilates therapy for the treatment of adult scoliosis. Journal of Manipulative and Physiological Therapeutics, 25(4), E1–E8

Casual research. (2017). Definition. Retrieved January 29, 2017, from Business Dictionary: http://www.businessdictionary.com/definition/casual-research.html

Conservative. (2018). Definition. Merriam-Webster. Retrieved August 6, 2018 from: https://www.merriam-webster.com/dictionary/conservative

Conservative treatment. (2018). Definition. Retrieved August 7, 2018, from: https://medical-dictionary.thefreedictionary.com/conservative+treatment

Consumer Reports. (2007). Too much treatment? Aggressive treatment can lead to more pain without gain. Retrieved January 20, 2017, from Consumer Reports.org: http://www.consumerreports.org/cro/2012/04/too-much-treatment/index.htm

Core Values. (2003). Retrieved January 22, 2017, from APTA: https://www.apta.org/uploadedFiles/APTAorg/About_Us/Policies/BOD/Judicial/ProfessionalisminPT.pdf

Cottingham, J. (1988). Shifts in pelvic inclination angle and parasympathetic tone produced by Rolfing soft tissue manipulation. Journal of the American Physical Therapy Association, 68, 1364–1370. Retrieved January 29, 2017, from Rolfing Wellness: http://www.rolfusa.com/research.html

Find a personal fitness trainer near me. (2017). Retrieved January 22, 2017, from National Register of Personal Trainers: http://www.nrpt.co.uk/find/index.htm

Harrison, D.E., Dennewald, A. (2013). 3-Point Bending Traction for Scoliotic Curvatures Using the New 3-D Denneroll Traction System: A Case Report. American Journal of Clinical Chiropractic, January 20, 2013. Retrieved August 6, 2018, from: http://www.chiropractic-biophysics.com/clinical_chiropractic/2013/1/20/3-point-bending-traction-for-scoliotic-curvatures-using-the.html

Henneman, E., Somgen, G., Carpenter, D.O. (1965) Functional significance of cell size in spinal motoneurons. Neurophysiology, 28(3), 560–580

Kane, W.J. (1977). Scoliosis prevalance: a call for a statement of terms. Journal of Clinical Orthopedics and Research, 126, 43–46.

Kendall, F.P., McCreary, E.K. (1993). Scoliosis. In: Kendall, F.P., McCreary, E.K., Provance, P. G., eds. Muscles: Testing and Function, 4th edn. Baltimore: Williams and Wilkins, Ch. 5, p. 129

Managing scoliosis with osteopathy. (2017). Retrieved January 29, 2017, from Lomax: bespoke wellness and nutrition: http://www.lomaxpt.com/managing-scoliosis-with-osteopathy_7585

Marty-Pourmarat, C., Scattin, L., Marpeau, M., Garreau de Loubresse, C. (2007). Natural history of progressive adult scoliosis. Spine, 32(11), 1227–1234; discussion 1235

National Register of Personal Trainers. (2017). Retrieved January 22, 2017, from: http://www.nrpt.co.uk/

Negrini, S., Donzelli, S., Aulisa, A. G. (2018). 2016 SOSORT guidelines: orthopaedic and rehabilitation treatment of idiopathic scoliosis during growth. Scoliosis and Spinal Disorders, 13: 3. Retrieved August 6, 2018 from: https://scoliosisjournal.biomedcentral.com/articles/10.1186/s13013-017-0145-8

PMA® Scope of Practice. (2015). Retrieved January 2017, from Pilates Method Alliance: http://www.pilatesmethodalliance.org/files/documentlibrary/Certification/Scope%20of%20Practice%20FINAL.pdf

Reamy, B.V., Slakey, J.B. (2001). Adolescent idiopathic scoliosis: review and current concepts. American Family Physician, 64(1), 111–116. Retrieved January 20, 2017, from: http://www.aafp.org/afp/2001/0701/p111.html

Romano, M., Negrini, A., Parzini, S. et al. (2015). SEAS (Scientific Exercise Approach to Scoliosis): a modern and evidence based effective approach to physiotherapic specific scoliosis exercises. Scoliosis, 10(3), 1–19

SpineCor® Training. (2013). Retrieved January 20, 2017, from SpineCor.com: http://www.spinecor.com/SpineCorTraining.aspx

Tanner Scale. (2011). Retrieved January 20, 2017, from Scientific Spine: http://scientificspine.com/spine-scores/tanner-scale.html

Tormenti, M.J., Maserati, M.B., Bonfield, C.M. et al. (2010). Complications and radiographic correction in adult scoliosis following combined transpsoas extreme lateral interbody fusion and posterior pedicle screw instrumentation. Neurosurgical Focus, 23(7), 1–7

US Registry of Exercise Professionals™. (2017). Retrieved January 22, 2017, from: http://www.usreps.org/Pages/exerciseprofessionals.aspx

Vibration platforms for scoliosis. (2016). Available online from: https://vibeplate.com/medical-rehabilitation/scoliosis-vibration-therapy/

Warburton, D.E.R., Charlesworth, S.A., Foulds, H.J., et al. (2013). Qualified exercise professionals: best practice. Canadian Family Physician, 59, 759–761. Retrieved January 29, 2017, from: http://www.cfp.ca/content/59/7/759.full.pdf+html

Weiss, H-R. (2011). The Method of Katerina Schroth – history, principles and current development. Scoliosis, 6(17), 1–21

Weistein, S.L., Dolan, L.A., Wright, J.G., Dobbs, M.B. (2013). Design of the bracing of adolescent idiopathic scoliosis trial. Spine, 38(21), 1832–41

Welcome to ICREPS. (2017). Retrieved January 22, 2017, from International Certified Registry of Exercise Professionals: http://www.icreps.org/

Wellness and cash-based services. (2013). Retrieved January 22, 2017, from WebPT: https://www.webpt.com/blog/post/wellness-and-cash-based-services-medicare

Being an influence: how Pilates instructors have a special place in scoliosis care

Scoliosis is a lifelong condition. A doctor's visit is limited in time and scope. A Pilates Method Movement Educator (PMME) can influence the details of the day-to-day physical and psychosocial challenges of scoliosis management through the life stages of this condition.

Establishing a relationship with the Pilates Method and an initial PMME, as part of a lifelong care team, gives a person with asymmetries time to learn the language of qualitative movement and to experience the plasticity of the effects of the Pilates environment, ultimately making it their own.

Over time, the Pilates Method can move clients with asymmetries through the phases of somatic training

Case example

I received a call from concerned parents about their adolescent son who had, surprisingly, developed a 60° left lumbar convexity over just two years. He was now about to go to university, having participated in a swim team along with extensive outdoor activities through his youth club. He had no pain except when wearing the recommended brace. Starting with education for the whole family, we worked with Arc, mat strength work with asymmetry cues (found in the SSPOT-2 in Chapter 7) along with eventual apparatus work. Now in his fourth year of the Pilates Method, we meet on every break in his schedule to progress him on his path. Now a strong young man, he has much more awareness of the need to continue his own management of his spine, and the tools to do this.

Table 3.1

Three phases of Pilates therapeutic application

Somatic	Corrective	Conditioning

where emotion, physical sensation and body awareness meet. From individualized correctives, we move into full conditioning, where the client moves onto acquiring the functionality of robustness for a fulfilling life.

Quality, not quantity

PMMEs have a unique potential to be leaders in quality of execution of movement. Friedman and Eisen, in one of the first books on the Pilates Method, summed the Pilates philosophy in a single sentence: "A few well-balanced movements, performed properly in a balanced sequence, are worth hours of doing sloppy calisthenics or forced contortions" (Eisen & Friedman, 1981).

The entire Method toolbox emphasizes whole-body commitment and self-awareness, with somatic, slow sensory work facilitated by imagery. The PMME and client both maintain motivation through intellectual engagement with the multiple foci and cues that address the imbalances in even the simplest of whole-body exercises.

Whether a PMME follows either classical or contemporary repertoires, both versions of the Pilates Method allow for adapted positions, correctives and movements designed for an individual's asymmetries.

Further, as a whole-body approach, the Pilates Method encourages awareness beyond the specific spinal and ribcage deviations of scoliosis into whole-body systems. This aspect is of primary importance since all systems receive influence from asymmetrical complexity, for better or for worse. Breaking down essential movements that integrate core control with appendage use allows time for neurological re-integration.

'All movements emanate from the torso' is a motto of the Method. Bringing attention into the spine along with its influence outwards into the rest of the body is critical in dealing with this client population.

Rhythmicity, precision, imagery, props and the plasticity of neurology bring movement education within the Pilates environment beyond the three-dimensional pull and push of simple de-rotation and spine correction. The Pilates environment embraces complexity of qualitative motion. Pilates is unique in its promotion of the spinal articulation in all planes.

Needless to say, spinal articulation is not suitable for everyone, especially for those with aging spines with osteoporosis or certain unstable spinal malalignments. Yet spinal awareness and relief techniques are appropriate for everyone.

The Pilates philosophy advocates small increments of change to add up to large changes. Small increments take time to develop and set. Learning takes place over time, in spaced repetition of the activity.

Confusion about what to do after bracing, initial physiotherapy or occupational therapy ends remains a primary issue for many young adults. Guiding a youth in the fragile initial years after revelation of the scoliosis onset takes time, often working through the completion of the growth spurt.

Adults with comorbidities of aging, such as hip replacement, cancer restoration and sarcopenia, require ongoing care due to overlapping conditions that often exacerbate the asymmetrical curve. Although it is well known that only a small percentage of those with scoliosis will require full medical management, making the Pilates environment a part of the lifelong plan through Lifestyle Medicine ensures daily maintenance and optimization of health (Abei, 2005).

The philosophy presented here does not imply that the Pilates environment is the only aspect of comprehensive asymmetric and scoliosis care. The Pilates Method is distinct from the scoliosis-specific physical therapy models, yet it is able to support them as part of the Scoliosis Team. It fills a gap and it enables a lifetime program, essentially a lifestyle component of the Lifestyle Medical Model (What is Lifestyle Medicine?, 2015).

Case example

I heard from a retired older adult interior designer who was shocked to receive a severe scoliosis diagnosis after meeting her physician for low back pain. She felt betrayal on several levels. She owned and had regularly used a high-quality weight resistance station in her home gym for many years. Upon viewing her significant right-thoracic convexity, body type and pelvic obliquity, my surprise caused me to inquire whether she noticed clothes measurement discrepancies or discomfort with long sitting due to her profession. She explained that her expensive ergonomic chair was fitted to her idiosyncrasies. She also wondered why the tailor always mentioned differences in pant leg lengths. In addition, her husband had never mentioned anything about her back. She also was under bone density supervision for osteoporosis.

Upon having her last test, unfortunately the technician asked her about having such severe scoliosis, an unprofessional comment that led her to seek legal advice about the possibility of negligence in not being alerted sooner by her general medical team. However, there is a happy ending: it is now five years since she started the Pilates Method, and she uses her home Reformer daily. Pleased with her progress, she has learned to manage her condition with Lifestyle Medicine.

Exerting influence through intention

Embracing a lifestyle approach takes faith in the process. Corrective alterations of fascial and movement patterns often feel unfamiliar to begin with, and then over time the new approach becomes automatic, thus creating a new normal for the individual.

The process of imagining a new way, thinking of the new way and then feeling how to incorporate the

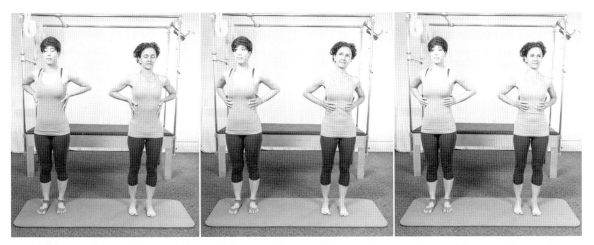

Figure 3.1
The three phases of movement acquisition: imagine, think, and feel.

new way is a recurrent theme throughout this book (Figure 3.1). Intention requires reflection. This reflection is a component of the Pilates Method principle of concentration.

Case study by an osteopath

An example of this possibility of intentional body guidance is a compelling presentation by osteopath Dr Peter Lewton-Brain from Monte Carlo. Presenting this interesting study at an IADMS meeting in 2008, his object was to determine the difference between a relaxed and an elongated spine, one of the principles of the Pilates Method. Presenting his own spine in three computed tomography images (CT scans), he examined the spinal differences in range when specific intention directs spinal positions, using spinal extension as an example.

He assumed three positions in prone, one of which was the spine in an arabesque. This position occurs in dance with one leg on the ground and the other suspended horizontally to the ground to the rear, creating substantial spinal extension. In prone (arched back into extension), the position is similar to the Swan in Classic Pilates or a Cobra pose in yoga.

The first image is a baseline image of neutral in prone. The next is a relaxed spinal extension position where his abdomen touched the bed. In the last he

consciously held an elongated spinal position, supporting the abdomen and elongating the spine for the duration of the imaging.

The second CT scan of elongation intent did indeed show that the spinal segments, particularly in the lumbar spine, appeared to have slightly more gapping between the vertebrae, achieving a cumulative elongating effect as measured by the researchers. However, Dr Lewton-Brain noticed that the soft tissue was the interesting element in the elongation of the second CT scan. He attributes the elongation effects to conscious decisions of the use of the soft tissue systems.

In the conclusions of the presentation, the lumbar spine in the back bend, performed with little elongation intent, indicates a more compressive force upon the spine than the intention test, measuring at a lumbar spine angle of 21°. The soft tissue shadows of the second CT scan indicate the guidance of the bones, through intent of action. When performed with no intent, in the back bend, the C1, the highest vertebra in the cervical spine, also became posteriorly displaced in the scan.

In Dr Lewton-Brain's words, "The findings showed visible changes in the soft tissue, seemingly little change to the vertebral column in individual segments but globally there were significant changes in angulation."

Furthermore, he offered that it was a quite strenuous activity to hold the elongation for such a duration, about 40 minutes, suggesting that elongation exercises do indeed challenge one's strength and muscular endurance (Lewton-Brain, 2008).

View this presentation showing how Pilates Method principles of elongation and concentration have a concrete effect upon spinal mechanics and human movement forms (Code 3.1).

Code 3.1 (free code)
Intentional vs non-intentional back extension

The PMME as leader

The PMME should be a leader in the client relationship, exerting influence to help the client and loved ones come to grips with a lifetime condition. Although the scoliosis condition is not curable, it is quantitatively changeable to a certain extent and qualitatively changeable to a much larger extent.

Do you know how to communicate with clients in such a situation? Every PMME wants to be heard by their clients. Before a client can hear what you know, they have to know that you care. Can you name four aspects of how to show you care, on an appropriate professional level?

Caring involves preparedness through your specialized training, commitment to integrity by not making false claims of cure, being interested during the process by inquiring in a friendly way about the client's life, showing why you are interested in spinal asymmetry and being comfortable with the topic.

Clients and their loved ones receiving difficult news of a spinal abnormality diagnosis find talking through difficult conversations about the options of management often brings enormous relief. Clients need to know if you can help them and if they can trust you. Trust is respect. Respect is earned. The PMME's role is both as a witness to the discomforts commonly experienced with asymmetries, and as a guide to offer

suggestions and concrete help with implementation of ergonomics, posture education, movement strategy, and general nutrition for health – all components in how to manage the condition in a practical way. However, it is always the responsibility of the PMME to work to support the Scoliosis Medical or Non-Medical Team, which varies as the client moves through life's stages.

Being a leader means exerting influence. Influence leans toward either a positive or a negative side. Becoming a reliable resource of positive influence is a process. A client may not remember what you said, but they will always remember how you made them feel.

Virtually no one is born with innate knowledge of how to lead a client through spinal asymmetry management without going through phases of growth. Use this book to identify where you are as a PMME in the phases of leadership growth and begin the process of professional growth:

Phase 1: *I don't know what I don't know*

Phase 2: *I know that I need to know*

Phase 3: *I know what I don't know*

Phase 4: *I know and grow, and it starts to show*

Phase 5: *I simply go because of what I know.*

Maxwell, 2007

This is not to say that intuition is not a part of the scenario in working with clients of this population. Intuition is knowing something without knowing how you knew it. Decision-making is best as a balance between deliberate and instinctive thinking.

Emotional acquisition of knowledge that turns into instinctual knowledge is quickly learned, such as when we learn as children to avoid hot flames by an adult yelling sharply at us.

Piecing together an asymmetry individual program is intricate and slow because it is a large collection of mini-skills. In good decision-making, frugality matters. That is why seeing the rule of threes in the big picture counts. *Ergonomics, exercise* and *emotion* guide the outline for what is necessary to learn. Exercise moves through *somatics, correctives* and *conditioning*. The way to learn is by *imagining, thinking* and *feeling*.

As you move on to exploring the leaves within the forest, keep referring back to the basics of what is important. Keep your eye on the prize: lifelong management. The PMME is a witness and a living log of the client's history and current status. Who better to notice changes as they arise? Through a balance of deliberate and instinctive thinking, the PMME is a prized influential participant in the Scoliosis Team.

A case for lifetime management and the influence of fascia

Why should one expect to manage a condition like scoliosis over a lifetime? A compelling story follows, related by Bonnie Thompson, a co-director of the Institute for Anatomical Research, a non-profit organization located in Colorado Springs in the USA. Their motto is, 'The human body is a priceless teacher.'

The Institute conducts cadaveric studies from donated bodies. Unusually, the Institute interviews the donors before their decease. In this way, information is obtained about lifestyle, nutrition, medical history, symptoms and quality of life. Of course, most of their donors are elderly.

Ms Thompson related a 2014 course featuring two women with scoliosis who donated their bodies. One woman was aged 79 at the time of passing. The other woman was in her early 90s. The younger woman had a severe scoliosis; she was in extreme pain yet did not try to manage it through exercise. The woman in her 90s, who should have been more fragile and symptomatic due to her older years, had less pain.

The older woman walked one mile per day until her death. Her scoliosis in standing was not very apparent. The younger woman's spinal asymmetry was very apparent when she was laid out on the dissection table, as one would expect.

Interestingly, the older woman showed little sign of the scoliosis when laid out prone upon the table. However, upon entering her body for study, the significant scoliosis became apparent. Is this observation contrary to what is usually believed, that a functional scoliosis normally subsides in a non-weightbearing position?

Of particular note, when the younger woman's body was opened for dissection, the researchers found a large thick band of connective tissue, essentially a fascial strap. It reached from the concave internal side of her pelvis and up toward the internal ribcage on the convex thoracic side, as if to attempt to pull the lateral prominence back toward a central line (Thompson, 2016).

Thompson's work is an important contemporary contribution to the body of knowledge surrounding the effect of fascia in an asymmetrical body. Fascia is our helper yet can also be our nemesis when fascia locks in compensatory asymmetries.

Chapter 4 explores the causes and dilemma of structural versus functional elements of spinal asymmetries. The two weave a tangled web. The PMME is the one to untangle it.

Bibliography

Abei, M. (2005). The adult scoliosis. European Spine Journal, 14(10), 925–938

Altan, L., Korkmaz, N., Bingol, U., Gunay, B. (2009). Effect of Pilates training on people with fibromyalgia: a pilot study. Archives of Physical Medicine and Rehabilitation, 90, 1983–1988. Retrieved January 26, 2017, from http://myalgia.com/PDF%20files/Pilates%20for%20Fibromyalgia%202010.pdf

Alves de Araújo, M.E. (2012). The effectiveness of the Pilates method: reducing the degree of non-structural scoliosis, and improving flexibility and pain in female college students. Journal of Bodywork and Movement Therapies, 16(2), 191–198

Asher, M.A., Burton, D.C. (2006). Adolescent idiopathic scoliosis: natural history and long term treatment effects. Scoliosis and Spinal Disorders, 1(2), 559–567

Balanced Body. (2014). Selected Research Bibliography. Retrieved September 2017, from www.pilates.com: https://www.pilates.com/BBAPP/V/pilates/library/bibliography.html

Balsamo, S., Willardson, J. M., Frederico Sde, S. et al. (2013). Effectiveness of exercise on cognitive impairment and Alzheimer's disease. International Journal of General Medicine, 6, 387–391

Betz, S.R. (2005). Modifying pilates for clients with osteoporosis. IDEA Fitness Journal, 2(4), 46–55. Retrieved January 29, 2017, from http://www.ideafit.com/fitness-library/pilates-osteoporosis

Bialek, M., Pawlak, P., Kotwicki, T. (2009). Foot loading asymmetry in patients with scoliosis. Scoliosis, 4(Suppl. 1): 19. doi:doi:10.1186/1748-7161-4-S1-O19

Blom, M.-J. (2012). Pilates and fascia: the art of 'working in'. In: Schleip, R., Findley, T.W., Chaitow, L., Huijing, P.A. eds. Fascia: The Tensional Network of the Human Body, Vol. 1. New York: Churchill Livingstone Elsevier, pp. 449–456

Borghuis, J., Hof, A.L., Lemmink, K.A. (2008). The importance of sensory-motor control in providing core stability:

implications for measurement and training. Sports Medicine, 38(11), 893–916

Chaitow, L. (2013). Breathing pattern disorders. Retrieved September 1, 2017, from www.leonchaitow: http://leonchaitow.com/2012/01/23/breathing-pattern-disorders-and-lumbopelvic-pain-and-dysfunction-an-update/

Czaprowski, D., Kotwicki, T., Pawlowska, P., L Stolinski, L. (2012). Joint hypermobility syndrome in children with idiopathic scoliosis. Scoliosis, 7 (Suppl. 1): O69. doi:10.1186/1748-7161-7-S1-O69

EDS International Classification. (2017). Retrieved September 1, 2017, from The Ehlers Danlos Society: https://www.ehlers-danlos.com/2017-eds-international-classification/

The Female Athlete Triad. (2011). Retrieved September 1, 2017, from: http://www.femaleathletetriad.org/wp-content/uploads/2010/03/FATC_Slideshow_2011.pdf

Friedman, P., Eisen, G. (1980). The Pilates Method of Physical and Mental Conditioning. Doubleday

Hawes, M.C. (2003). The use of exercises in the treatment of scoliosis: an evidence-based critical review of the literature. Pediatric Rehabilitation, 6(3–4), 171–182

Jaroszweski D, Notricia, D., McMahon, L., et al. (2010). Current management of pectus excavatum: a review and update of therapy and treatment recommendations. Journal of American Board of Family Medicine, 23(2), 230–239

Kaya, D.O., Duzgun, I., Baltaci, G. et al. (2012). Effects of calisthenics and Pilates exercises on coordination and proprioception in adult women: a randomized controlled trial. Journal of Sport Rehabilitation, 21(3), 235–243. Retrieved September 1, 2017, from http://www.academia.edu/1123285/Effects_of_Calisthenics_and_Pilates_Exercises_on_Coordination_and_Proprioception_in_Adult_Women_Randomized_Controlled_Trial

Kendall, F.P., McCreary, E.K., Provance, P. G., eds. (1993). Muscles: Testing and Function, 4th edn. Baltimore: Williams and Wilkins

Key, J. (2010). The pelvic crossed syndromes: a reflection of imbalanced function in the myofascial envelope; a further exploration of Janda's work. Journal of Bodywork and Movement Therapies, 14(3), 299–301

Kirkwood T. (2010). Why women live longer. Scientific American, pp. 34–36. Retrieved February 5, 2017, from https://www.scientificamerican.com/article/why-women-live-longer/

Klippinger, K. (2017). Interview with K. Klippinger, Professor of Anatomy. (S. Martin, Interviewer)

Larsson, M. (2013). All about Eve. Retrieved August 13, 2018, from: http://coredynamicspilates.com/wp-content/uploads/2014/10/AllAboutEve-SantaFe-NM.pdf

Levine B., Kaplanek, B., Jaffe, W.L. (2009). Pilates training for use in rehabilitation after total hip and knee arthroplasty. Clinical Orthopaedics and Related Research, 467, 1465–1475. doi:10.1007/s11999-009-0779-9

Lewton-Brain, P.A. (2008). Back-bend or spinal extension? Biomechanics and multi-sliced computed tomography and movement intention. Centre Hospitale de Princesse Grace. Monaco: Centre Hospitale de Princesse Grace

Lin, J.J., Chen, W.H., Chen, P.Q., Tsauo, J.Y. (2010). Alteration in shoulder kinematics and associated muscle activity in people with idiopathic scoliosis. Spine, 35(11), 1151–1157. doi: 10.1097/BRS.0b013e3181cd5923

Lowe T.G., Burwell, R.G., Dangerfield, P.H. (2004). Platelet calmodulin levels in adolescent idiopathic scoliosis (AIS): can they predict curve progression and severity? European Spine Journal, 13(3), 257–265. doi: 10.1007/s00586-003-0655-3

Maxwell, J. (2007). 21 Irrefutable laws of leadership. Chapter 3. Nashville: Thomas Nelson

Mayo, N.E., Goldberg, M.S., Scott, S., Hanley, J. (1994). The Ste-Justine Adolescent Idiopathic Scoliosis Cohort Study. Part III: Back pain. Spine (Phila Pa) 1976, 19(14), 1573–1581

McNaughton, S., Farley, D., Staggs, R. et al. (2008). Pregnancy, fertility, and contraception risk in the context of chronic disease: scoliosis. Journal for Nurse Practitioners, 4(5), 370–376.

Myers, T.W. (2014). Anatomy Trains: Myofascial Meridians for Manual and Movement Therapists, 3rd edn. Edinburgh: Churchill Livingstone

National Center for Chronic Disease Prevention. (2013). The state of aging and health in America. Retrieved February 5, 2017, from Center for Disease Control; cdc.com: https://www.cdc.gov/aging/pdf/state-aging-health-in-america-2013.pdf

Negrini, A., Parzini, S., Negrini, M.G. et al. (2008). Adult scoliosis can be reduced through specific SEAS exercises: a case report. Scoliosis and Spinal Disorders, 3(20), 1–11

Osteoporosis in men. (2015). Retrieved September 1, 2017, from www.nih.gov: https://catalog.niams.nih.gov/detail.cfm?pubid=1595

Phrompaet, S., Paungmali, A., Pirunsan, U., Sitilertpisan, P. (2011). Effects of Pilates training on lumbo-pelvic stability and flexibility. Asian Journal of Sports Medicine, 2(1), 16–22

Pilates Method Alliance. (2017). The 2016 Pilates In America Study. Retrieved from: https://www.pilatesmethodalliance.org/i4a/pages/index.cfm?pageID=3821

Pilates, J.H. (1945) [2010]. Return to Life Through Contrology. Miami, Florida: Pilates Method Alliance

Rabago D., Slattengren, A., Zgierska, A. (2010). Prolotherapy in primary care practice. Primary Care, 37(1), 65–80

Rapoport, I.C. (2016). A Day with Joseph Pilates. Retrieved January 27, 2017, from: http://icrapoport.com/category/onassignment/sports-illustrated/

Richardson C., Jull, G., Hodges, P.W., Hides, J. (2004). Therapeutic exercise for spinal segmental stabilization in low back pain: scientific basis and clinical approach. Edinburgh: Churchill Livingstone

Rock, J.A., Roberts, C.P., Jones, H.W., Jr. (2010). Congenital anomalies of the uterine cervix: lessons from 30 cases managed clinically by a common protocol. Fertility and Sterility, 94(5), 1858–1863

Saccuci, M., Tettamanti, L., Mummolo, S. et al. (2011). Scoliosis and dental occlusion: a review of the literature. Scoliosis, 6(15), 1–12.

Schoeneman, S. (2007/2008). Implementing Pilates into my practice. Retrieved August 7, 2018 from Balanced Body: http://www.pilates.com/BBAPP/V/pilates/library/articles/implementing-pilates-into-my-practice.html

Silva, F.E., Lenke. L. (2010). Adult degenerative scoliosis: evaluation and management. Neurosurgery Focus, 28(3), E1: 1–10

Svantesson H., Marhaug, G., Haeffner, F. (1981). Scoliosis in children with juvenile rheumatoid arthritis. Scandinavian Journal of Rheumatology, 10(2), 65–68

Tate, L. (2015). Prevalence of scoliosis in a Pelvic Pain Cohort. Journal of Women's Health Physical Therapy, 39(1), 3–9

Thompson, B. (2016). Case of 2 female elderly cadaver donors with scoliosis. (S. Martin, Interviewer). Retrieved February 2, 2017, from: http://www.anatomicalresearch.org/

van der Linden, M.L., Bulley, C., Geneen, L.J. et al. (2014). Pilates for people with multiple sclerosis who use a wheelchair: feasibility, efficacy and participant experiences. (PubMed, Ed.) Disability and Rehabilitation, 36(11), 932–939

Virginia Spine Institute. (2017). Flat back syndrome. Retrieved February 4, 2017, from Spine MD: http://www.spinemd.com/symptoms-conditions/flat-back-syndrome

Watson, J. (2012). Sarcopenia in older adults. Current Opinions in Rheumatology, 24(6), 623–627

Weinstein, S.L., Dolan, L.A., Spratt, K.F. (2003). Health and function of patients with untreated idiopathic scoliosis: a 50-year natural history study. JAMA, 289(5), 559–567

What is Lifestyle Medicine? (2015). Retrieved January 26, 2017, from American College of Lifestyle Medicine: https://www.lifestylemedicine.org/What-is-Lifestyle-Medicine/

Which Pilates exercises are good for someone with Parkinson's disease? (2017). Retrieved January 29, 2017, from MedicineNet.com: http://www.medicinenet.com/script/main/art.asp?articlekey=78165

Women's International Pharmacy. (2013). Pelvic organ prolapse: what can be done to prevent it? Retrieved February 5, 2017, from Connections: An Educational Resource of Women's International Pharmacy: http://womensinternational.com/connections/prolapse.html

Looking at the causes of scoliosis

The causes of spinal asymmetry and scoliosis break down into two main categories: structural and functional. The purpose of this book is to address functional solutions, yet the structural components deserve attention in order to understand what is changeable and what is not (see Table 4.1). A podiatrist explained to me once that in foot care, the goal is to change the structural problem into a functional problem. Is this possible with scoliosis?

Neuromuscular scoliosis

First consider that most spinal asymmetry cases seen in medical clinics and in our studios do not come from congenital/birth issues, nor are they true genetic neurological conditions, called neuromuscular scoliosis.

Neuromuscular scoliosis conditions involve paralysis or partial paralysis due to myriad issues, which eventually result in an unbalanced skeleton with more or less ability to recruit and use appropriate musculature, and sometimes involve cognitive (thinking) difficulties. As a result, the spinal asymmetry is created by default due to deficiencies. Review Table 4.1 to better understand common neurological scenarios.

Other connections: nationality

Scoliosis is connected to other chromosomal tendencies according to nationality: a 10-year study through the RIKEN Institute in Japan recently identified a gene found in Asian and Caucasian populations. The genes of 1819 Japanese individuals with scoliosis were compared to 25 939 Japanese individuals over a 10-year period. The gene associated with a susceptibility to develop scoliosis is on chromosome 6.

The hypothesis is that gene 'GPR126' affects not only susceptibility to adolescent idiopathic scoliosis (AIS), but also impacts full-grown height through abnormal spinal development and growth. It is unclear

what turns on these genes environmentally, the focus of a field called epigenetics (Ikegawa, 2016).

ScoliScore® is a genetic test specific for scoliosis; however, it is experimental in predicting actual progression, the worsening, of AIS, so it needs to be used cautiously and under supervision of interpretation (Carlson, 2011).

Eighty percent of clinical scoliosis-diagnosed cases are idiopathic, meaning from an unknown cause. The focus of this book addresses mostly those members of the 80% who come to our studios.

As mentioned in Chapter 1, please keep an open mind and work with the client who has neurological issues. When working with these individuals, it helps to be part of a team with other healthcare givers that explain the condition and guide the Pilates Method Movement Educator (PMME).

Neurological conditions are baffling and often frustrating for both the client and the PMME since this type of client does not follow a common trajectory of response, as with typical injury rehabilitation or scoliosis training. Gains are often slow and hard-won. Although improvement is a rollercoaster ride of ups and downs, the client will benefit from the Pilates environment.

One mentee showed up to a mentoring session with her daughter, who was almost at university age. The young woman had seizures in early life that left her with spinal asymmetry and impairments on her dominant arm and leg side. A beautiful young woman, she hid it well, at one point relating to us how she changed schools due to bullying. The intensive weekend mentoring session included her care, as a model patient; she was very willing to try. It opened windows of possibility for her. The work was not going to cure her, but she saw hope for improvement.

Table 4.1

Less than 10% of scoliosis results from neurologic, congenital, and genetic conditions such as those listed, which are associated with spinal asymmetry and scoliosis (Soutanis et al., 2007)

Neurologic	Congenital	Genetic
Cerebral palsy A one-time birth incident that deprives the baby of oxygen resulting in the inability to develop normally	**Spinal cord cysts** Cysts in the cord cause abnormal pressures against the spinal column	**Down syndrome** A chromosomal defect that causes hypermobility in the upper cervical spine along with other spinal issues
Muscular dystrophy A defect in the nerve conduction of muscle physiology that creates intermittent to permanent severe weakness	**Dural cysts** Cysts in the coverings of the spinal cord cause abnormal pressures and growth along the spinal column	**William syndrome** A genetic condition that causes growth disturbances
Charcot–Marie–Tooth disease A neurological disorder that usually gives an unbalanced gait and weakness that is difficult to strengthen	**Non-closure of the vertebral column**	**Chromosome 19p defect** Associated with causing adolescent idiopathic scoliosis in Caucasians and Asians
Traumatic brain injury A neurological brain trauma that affects both mood and executive thinking impacting both emotional control and motor control; concussion is included in this category	**Shortened (tethered) cord**	
Multiple sclerosis A special nerve and muscle condition that slows down movement ability in an unbalanced way		**POC5 gene** Causes familial scoliosis for unknown reasons
Post-polio syndrome The aftermath of the infection leaves partial paralysis and can worsen with over-exertion or even simple exercise		
Stroke Stroke results from brain blockage or blood hemorrhage where both deprive certain areas of the brain of oxygen, giving partial or extreme varied paralysis and motor control dysfunction (I worked with a stroke patient for 25 years who benefited tremendously from the Pilates environment)		
Parkinson's disease A problem of motor control causing stiffening, repetitive tremors (shaking)		

Structural curves

Structural curves do not usually straighten out when lying down but remain fixed in their shape. A structural curve is most evident in the prone position. Structural scoliosis has an irreversible lateral spinal curve, involving rotation in the spine, ribcage and often the pelvis. The spinous processes become permanently bent and rotated in the direction of the concave side of the lateral curve. The bodies of the vertebra rotate in the direction of the convex portion of the curve and are often irregularly shaped.

The Major Curve is the largest structural curve. One or more Compensatory Curves occur above or below the Major Curve, attempting to maintain a normal vertical body alignment. The structural element of scoliosis, once set at maturity, is a true skeletal deformity that does not change.

Early intervention

This concrete element of structural spinal asymmetry is the reason for early intervention, when there is a possibility of lessening or even eradicating the curves.

An international call for screening and research into what is called scoliogeny, the early onset of spinal asymmetry, is underway. Initiated by the International Research Society of Spinal Deformities, it calls for more research and vigilance. Although spinal asymmetry and scoliosis is not in and of itself life-threatening in most cases, its likely progression into adulthood warrants young life care (Burwell et al., 2013; Grivas et al., 2013b).

One problem is that the beginning of the asymmetry often develops very quickly, reported as within a few months, before the youth or the parents realize what is happening. PMMEs help enormously in monitoring the improvement or progression of asymmetry through their observation skills.

Worsening of the curves or collapse of the spine in adulthood is just as alarming and distressing. Several of my adult clients experienced shock and dismay over finding that their back pain is a spinal curve, some surprised at even a 60° Cobb angle curve!

Adult clients sent to me as a last-ditch effort to stem the collapsing waist are often shocked at what it takes to prevent full collapse, possibly requiring surgical intervention. Older adults with a high-functioning lifestyle often do not want to change, just trying to get through each day. The benefits of establishing reasonable lifetime management habits for this condition cannot be overstated. No money or entitlement in the world is a substitute for functional spinal health.

Structural causes

Structural causes for idiopathic (unknown) reasons of spinal asymmetry development break down into two major divisions. The first is *neurophysiology*, also called *pathophysiology*, which involves growth hormones and reproductive hormones in the endocrine system that interact with the nervous system.

The second component, *bone physiology*, involving *pathomechanics*, describes how the bones develop into an adaptive, asymmetrical curve. It is unsure where

one begins and the other stops. Is it the chicken or the egg coming first?

It is easier to pinpoint the origin of the cause in true neurological, genetic or disease conditions.

The two components of pathophysiology and pathomechanics derive from several main theories for structural spinal asymmetry development in the study of especially unknown cause cases. They are the Neuro-osseous Theory, the Hueter–Volkmann law of Bone Modulation (H–V law), and the Vicious Cycle, all culminating in the Cascade Concept. Cases with neurological cause also follow the H–V law and Vicious Cycle theoretical models of asymmetrical development.

Foundations of the Neuro-osseous Theory

Milan Roth, a Czech scientist from Brno, developed his concepts on the neurovertebral (spinal cord lengthening) and neuro-osseous (bone growth stimulated by the endocrine system) systems, between 1960 and 1985. These systems relate during growth in reciprocal influence between the two tissues of bone and spinal cord.

Roth's basic premise is a result of the many mechanical models he constructed based on a multitude of experiments that demonstrate the need for the neurological development of the spinal cord and central nervous system to coordinate with the osseous growth of the spinal column. This discovery is the foundation for the current pathophysiological hypotheses on the development of AIS (Loon, 2012).

The Neuro-osseous Theory

The Neuro-osseous Theory, postulated by Dr Burwell in 2009, is also labeled the neuro-osseous timing of maturation (NOTOM). The hypothesis is that normal skeletal growth and maturation depend upon a physiological balance between the growth hormones and musculoskeletal development, by way of biological factors called 'escalators.' Here the term 'escalator' means a process of biological factors which allow normal growth when present or abnormal growth when deficient.

Dr Burwell describes two escalators, one associated with bone, the other with nerves. The first escalator is the 'osseous (bony) escalator,' responsible for increasing skeletal size and shape, which in turn promotes sensory, proprioceptive inputs to the 'neural escalator' in the brain.

The second escalator, the 'neural escalator' constitutes the re-calibration and interaction between the brain and the central nervous system body scheme to constantly adjust skeletal enlargement, shape and relative mass changes, ultimately coordinating motor actions.

The Neuro-osseous Theory states that AIS, which occurs mostly in girls, results from a developmental discrepancy between the spine and the physiological systems controlling autonomic and somatic nervous systems.

Autonomic systems are the relatively automatic systems that regulate heart rate, blood pressure, breathing, as well as the timing of maturation and the growth spurt. The somatic nervous system is the sensory-motor system, which receives input from the brain, and the spinal cord, which produces output to stimulate bone growth. This is a reciprocal relationship where the sensory-motor system then also gives information to the spinal cord and brain to produce either more or less development.

A dysfunction in circulating hormones, including ghrelin, the hormone for appetite, and leptin, the hormone responsible for the deposition of fat, is necessary for the production of estrogen, promoting reproductive maturation. This aspect of the theory is consistent with other researchers that note a low BMI (basal metabolic index – a height and weight scale to determine expected averageness) is related to truncal asymmetry.

The focus is the female in these studies because the majority of those with spinal asymmetry that goes on to progress to severity are female. However, males also need estrogen for bone growth. This theory tells us that nutrition is an important component of normal maturation and health (Burwell et al., 2009; Grivas et al., 2013a).

The Hueter–Volkmann law

The next theory is called the Hueter–Volkmann law (H–V law), which relates to the escalators of the

NOTOM. The H–V law states that increased pressure on the vertebral growth or end plates retards the bone's vertical growth (Hueter), and conversely, when mechanical pressure is reduced or unloaded, longitudinal growth rate accelerates (Volkmann) (Figure 4.1).

Dr Ian Stokes researches the uncoupling patterns of the spine involved with lateral curvature of the spine, as theorized by the H–V law. His work explores the reason and effects of the progression of the lateral curvature in scoliosis. He created various computer-generated models to better understand how instability, true unraveling of the spine, occurs. He verified that when the spine begins to form a lateral curvature, one side of the vertebra receives more force upon it than the other. Do not confuse this theory with Wolff's law which states that increasing mechanical stresses upon bone increases bone density.

Note the difference between the two. According to Dr Stokes, "Bone remodeling (basic bone growth) is

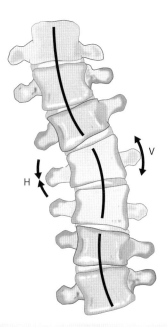

Figure 4.1

The Heuter–Volkman law of spinal growth: increased pressure inhibits growth on the concave side (H) and decreased pressure on the other side increases growth (V).

said to be governed by Wolff's Law, while mechanical influence on longitudinal bone growth (vertical growth height) is said to be controlled by the Hueter–Volkmann Law."

This means that bone is deposited, remodeled, in response to stresses placed upon it according to Wolff's law, but that the height of the vertebrae as well as long bone growth are modulated, or altered, due to stress or the removal of stress upon them. This information tells us that balancing posture in verticality is important.

One reason why this change in vertebral shape often goes unnoticed is that the spine is usually growing longer in general. Both sides are growing vertically, but just at different rates.

The Vicious Cycle

Stokes also explains that a Vicious Cycle then begins (Figure 4.2). The main driving factor for asymmetry is the onset and development of deformities created by the altering vertebral growth dynamics. Once a critical threshold of gravitational asymmetric load occurs, the deformity progresses, and is unavoidable (Figure 4.3). Only a compensatory force applied to offset the biomechanical effects will counteract such abnormal bone growth. Stokes also contributes a simulated model of muscle stresses showing how altered and asymmetrical muscle loads about the asymmetrical spinal column have difficulty in achieving stability about the spinal column (Figure 4.4) (Stokes,

2007). However, Stokes' multiple research works show that muscle activation indeed aids spinal stability and general ability to recover from uneven outside forces using spinal activation techniques.

The work of Dr Stokes is of utmost importance to PMMEs, indicating that the judicious and timely use of exercise is potentially helpful (Stokes, 2002; Stokes, 2018).

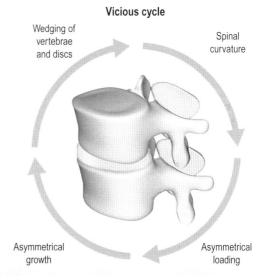

Figure 4.2

Stokes' Vicious Cycle model of asymmetrical spine growth. Reproduced with permission.

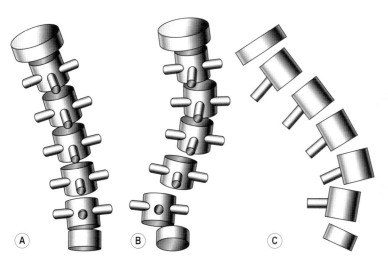

Figure 4.3

Stokes' Predicted Buckling Models of asymmetrical lumbar spine forces. Reproduced with permission.

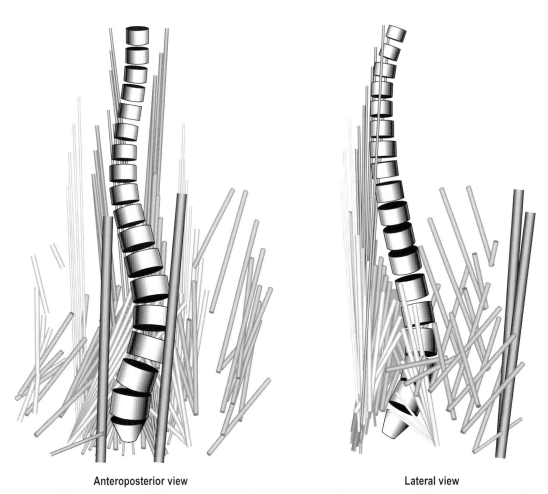

Anteroposterior view   **Lateral view**

Figure 4.4
Stokes' asymmetrical muscle loading with asymmetrical spine. Reproduced with permission.

The Cascade Concept

The Cascade Concept is a hypothesis for the development of AIS. It states that fat deposition and metabolism issues, especially at 10 years of age, predispose certain adolescents toward spinal asymmetry.

Although uncertain, leptin is somehow necessary to human central nervous system development and its lack alters the spinal cord growth mechanism. There is reason to believe that low body fat quantities impair the proper growth of the spinal cord, especially if environmental factors such as Vitamin D or calcium deficiency exist.

Once these deficits take hold and the vertical spinal column development starts to become asymmetrical, the scenario enters the Vicious Cycle of lateral curvature development (Burwell et al., 2016).

Although these concepts and theories center on youth, they highlight the necessity for bone health and nutrition that supports bone health practices for all age groups.

Besides misshapen vertebrae, research indicates that other distinct structural changes happen over time, such as the asymmetry in length of especially the 12th rib, which is associated with the length and use of the quadratus lumborum, the muscles that attach the ribs to the pelvis. In addition, the ribs on the convex side at the apex of the lateral prominence become longer than the other (Stokes, 1989; Grivas et al., 2016).

The scapulothoracic joint is considered a functional rather than an anatomic joint, such as the glenohumeral joint where the humerus abuts to the scapula. However, it can be included with structural changes revealing the alteration of shoulder kinematics, where the scapular positioning is unusual. The scapula on the convex side of the rib cage tips anteriorly and the concave side rotates relatively upwards, affecting function of the lower trapezius on the convex side interfering with scapular tipping (Lin et al., 2010).

In addition, observations include an anterior protrusion in the mid-rib area, often associated with the concave side. Ribs 8–10 are called the false ribs since they connect to the sternum only through the cartilage of the 7th rib. When the ribcage begins to twist as a result of the spinal asymmetry, the cartilage is dragged along, creating imbalances. The internal obliques dominate, flaring the ribs upwards in elevation toward the head, creating changes in diaphragm, intercostals and external oblique functioning. The deep and superficial front and back arm fascial lines are then affected as well. Review the bone alterations image in Chapter 1 (see Figure 1.9).

Leg length discrepancy is another structural or functional issue. It most often is functional, which then causes a pelvic obliquity. To be purely structural, the difference needs to be greater than 1.0 cm (Landauer, 2013).

Even if the person does not exhibit true pelvic obliquity, evidence suggests that uneven leg loading in gait occurs in those with spinal asymmetry (Bialek et al., 2009). See Table 4.2 for a summary of the potential anatomic changes caused by spinal assymetry.

Asymmetry in gait pattern occurs in the next section since functional forces also occur due to natal patterning, life experiences, laterality and preferences.

The head is not mentioned much in the scoliosis literature yet all humans have a tendency to experience cranial (head) asymmetry due to exit from the birth

Table 4. 2
Summary of potential anatomic changes due to spinal asymmetry

Spine	Ribcage	Shoulder girdle	Pelvis	Legs
Major and compensatory adapted curves	The rib lengths at the apex of the convex side are longer than the other side	The shoulder girdle relationship to the ribcage is shifted causing a potential humeral length difference	The pelvis is often oblique with all three bones of the pelvis malaligned in a domino effect due to the closed system of the pelvic ring potentially causing bone shape irregularities	A leg length discrepancy due to either a functional pelvic obliquity or a true developed or acquired inequality
The spinous processes bend toward the concave side	The 12th ribs are different lengths	The scapula on the convex side is anteriorly rotated (forward and tipped)		The ankles are pronated on one side and supinated on the other in response to the oblique pelvis and/or leg length discrepancy giving potential bone shape differences
The bodies of the vertebrae are larger in width on the convex side	The costal cartilage on ribs 8–10 is possibly misshapen, causing a protrusion	The scapula on the concave side is upwardly rotated		

canal. Natal asymmetry impacts the body in general creating potential lifelong compensatory patterns. Compensatory pattern discussion appears in the next section.

It is important to intervene during youth to help establish the strongest skeleton possible to attempt to diminish impending structural skeletal deformities.

The Scoliosis Specific Physical and Observational Test (SSPOT) in Chapter 7 (Assessments) is both a test of strength and flexibility for youth and also provides a framework of goal accomplishment for youth. SSPOT provides spinal stability, bone-building and functional flexibility through a series of modifications of the Pilates Method Mat Series, emphasizing weight-bearing exercises. While specifically made for youth, adults also benefit and improve from many elements.

Chapter 5 details both the medical and the physical therapy classifications used in diagnosing the tendencies and types of the actual curve.

On the way to function

Non-structural curves are functional curves that tend to straighten out when the person lies supine on their back or prone on the front of their body. The functional type and/or aspect of a structural scoliosis has some flexibility for change.

It has a reversible element to its lateral curve, or other postural deviations. Non-structural curves also have Major and often Compensatory Curves. These curves usually straighten out when the muscles, joints and fascia are balanced by lying down, body work or exercise.

The functional layers

Functional, adaptable elements are layers that start at the skin and superficial fascial matrix just underneath the skin. Next are muscles with their inter- and intra-muscular fascia, connective tissue matrices within and outside of the muscles, tendons, and ligaments. More soft tissue structure occurs with aponeuroses, the flat planes of fascia that encase the cylinders of the legs and pelvis as well as wrap the torso.

Visceral fascia encapsulates our internal organs while proper fascia connects many internal to external body areas. Even structural scoliosis can change some of its compensatory elements that are not fixed or irreversible due to the enormity of the soft tissue systems.

Fascial restrictions are both a help and a hindrance, as covered later in this chapter. Davis's law of soft tissue deposition states that soft tissue remodels because of imposed demands in a similar way that Wolff's law states that bone is deposited due to imposed stress.

Bonnie Thompson's account at the end of Chapter 3 supports this idea of fascial generation in spinal asymmetry. Fascia has a great impact in the body with asymmetries, either helping to hold an asymmetrical body together or restricting a body's ability for motion when over-developed or adherent.

Buckminster Fuller introduced the concept of tensegrity in 1916 that, when applied to biology, explains architecturally the nature of the fascial bodily infrastructure. The cell architecture has mechanical behavior resulting from physical interactions between environmental and differing molecular filament systems, which form the cytoskeleton (internal cell scaffold) and the nucleus. Tensile elements of the connective tissues are fluidly countered by compressive elements creating ultimate flexibility and balance in an unequal three-dimensional system (Loghmani & Whitted, 2016).

The fourth dimension

Ultimately a fourth dimension exists within and beyond the traditional three-dimensional planar model of the body.

Evidence shows it is possible that the client with functional spinal asymmetry may be fully reversible; however, structural spinal asymmetries also have a malleable component due to the variability of the neuromusculofascial sling systems.

A study by Duval-Beaupère et al. (1985) illustrates plasticity between the rigid/structural to functional systems. A client with a structural/rigid 20° right thoracic convexity appears in both a supine, non-weight-bearing position and a standing gravitational position. Figure 4.5 shows the supine client with the rigid brace indicating that the 20° curve is rigid.

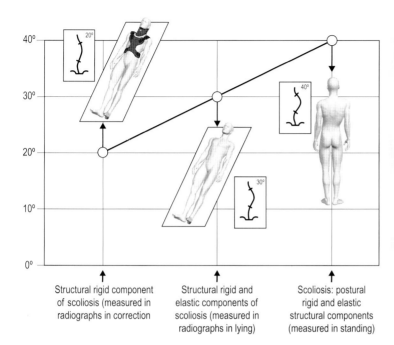

Figure 4.5
Functional changes are seen in a standing position. The standing position shows the summation of structural and functional components of spinal asymmetry. Adapted from Duval-Beaupère et al. (1985).

Structural rigid component of scoliosis (measured in radiographs in correction)

Structural rigid and elastic components of scoliosis (measured in radiographs in lying)

Scoliosis: postural rigid and elastic structural components (measured in standing)

The same client once again assumes a supine position but without the brace to show that the curve now registers 30°. In standing without the brace, the same client measures 40° at the same spinal curve measure and displays an impressive regression in neutral posture. This study shows the great effect that gravity has upon the functional adaptable elements of those with bodily asymmetry (Duval-Beaupère et al., 1985)

The physiotherapy (PT) treatment of scoliosis, the SEAS method, promotes use of the functional systems with re-training in everyday activities. The hypothesis provided by the PT SEAS method promises that positive influence upon the neuromotor systems for those with asymmetrical spines and bodies is possible with re-learning and re-training, corroborating with Duval-Beaupère et al.'s study that functional impact matters. Functional solutions also address these connective tissue and neuromotor elements (Negrini et al., 2008).

There are several points where it is important to understand which parts are rigid and which parts are changeable. It helps to decide how and when to add intensity to an exercise, how realistic postural change is, and predicts whether instruction potentially affects the curve or affects the compensations associated with the curve. The compensatory aspects are most changeable.

An Australian woman on one of my courses explained that her athletic teenage son received school screening where a forward bend test showed he had a back asymmetry. She brought him to physiotherapists who are certified in Schroth Method® assessment and training. They revealed that he merely had a hamstring imbalance and not a true spinal curve!

Good for them! Not everyone exhibits reversible curves, but they do exist.

From structural to functional

Numerous functional causes enter the mix of where the structural aspect ends and where the functional aspect begins.

Laterality: vertical and side symmetry

As mentioned earlier, structural asymmetry leading to functional asymmetry starts in the womb. Lateralization begins due to positioning around the mother's internal organs. As the infant arrives, often with a misshapen cranium, the labyrinthine reflex that dictates vertical head position comes into play.

The head position stimulates our balance system, the vestibular system, involving coordination of vision, inner ear (semi-circular canals and otolith organs), and joint position sense (proprioception). The vestibular system is responsible for stabilizing the position of the body, head and eyes in space.

Each side of the body has a separate vestibular apparatus that stimulates the ipsilateral, same-side extensors of the body, the back muscles, gluteal muscles, hamstrings, and calves. Evidence shows that unequal vestibular use, an alteration from what is expected, is common in those with scoliosis (Lambert et al., 2009).

Posture and vestibular control function to enable us to maintain an upright position and orientation due to the body's creation of anti-gravitational forces. Research indicates that there is a left vestibular dominance in approximately two-thirds of the general population (Pope, 2003).

When the head begins to select one side of the body versus the other, the anti-gravitational extensors then begin to dominate on that side, affecting how much body weight goes down into that side of the body.

Laterality: postural sway

In addition to natural tendencies experienced by the general populace, evidence shows that those with spinal asymmetry also exhibit issues of increased postural sway in quiet stance and being pushed off balance. Visual control issues in reflex reaction times after being thrown off balance suggest problems in coordination of the eyes with other components of the vestibular and musculoskeletal system, particularly the axial, spinal motor system (Herman, 1985; Pialasse et al., 2015).

Postural sway is an element of laterality that is re-trainable. Increased postural sway correlates with low back pain in general so it is wise for the PMME to include use of the PM principle of centering and standing shift activities to address these issues (Walker et al., 2012).

Chapter 1 discussed a right-handed world and the development of biased tasks and skills, developing preferences that create motor patterns of ease and efficiency in performing tasks.

Laterality: vestibulo-ocular control

Research shows that the processing of space perception, a task of the vestibulo-ocular reflex in those with spinal asymmetry, is different in the scoliosis population. When the whole body is moved, the eye spatial coordination is accurate, but when only the eyes are moved to a target, a rotational muscular activity of the eyes, there is an imprecision, an undershooting the mark, in the task. The cerebellum of the brain regulates precision. The implications in the functional aspects of spinal asymmetry is that the vestibulo-ocular systems play an important role in either the development of spinal asymmetry, or the perpetuation of it (Simoneau et al., 2009).

Eye dominance

Eye dominance is a phenomenon used, and promoted, in many sport-specific activities such as archery. Eye dominance and laterality were considered in a study that linked the two variables in people with AIS. More individuals exhibited crossed eye-hand laterality (63%) than the control group, meaning the right hand was dominant and the left eye was dominant (Catanzariti et al., 2014). Goldberg and Dowling also found a significant amount of right-handedness in a group of girls with right ribcage convexities (Goldberg & Dowling, 1990).

The three functional elements relating to laterality, limb dominance and bias found in those with spinal asymmetry covered so far are: 1) vertical spinal anti-gravitational side symmetry; 2) postural sway; and 3) vestibular and eye control. Each subject warrants more research into the role each plays as a potentially plastic element to manage lifelong spinal asymmetry. Chapter 6 outlines a framework to attend to these issues.

Other functional aspects

There are three more functional aspects to consider: first is the role of posture, especially spinal flexion, on the development of spinal asymmetry. Secondly, the role of fascia, how fascial compensatory and restrictive patterns affect posture and recoil ability in function. And thirdly, the influence of emotion, specifically the role of interoception, a personal view of body sensations.

Posture

Posture control is a major contributor to the development of AIS as well as adult spinal asymmetry. Evidence suggests that prolonged sitting strongly contributes to spinal abnormalities.

As early as 1912, Dutch orthopedic surgeon Marc Jansen conducted studies that show that the anatomic and physiologic asymmetries of the right versus left crurae of the respiratory diaphragm create asymmetrical rotational forces around the thoracolumbar area in respiration. Jansen hypothesized that prolonged sitting allows the thoracolumbar junction to stiffen thereby creating a leverage that then begins the curve pattern. This curve pattern then creates the right-sided thoracic and left lumbar convexities commonly seen in scoliosis. He advised the restriction of passive sitting and concluded that a flexion-dominant sitting lifestyle is conducive to spinal growth abnormalities. For this reason, the astute PMME fosters new strategies with their clients of posture control and sitting habits for spine health.

Even as far back as 1792, the Dutch surgeon van Gessher formed the concept of the head centering over the center of gravity as a postural device. He found that the head and shoulders balanced in an energy saving way above the hips in stance and was necessary during walking (van Loon, 2012).

Fascia

In addition to general vertical skeletal posture control, a general postural model gives insight on the influences that fascia convey on the volumetric body.

Not only does the person with spinal asymmetry have certain typical fascial compensatory human propensities due to laterality and typical spinal junction transition points, they also have their own individualized asymmetrical curve spinal transition points and fascial compensatory pulls.

Figure 4.6 shows the transition points between the spinal regions in a typical spine. The vulnerable points lie where the head meets the cervical spine (atlanto-occipital, AO), the flexible neck meets the

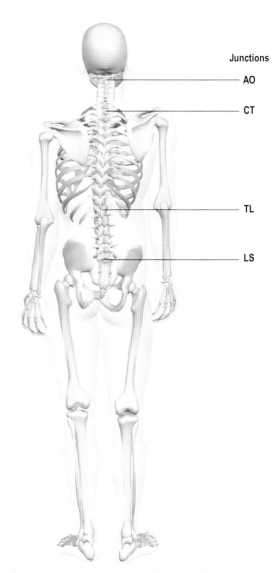

Figure 4.6
Vulnerable transition points in the junctions between spinal regions. Adapted with permission from Ross Pope, DO.

stiff ribcage (cervicothoracic, CT), the rigid ribcage meets the top of the flexible waist (thoracolumbar, TL), and the flexible low back meets the bony pelvis (lumbosacral, LS). These junctions are at prey to the functions of motor control and soft tissue pulls.

Figure 4.7 shows the manifestation of a hypothetical asymmetrical body combining the typical skeletal

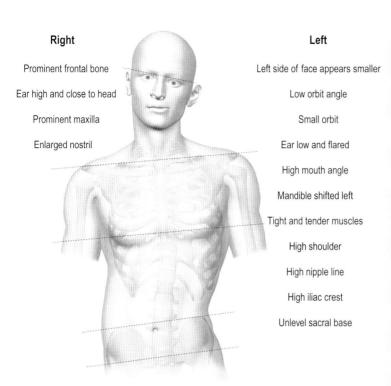

Right

Prominent frontal bone

Ear high and close to head

Prominent maxilla

Enlarged nostril

Left

Left side of face appears smaller

Low orbit angle

Small orbit

Ear low and flared

High mouth angle

Mandible shifted left

Tight and tender muscles

High shoulder

High nipple line

High iliac crest

Unlevel sacral base

Figure 4.7
Typical short right leg asymmetry findings. Adapted with permission from Ross Pope, DO.

vulnerable points with a multi-curve model. Note in this case, a relatively minor high right thoracic convexity is altering the cervicothoracic alignment, and creating a more major left lower thoracic convexity, shifting at the thoracolumbar junction to create a relatively strong right lumbar curve, and then altering the horizontal line of the iliac crest, creating an unequal sacral base. Chapter 5 lists the classifications of typical asymmetrical spinal curve models in more detail.

An ideal fascial pattern

Posture is categorized into ideal, compensated and uncompensated patterns (Figure 4.8). An ideal fascial postural pattern displays equal fascial glide in the side-to-side and longitudinal directions. In an ideal yet seldom clinically seen model no preference exists for fascial rotation or side-bending to either right or left in any of the transitional zones.

The compensated pattern is an alternating pattern of fascial ease and restriction that assumes a balanced rotational bias from one transitional zone to

the next. This pattern, possible in the person with spinal asymmetry, most likely finds the head position over the pelvis, close to the center of gravity (COG) at S2. This system of counterbalanced pulls shows adaptability, a possible sign of resilience for general health.

Therefore teaching the body skill of 'head over COG' is a favorable skill to attain. The uncompensated pattern with the head likely off-center of the COG, due to non-alternating rotational patterns, shows possible additional signs of trauma, accidents and probably a slower recovery, indicating more difficulty in resilience. Note that Figure 4.7 is a non-compensated model.

The bias of the fascias creating these patterns starts from the ground up in most functional activities, indicating the importance of the posture and architecture of the feet. The most common compensated pattern, L/R/L/R, due to the general lateralization of birth and right-handed development, finds a series of transverse plane rotations that start at the feet upwards to a rotated right, the pelvic girdle to a left

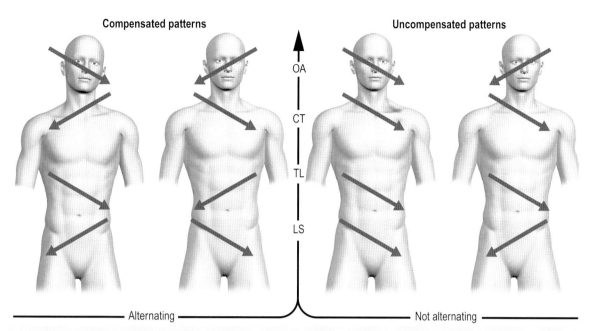

Figure 4.8
Compensated and uncompensated patterns. Adapted with permission from Ross Pope, DO.

lower thoracic outlet (waist-level), to a right upper thoracic outlet (clavicle region), to a left craniocervical junction. Developing the eye for these lines of pull and rotation greatly aid the PMME in working with those with spinal asymmetry.

Compensations in leg loading

Earlier in this chapter, we saw that the typical leg weightbearing pattern of those with spinal asymmetry is that one foot is not as loaded as the other in weightbearing, giving at least a functional leg length difference.

Pronation and supination

Pronation usually accompanies a shorter leg and supination usually accompanies a longer leg. These foot and ankle positions produce rotations up the leg which produces rotation of the pelvis.

Foot/ankle supination usually results in femoral external rotation causing ipsilateral (same side) rotation of the pelvis. In opposition, foot/ankle pronation runs upwards into internal rotation of the femur causing a contralateral rotation of the pelvis.

In addition, the position of the femoral heads alters so that with forward position of one femoral head combined with posterior position of the opposite an overall rotation of the bony pelvis occurs. See Figure 4.9 for a visual explanation of counter-rotations (Pope, 2003).

Walking in general is not a symmetric activity even if stride distance and duration are equal for a stride length. Evidence on those with spinal asymmetry shows that significant asymmetric pelvic side-to-side bony measurements occur in 15 variables correlated with the right versus left sides for the following anatomical regions: sacrum, iliac blades, iliac width, acetabulum and the superior lunate surface of the acetabulum.

However, still other researchers show that functional aspects of range of motion of the lower limb joints and muscle activity, particularly the soleus during the propulsion phase, explain a functional aspect to an asymmetric walking cycle. Although kinetic analysis of strictly right-handed people shows that the dominant lower limb has a greater role in propulsion and the non-dominant lower limb has a greater role in the

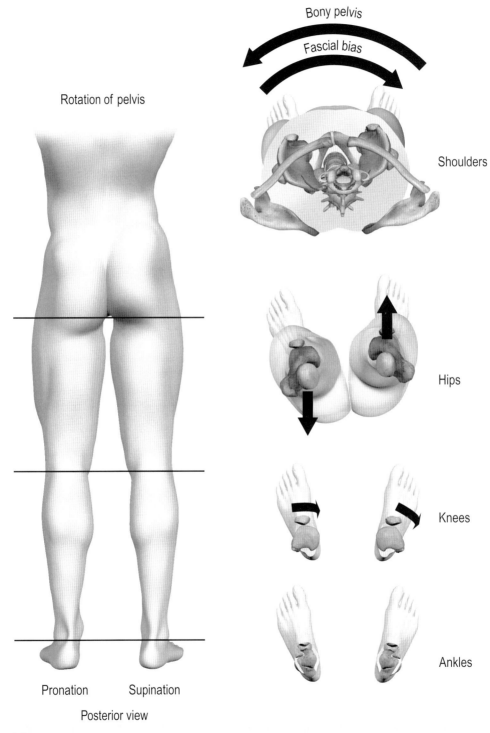

Rotation of pelvis

Bony pelvis

Fascial bias

Shoulders

Hips

Knees

Ankles

Pronation   Supination

Posterior view

Figure 4.9
The relationship between pelvic rotation and foot postures. Adapted with permission from Ross Pope, DO

kinetic loading response at heel-strike, each individual develops strategies in which dominance varies (Boulay et al., 2006).

A general postural model

A general postural model developed by osteopath Dr Pope helps to understand how the asymmetrical body emerges from an amalgam of genetic, developmental, functional, structural and outer boundary (braces, lifts, appliances) parameters (Pope, 2003). The wise PMME takes this general model into account when working with clients.

Dynamic posture

Beyond static skeletal and fascial posture is the use of dynamic posture.

Research indicates that mammals need movement and benefit from rhythmic motion. Animal experiments show how quickly a lack of movement instigates development of additional cross-links, the bindings of cells, in fascial tissues, causing thickening and adhesions.

When fascial fibers lose the elasticity to glide past each other, adhesions form to become not only stuck together but also, in the worst cases, matted together. It is detrimental enough to have fascial restrictions due to an asymmetric waist and shoulder and much worse to add fascial restrictions through sedentary or repressed living.

It is unfortunate that some clients with asymmetry received advice not to pursue their activity dreams. A critical characteristic of youthful fascia is its ability to create a stored energy recoil motion which is an oscillatory movement, like a pendulum motion, with an elastic spring quality. This ability has the possibility of re-training if it becomes diminished. Interestingly, muscle biology now in conjunction with new fascial findings reveals that in this type of motion, the length of the muscle fibers does not change appreciably.

This phenomenon accounts for why a kangaroo jumps higher than its musculature allows. As the muscle fibers contract in an almost isometric fashion, they stiffen temporarily without any significant change of their length. Isometric contractions use more of their cross-bridges, the ratchets that produce muscle contraction, than other types of muscle contractions such as isotonic, used in traditional weight training.

The fascial elements take more action than the muscle fibers to produce the actual movement in an elastic fashion similar to the pendulum motion of a swinging yo-yo. This recoil qualitative aspect of movement shows promise to allow those with low or altered muscle tone to participate and even excel in many activities (Schleip & Müller, 2012).

Clients and asymmetry: interoception

Clients with asymmetrical issues need encouragement to strive toward resilience, go beyond or into the limitations of their condition to see where their capabilities lie and develop true robustness. A recurrent theme in this book is to move the client from the somatic, guide them through the correctives and onto conditioning, not only for daily life but also to include higher functioning goals. To this end is the development of emotional stability through interoception.

Interoception is an internal listening skill, focusing on visceral sensations such as a gut feeling of empathy, muscular effort, tickling or blushing. It is not only registering the kind of sensation felt, such as heat, pressure, pain, but also how you feel about feeling the sensation.

Research shows these receptors bypass the normal sensory area of the brain (somatosensory area) and go straight to the deeper part of the brain (insula), registering an enormous variety of situations involving the processing of visceral sensory, visceral motor, vestibular, attention, pain, emotion, verbal information, motor information, inputs related to music and eating, such as gustatory, olfactory, visual, auditory, and tactile data. It essentially helps one perceive and interpret personal physical sensations.

Clients with spinal asymmetry need encouragement to find good meaning in physical sensations. Chronic pain, distress or disappointment causes stressful conditions for a person. The wise PMME emphasizes self-perception along with bodily perception of finer sensations in a training approach integrating minute movements of vertebra with larger movements. Using guidance with imagery and breathing along with internal monitoring and organization helps a client reach deeper into observation of subtle integrative sensory changes such as inner spaciousness, aliveness, home-coming, or inner silence. The sections on breathing in Chapter 6 explore this possibility further (Schleip & Jäger, 2012; Payne et al., 2015).

Conclusion

In concluding this chapter on the two main categories of causes of spinal asymmetry and scoliosis, structural and functional, an interwoven theme becomes apparent. Due to the diminishment of polio and tuberculosis in modern society, most spinal asymmetry is likely due to functional development manifesting at a particular point in an individual's development in response to a combination of environmental, functional and genetic influences. The work of researchers mentioned in this chapter, along with others in the medical community, gives insight in supporting early detection and early treatment, including exercise to help avoid the development of spinal rigidity, the cornerstone definition of structural scoliosis. Research reveals that thoracic flexibility, shifting and side-bending exercises particularly help when the exercises are not forceful and the spine is not placed into prolonged stretching, especially at an end of spinal range (Hawes, 2003).

PMMEs benefit from the work of the medical field using its insights, clinical and analytical knowledge to take the client one step further, bringing art into the science of exercise.

Bibliography

Bialek, M., Pawlak, P., Kotwicki, T. (2009). Foot loading asymmetry in patients with scoliosis. Scoliosis, 4 (Suppl. 1): O19. doi:10.1186/1748-7161-4-S1-O19

Boulay, C., Tardieu, C., Benaim, C., et al. (2006). Three-dimensional study of pelvic asymmetry on anatomical specimens and its clinical perspectives. Journal of Anatomy, 208(1), 21–23. doi: 10.1111/j.1469-7580.2006.00513.x

Burwell, R.G., Aujla ,R..K, Grevitt, M.P., et al. (2009). Pathogenesis of adolescent idiopathic scoliosis in girls – a double neuro-osseous theory involving disharmony between two nervous systems, somatic and autonomic expressed in the spine and trunk: possible dependency on sympathetic nervous system and hormones. Scoliosis and Spinal Disorders, 4: 24, doi: 10.1186/1748-7161-4-24.

Burwell, R.G., Clark, E., Dangerfield, P.H., Moulton, A. (2016). Adolescent idiopathic scoliosis (AIS): a multi-factorial cascade concept for pathogenesis and embryonic origin. Scoliosis and Spinal Disorders, 11: 8. doi:10.1186/s13013-016-0063-1

Burwell, R.G., Dangerfield, P.H., Moulton, A., Grivas, T.B. (2013). Whither the etiopathogenesis (and scoliogeny) of adolescent idiopathic scoliosis? Incorporating presentations on scoliogeny at the 2012 IRSSD and SRS meetings. Scoliosis, 8: 4. doi:10.1186/1748-7161-8-4

Carlson, B. (2011). ScoliScore AIS Prognostic Test personalizes treatment for children with spinal curve. Biotechnology Healthcare, 8(2), 30–31. Retrieved September 2, 2017, from https://www.ncbi.nlm.nih.gov/pmc/articles/PMC3138384/

Catanzariti, J.-F., Guyot, M.A., Agnani, O. et al. (2014). Eye-hand laterality and right thoracic idiopathic scoliosis. European Spine Journal, 23(6), 1232–1236. doi:10.1007/s00586-014-3269-z

Collins, D. F. (2017). Scoliosis traced to problems in spinal fluid flow. Retrieved September 8, 2017, from National Institutes of Health: https://directorsblog.nih.gov/tag/adolescent-idiopathic-scoliosis/

Duval-Beaupère, G., Lespargo, A., Grossiord, A. (1985). Flexibility of scoliosis. What does it mean? Is this terminology appropriate? Spine (Phila Pa 1976), 10(5), 428–432

Goldberg, C., Dowling, F.E. (1990). Handedness and scoliosis convexity: a reappraisal. Spine, 15(2), 61–64. doi:10.1097/00007632-199002000-00001

Grimes, D.T, B.C. (2016). Zebrafish models of idiopathic scoliosis link cerebral spinal fluid flow defects to spinal curvature. Science, 352(6291), 1341–1344

Grivas, T.B., Burwell, R.G., Dangerfield, P.H. (2013a). Body mass index in relation to truncal asymmetry of healthy adolescents, a physiopathogenetic concept in common with idiopathic scoliosis: summary of an electronic focus group debate of the IBSE. Scoliosis, 8: 10. doi:10.1186/1748-7161-8-10

Grivas, T.B., Hresko, M.T., Labelle, H. et al. (2013b). The pendulum swings back to scoliosis screening: screening policies for early detection and treatment of idiopathic scoliosis - current concepts and recommendations. Scoliosis, 8: 16. doi:10.1186/1748-7161-8-16

Grivas, TB., Burwell R.G., Kechagias V. et al. (2016). Idiopathic and normal lateral lumbar curves: muscle effects interpreted by 12th rib length asymmetry with pathomechanic implications for lumbar idiopathic scoliosis. Scoliosis and Spinal Disorders, 11(Suppl. 2): 35. doi:10.1186/s13013-016-0093-8

Hawes, M.C. (2003). The use of exercises in the treatment of scoliosis: an evidence-based critical review of the literature. Pediatric Rehabilitation, 6(3–4), 171–182

Herman, R. (1985). Idiopathic scoliosis and the central nervous system: a motor control problem. The Harrington lecture, 1983. Scoliosis Research Society. Spine (Phila Pa 1976), 10(1), 1–14. Retrieved September 3, 2017, from: https://www.ncbi.nlm.nih.gov/pubmed/3885413

Ikegawa, S. (2016). Genomic study of adolescent idiopathic scoliosis in Japan. Scoliosis and Spinal Disorders, 11: 5. doi:10.1186/s13013-016-0067-x

Lambert, F.M., Malvinaud, D., Glaunes, J. et al. (2009). Vestibular asymmetry as the cause of idiopathic scoliosis: a possible answer from Xenopus. Journal of Neuroscience, 29(40), 12477–12483

Landauer, F. (2013). Diagnosis and treatment of leg-length discrepancy in scoliosis. Scoliosis and Spinal Disorders, 8(Suppl. 2): O41. doi:10.1186/1748-7161-8-S2-O41

Lin, J.J., Chen, W.H., Chen, P.Q., Tsauo, J.Y. (2010). Alteration in shoulder kinematics and associated muscle activity in people with idiopathic scoliosis. Spine, 35(11), 1151–1157

Loghmani, M.T., Whitted, M. (2016). Soft tissue manipulation: a powerful form of mechanotherapy. Journal of Physiotherapy and Physical Rehabilitation, 1(4), 1–6

Negrini, A., Parzini, A., Negrini, M.G. et al. (2008). Adult scoliosis can be reduced through specific SEAS exercises: a case report. Scoliosis, 3: 20. doi:10.1186/1748-7161-3-20

Payne, P., Levine, P., Crane-Godreau M. (2015). Somatic experiencing: using interoception and proprioception as core elements of trauma therapy. Frontiers in Psychology, 6: 93. doi:10.3389/fpsyg.2015.00093

Pialasse, J.-P., Descarreaux, M., Mercier, P. et al. (2015). The vestibular-evoked postural response of adolescents with idiopathic scoliosis is altered. PLoS ONE 10(11), e0143124. doi:10.1371/journal.pone.0143124

Pope, R. (2003). The common compensatory pattern: its origin and relationship to the postural model. American Academy of Osteopathy Journal, Winter, 2003, 19–40

Schleip, R., Jäger, H. (2012). Interoception. In: Schleip, R., Findley, T.W., Chaitow, L., Huijing, P.A. eds. Fascia: The Tensional Network of the Human Body. Edinburgh, UK: Churchill Livingstone, pp. 89–94

Schleip, R., Müller, D.G. (2012). Training principles for fascial connective tissues: Scientific foundation and suggested practical applications. Journal of Bodywork and

Movement Therapies, 17(1), 103–115. doi:10.1016/j.jbmt.2012.06.007

Simoneau, M., Lamothe, V., Hutin, E., et al. (2009). Evidence for cognitive vestibular integration impairment in idiopathic scoliosis patients. BMC Neuroscience, 10: 102. doi:10.1186/1471-2202-10-102

Soutanis, K.C., Payatakes, A.H., Chouliaris, V.T. (2007). Rare causes of scoliosis and spine deformity: experience and particular features. Scoliosis, 2: 15. doi:10.1186/1748-7161-2-15

Stokes I.A. (1989). Rib cage asymmetry in idiopathic scoliosis. Journal of Orthopedic Research, 7(4), 599–606. doi:10.1002/jor.1100070419

Stokes, I.A. (2002). Mechanical effects on skeletal growth. Journal of Musculoskeletal and Neuronal Interactions, 2(3), 277–280

Stokes, I.A.F. (2018). Evaluation of the role of the biomechanical 'vicious cycle' in progression of scoliosis during growth. Orthopaedic Proceedings. A supplement to The Bone & Joint Journal, 90-B(Supp_III), 429–430

van Loon, P.J.M. (2012). Scoliosis idiopathic? The etiologic factors in scoliosis will affect preventive and conservative therapeutic strategies. In: Grivas, T. (ed.) Recent Advances in Scoliosis. InTech, pp. 211–234. Retrieved August 13, 2018, from: http://www.intechopen.com/books/recent-advances-inscoliosis/changes-in-conservative-treatment-of-spinal-deformities-based-on-increased-knowledge-on-etiology

Walker, A, Ruhe, R., Feher, B. (2012). Pain relief is associated with decreasing postural sway in patients with non-specific low back pain. BMC Musculoskeletal Disorders, 13(39), 1–12

Learning from the medical field: diagnosis, classifications

The PMME will rely heavily upon the diagnosis and observations of the medical professionals on the Scoliosis Team. This chapter describes these processes and introduces the reader to some useful terminology and concepts.

Observation and diagnosis

Spinal asymmetry and the diagnosis of scoliosis begins through observation. Curve is measured by X-ray imaging. Progression is followed through observation via imaging for adults, or for youth, by imaging plus measurement of bone growth, most commonly, pelvic growth or wrist growth.

In either case, a radiologist identifies and classifies the types of curves and the presence of pathology such as *spondylolisthesis* (where one vertebra slips out of the expected gravitational curve pattern) or an abnormal vertebral shape such as a wedged vertebra.

Please use caution with your words! For sensitivity, use the term *lateral prominence* in place of 'hump.' 'Lateral prominence' is also more accurate than the word 'curve.'

Stages of life

Diagnosis in youth

A family physician, parent or school screening usually detects spinal asymmetry in infants, children and adolescents. The general test is the Adam forward bend test, performed with a Scoliometer®, as shown in Chapter 7 (Figure 5.1).

Direct observation without the use of a measuring tool, called *surface topography*, is also a valid method described in Chapter 7 (Chowanska et al., 2012).

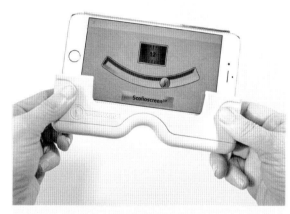

Figure 5.1
A Scoliometer®.

Measurement: Cobb angle

If screening tests indicate a need, the medical team, along with a radiologist, determine the Cobb angle by a full-length frontal X-ray to measure and quantify spinal deformities.

Analyzing the number, direction and severity of each curve veering from a normal straight line, the radiologist draws two perpendicular lines, one from the upper end and one from the lower end of the curve. The lines that intersect give the degree of spinal curvature, the Cobb angle (Figure 5.2).

Treatment of a curve greater than 10° might include bracing, exercise prescription, physical therapy or, typically, simply a 'wait and see' approach to see if the

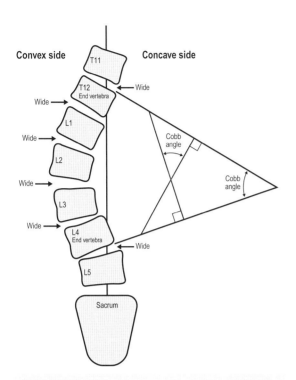

Convex side   Concave side

T11

T12
End vertebra   ← Wide

Wide →

L1

Wide →   Cobb
                               angle

L2
                                        Cobb
Wide →   angle

L3

Wide →

L4
End vertebra   ← Wide

L5

Sacrum

Figure 5.2
The Cobb angle is measured from the top vertebra of the curve to the bottom vertebra. These two lines meet at a perpendicular point, called the Cobb angle.

curve progresses. Bracing for youth is recommended at about 22°.

Measurement: axial trunk rotation and the Scoliometer®

When I am asked in courses what the Scoliometer® measures exactly, and why measurement with a Scoliometer® is of value to a PMME, I always point out that it only measures one thing – *axial trunk rotation*.

Axial trunk rotation is not the same as the Cobb angle; however, it is correlated with it. The Cobb angle measurement is a two-dimensional measurement, not fully revealing the rotation dimension of each vertebra. Scoliosis is at least three-dimensional and is easily four-dimensional given the fascial component. Surgeons use multiple resources to ascertain more precise readings, such as using

computerized tomography (CT scans) (Lam et al., 2008; Doi et al., 2011).

The biggest reason a PMME needs the Scoliometer® is not to measure axial rotation per session, but to observe the actual spinal variations in rotation from region to region. Watch the video demonstration in Chapter 7 (Code 7.2).

Done periodically, a Scoliometer® reading provides insight as to the functional strategy of the client. Many clients have a structural, non-changeable component to their spinal asymmetry, along with a functional component, so improvement seen with the Scoliometer® potentially shows both. Research suggests that the spinal forward bend is more appropriately performed in the sitting position; however, for the PMME standing is better to see the lower body influence upon the spinal asymmetry (Grivas et al., 2006).

Diagnosis in adults

Adults seek a spinal medical diagnosis involving imaging when pain becomes worrisome. Adults experience pathology associated with aging, including degenerative joint disease (arthritis), vertebral slippage (spondylolisthesis) from other disease states or life traumas.

The medical assessment determines the level and severity of pathology and is matched up with an appropriate medical intervention.

X-rays and other tests

Bone density screening to detect bone thinning called a *DEXA* X-ray is another way for adults to discover a spinal asymmetry.

The DEXA is a standard test at age 60 to determine the presence of osteoporosis. Not technically a screening for scoliosis, a DEXA image surprised several of my clients when it revealed spinal asymmetry. One client thought her primary medical team withheld information about her scoliosis on the basis that her DEXA image predated her spinal pain episode and ensuing issues.

The scope of the PMME is not technically to read or decipher an X-ray for a client, although many clients wish to show the X-ray to the PMME, and it can

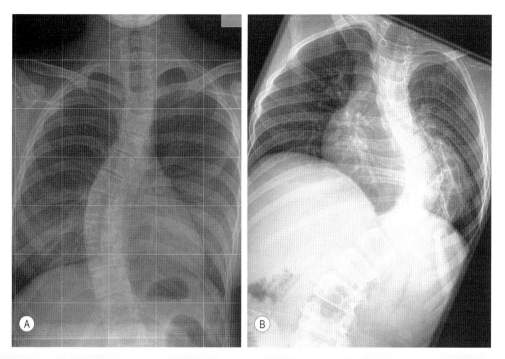

Figure 5.3
(A) A compensated left thoracolumbar main curve from T2 to L1 with minor rib alterations. (B) An uncompensated right thoracic main curve with major rib involvement.

provide you with very useful information. Here are some details in how to decipher the X-ray for your own needs. Study the image in Figure 5.3 along with Figure 1.9, showing the changes in the asymmetrical skeleton along with the drawing of vertebral rotation analysis later in this chapter (see Figure 5.6). Scan the central spinal line, the distances between vertebrae and note any wedging of vertebrae and see the basic shape, how it veers from a vertical line. Then, note the ribs.

The areas where the ribs are further apart indicate convexity, a lateral prominence. These ribs are longer than the ribs on the other side. The muscles in this area are elongated and the fascia could be either stretched or actually thickened due to the pressure exerted upon the area. The area is usually stiff.

The area where the ribs are closer together indicate concavity. The muscles here are short, and probably weak. The ribs in front are usually pushed anteriorly, called an anterior protrusion. The biggest area of

spinal shift from the central vertical line is the major curve, here above at the left thoracolumbar region, showing a 70°, severe, Cobb angle.

In this X-ray, look closely at the largest area of concavity, see how the spinous processes are tilting toward the concave side. If it is difficult to find the spinous processes, find the two dots on each vertebra, indicating the *pedicles*, the feet of the interlocking facet joints. Follow the center area between these two dots to find the rotations.

Note the lumbar area. Find the transverse processes, deeper into the hazy gray areas. See how they change in perspective, enlarging as one side moves away from the camera, and disappearing as one comes closer. Look at the end plates of the vertebrae and see if they are smooth or irregular indicating disc disease.

Look at the *ilia* of the pelvis (see Figure 1.2), the large bones at the top that look like a butterfly's wings. Is one side higher than the other, indicating a pelvic obliquity? Notice the shape of the ilia. One side is enlarging, twisting backwards on itself (flaring out) and the other is narrowing, twisting forward on itself (flaring forward), along with a global pelvic transverse (horizontal) plane rotation. Look at the tilt of the sacral base, and the asymmetry of the pubic symphysis. Keep an open mind. Nature is asymmetrical. Everyone is perfect in our imperfections. Remember the PMME scope of practice. Use discretion in discussing these features with your client (Magee, 2016).

Progression in youth and adults

Progression is of major concern in scoliosis management. A physician estimates future changes (called a *prognosis*) statistically calculating the likelihood to progress.

Surgical intervention is serious, usually involving insertion of a vertical rod or cables and screws to hold the rod or cables in place until bone chips fuse the vertebra over the desired area. Some countries give this choice to minors. In other countries, parents choose. It is controversial for older adults because of the fragility of bone and the client's ability to withstand spinal surgery (Silva & Lenke, 2010).

Youth progression potential is a combination of the current and subsequent Cobb measurements, the maturation Tanner Score and the skeletal closure Risser Score. The Tanner maturation score lists how many secondary sex characteristics are apparent. The Risser Score analyzes the cartilage mineralization of the pelvis (Figure 5.4).

The *apophyses*, long pieces of cartilage in the immature ilia, mineralize with calcium from the anterior toward the posterior. The score scale ranges from 0 to 5, where zero indicates no sign of the *apophysis*, typical of prepubescence, to a score of 5 indicating completion of mineralization. A low scale suggests more chance for deformation before growth ends. Female skeletons complete with calcium about age 16 years and males about age 17.

Known risk factors for progression include low bone mineral density, which may be due to nutritional issues as well as genetics. The longer a youth with a progressing curve continues to grow skeletally before the skeleton completes mineralization, the more chance the curve will increase.

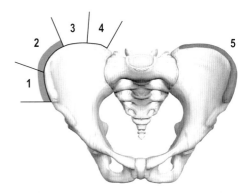

Figure 5.4

Risser Progression Scale model. A scale of 0 to 5 measures the progression of bone formation (5 means that skeletal maturity is reached).

Other risk factors

Other risk factors for progression include: any underlying neurological or congenital condition that might cause musculoskeletal underdevelopment, such as cerebral palsy; a pathological degenerative condition, such as muscular dystrophy; the patient's BMI (basal metabolic index) or family background; and female gender in particular.

Females are eight times more likely to experience rapid and severe curve progressions, usually a year before the onset of menses (Heary & Todd, 2016). One problem is that this time of budding sexuality is also a time of more desire for individual privacy, preventing observation of an oncoming curve. This is a good argument for school screening.

Adult skeletons are mostly non-changeable except by toxicity, trauma or disease. Although adult skeletons are more stable, fragility and bone thinning come with age. Comorbidities such as duration and stringency of cancer treatments, joint replacement, loss of mobility due to accidents, and even dental work have the potential to accelerate, or begin, the progression of an existing spinal asymmetry (Saccucci et al. 2011; Walston, 2012; Levine et al. 2009).

The good news is that research indicates a positive effect using the Pilates Method for these occurrences. More research is needed to see the effect of the Method on the combination of spinal asymmetry and each comorbidity, yet the outlook remains promising.

Other medical classifications

Medical classifications extend beyond the measures of Cobb angle and Risser Score to include the characteristics of structural/functional, compensated/uncompensated, and the general C and S curve designations.

Discussions of structural/functional and compensated/uncompensated appear in more detail in Chapter 4, and continue below. These characteristics help to gain a basic understanding of the client. The 'C' and 'S' curve designations are similar to the terms 'compensated' and 'uncompensated.'

In compensated scoliosis, the head finds a central point over the center of gravity in the pelvis. This center of gravity is approximately three inches below the navel and three inches inwards from the front to the back.

In uncompensated scoliosis, the head is off the central line either to the right or the left. This observation helps us understand a client's pain or dysfunction in the neck, shoulders and arms.

The 'C' shape is generally one major, long, single curve that traverses several regions of the spine. Regions are cervical, thoracic, lumbar, sacral. The C is perhaps only postural in nature, due to handedness. A *levoscoliosis* curves to the left. A *dextroscoliosis* curves to the right.

The 'S' shape has two major curves with the possibility of a number of variations: for example, curves occurring on one side of the central vertical spinal line (CVSL) with counter-balancing minor curves. Another variation is each major curve occurring on opposite sides of the CVSL, allowing for better balance and equilibrium. Each curve of the S tends to occur mostly in one region. The S indicates that the lateral bending of the spine accomplished a full equilibrium.

The 'C' and 'S' shapes are general classifications, sometimes referred to as a 2-curve and a 3- or 4-curve respectively, part of a basic 2-, 3- or 4-curve system.

The 3-curve and 4-curve labels both refer to an S curve where a 3-curve has a right thoracic primary curve and 4-curve is an S with a left thoracolumbar primary curve. Each of these shapes receives, and

deserves, more intricate classification by surgeons, and warrants closer inspection by PMMEs.

Understanding and respecting the classic information of the individual skeleton helps before attempting individual functional asymmetrical alterations.

This is how art happens. Classicism (learning the rules) precedes creativity.

Deviations from a CVSL

Each case of scoliosis has characteristic deviations from a CVSL in terms of location, direction and magnitude, which surgeons use to classify the characteristics of the curves.

Dr Lenke's 2005 Classification System (LCS), highlighted here (Figure 5.5), reveals the complexity involved with the spine. The systems apply to both adolescent idiopathic scoliosis and adult scoliosis.

The Lenke system addresses six different curve types, modifiers for thoracic kyphosis, the amount of lateral (and so rotational) lumbar involvement, a sagittal gravitational curve modifier, and structural/functional qualifications.

Part 1 describes the six types (1–6) of curves of the Lenke system. The bottom part addresses possible sagittal variations. Part 2 shows the lumbar spine modifier (A, B or C) as well as a mid-line (sagittal) thoracic modifier (–, N or +).

The lumbar spine and thoracic spine modifiers indicate whether the spine has veered from the favorable apices of L3 and T8 respectively (Lenke et al., 2001).

Classifying curves in three dimensions

It is important to note that classifying the curves begins as a visual two-dimensional description, a major limitation cited by researchers of the Cobb angle. The Cobb angle individual vertebral rotation score is measured on the radiograph measuring the distance of the spinous process to the lateral side of the body of the vertebra (Stokes et al., 1986).

Due to the typical distortion of the vertebrae impacted by the curves, actual rotational values are difficult to accurately analyze. For this reason, numerous researchers found the newer technology of digital

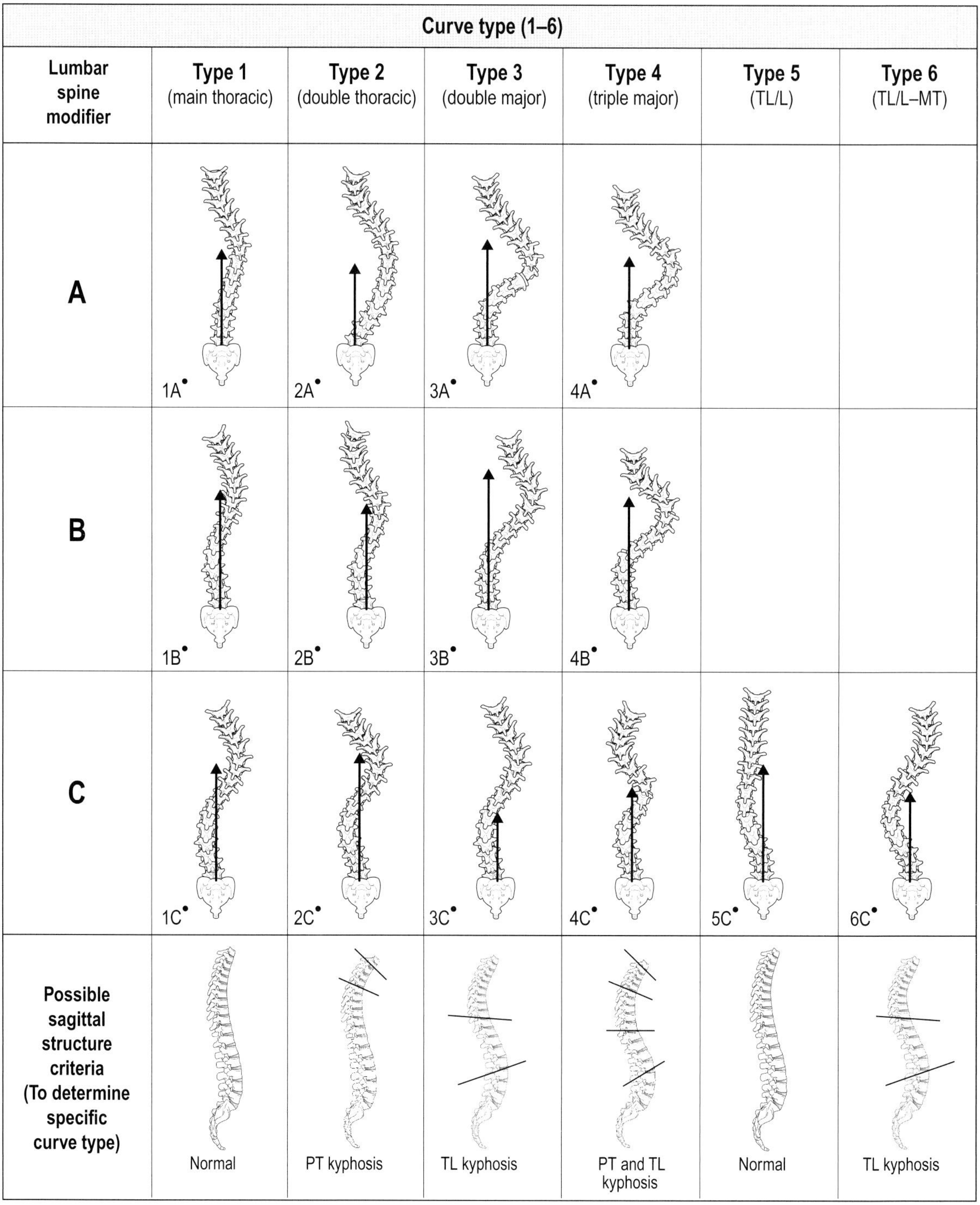

Curve type (1–6)						
Lumbar spine modifier	**Type 1** (main thoracic)	**Type 2** (double thoracic)	**Type 3** (double major)	**Type 4** (triple major)	**Type 5** (TL/L)	**Type 6** (TL/L–MT)
A	1A●	2A●	3A●	4A●		
B	1B●	2B●	3B●	4B●		
C	1C●	2C●	3C●	4C●	5C●	6C●
Possible sagittal structure criteria (To determine specific curve type)	Normal	PT kyphosis	TL kyphosis	PT and TL kyphosis	Normal	TL kyphosis

● T5–12 sagittal alignment modifier: **–**, **N**, or **+**   **–**: <10°   **N**: 10–40°   **+**: >40°

Figure 5.5
Lenke Classification System for Scoliosis Part 1 and Part 2. Reprinted with permission.

Curve type				
Type	**Proximal thoracic**	**Main thoracic**	**Thoracolumbar/lumbar**	**Description**
1	Non-structural	Structural (major)[*]	Non-structural	Main thoracic (MT)
2	Structural	Structural (major)[*]	Non-structural	Double thoracic (DT)
3	Non-structural	Structural (major)[*]	Structural	Double major (DM)
4	Structural	Structural (major)[*]	Structural (major)[*]	Triple major (TM)[†]
5	Non-structural	Non-structural	Structural (major)[*]	Thoracolumbar/lumbar (TL/L)
6	Non-structural	Structural	Structural (major)[*]	Thoracolumbar/lumbar-main thoracic (TL/L-MT)

Structural criteria
(Minor curves)

Proximal thoracic (PT) Side-bending Cobb ≥ 25º
T2–T5 kyphosis ≥ +20º

Main thoracic Side-bending Cobb ≥ 25º
T10–L2 kyphosis ≥ +20º

Thoracolumbar/lumbar Side-bending Cobb ≥ 25º
T10–L2 kyphosis ≥ +20º

[*]Major = largest Cobb measuremant, always structural
Minor = all other curves with structural criteria applied
[†]Type 4 – MT or TL/L can be major curve

Location of apex
(SRS definition)

Curve	Apex
Thoracic	T2–T11/12 disc
Thoracolumbar	T12–L1
Thoracolumbar/lumbar	L1/2 disc–L4

Modifiers				
Lumbar spine modifier	**CSVL to lumbar apex**		**Thoracic sagittal profile T5–12**	
A	CSVL between pedicles		− (Hypo)	< 10º
B	CSVL touches apical body (bodies)		**N** (Normal)	10º–40º
C	CSVL completely medial		**+** (Hyper)	> 40º

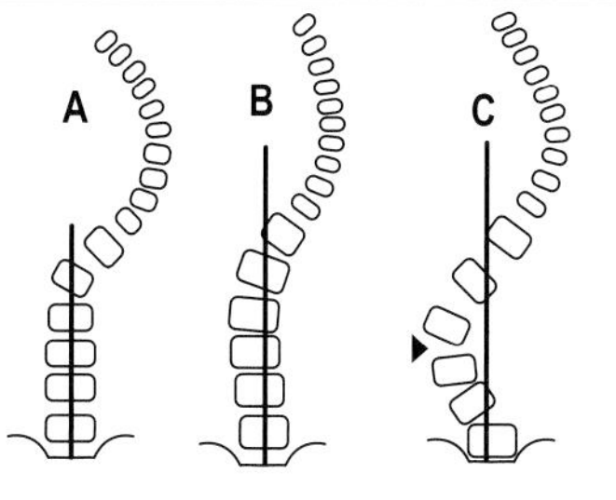

Curve type (**1–6**) + lumbar spine modifier (**A B C**) + thoracic sagittal modifier (**– N +**)   Classification (e.g. **1B+**): _____

Figure 5.5
Continued

imaging to help surgeons and *orthotists* (those who make *orthotics*, or braces) with their need for precision. The chart in Figure 5.6 shows the various methods used to determine detailed individual rotations (Lam et al., 2008).

In functional work, look at the rotations, lines of force, muscle tone and movement strategy. However, a physician's skill extends to the ability to decipher three-dimensional activity in a two-dimensional image, an inspiration for PMMEs to attempt a level of this skill.

Method	Method description	Diagram
Cobb (24)	The vertebral body is divided into six sections; the region in which the spinous process is aligned determines the grade assigned	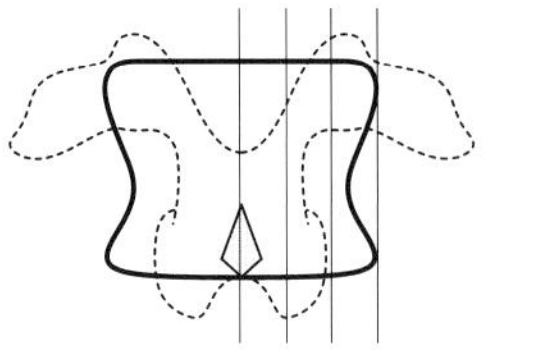 Position of spinous process A B C D Beyond D Grading 0 1+ 2+ 3+ 4+
Nash–Moe (25)	The percentage displacement of the convex pedicle with respect to the vertebral body width is used to approximate the angle of vertebral rotation	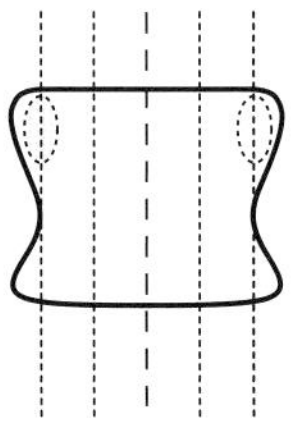 Percentage displacement 0% 50% 100% Approximate rotation angle 0° 50° 100°
Perdriolle (10)	The edges of the nomogram are aligned with innermost points on the vertebral margin (A and B); rotation angle is read from a vertical line drawn through the convex pedicle (C)	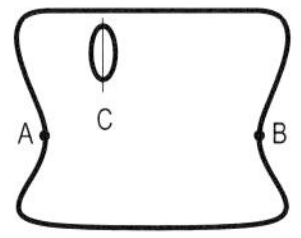 A C B
Stokes (27)	The projected distances of both pedicles from the vertebral center (a and b) are measured from the radiographic film; fixed width-to-depth ratios for each vertebral level are applied to Stokes' formula to determine rotation angle	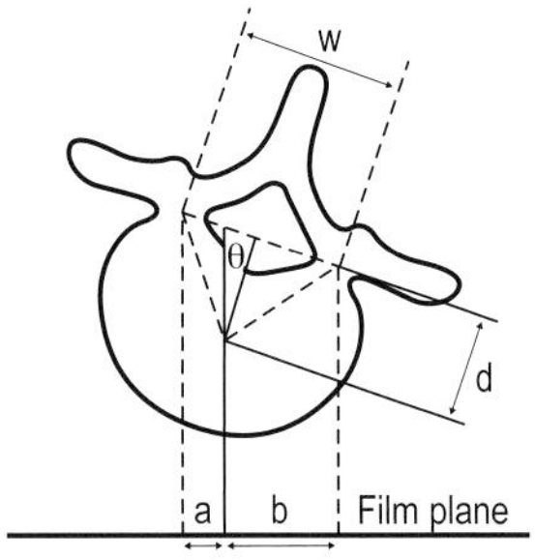 W θ d a b Film plane

Figure 5.6

Vertebral rotation analysis. Open access. Lam, G.C., Hill, D.L., Le, L.H. (2008). Vertebral rotation measurement: a summary and comparison of common radiographic and CT methods. Scoliosis, 3: 16. doi:10.1186/1748-7161-3-16

Bracing

A knowledge of the conservative method of bracing is another medical practice that PMMEs need in their tool box. Braces prevent potential progression in youth and in adults, mostly for posture and pain control.

Published in 2013, the BrAISt Study (Bracing in Adolescent Idiopathic Scoliosis Trial) showed that a hard orthotic brace helps stop progression to the level necessary for surgery in adolescents still growing with a 50° Cobb angle (Weinstein et al., 2013).

Bracing generally does not eradicate the deformity; it just stops it from getting worse.

The National Institutes of Health (NIH) brace classifications of orthosis prescription offer PMMEs a closer look at curve classifications. Their analyses show how differing medical professionals explain the 2-, 3- or 4-curve basic system, offering PMMEs another way to learn observation skills.

Compliance is often difficult as braces are hot, uncomfortable, chafe skin, are embarrassing and are difficult to wear under clothing.

Clothing items, such as Brace Buddies Scoliosis Body Sock, hide the brace. Corn starch (corn flour) underneath the brace prevents *maceration* (breakdown) of the skin.

A couple of years of bracing is worth a lifetime of surgery. Unfortunately, a certain percentage of brace wearers still warrant surgery. Our ethical standards dictate that we support a client's decision for surgery and do the best to prepare the client for such an event.

Braces are customized for each client and include padding in critical areas of pressure that usually needs to be changed if uncomfortable or as growth occurs. A hard brace is usually not worn during exercise, including Pilates, in order to maximize muscle use.

Typically, a brace must be used to stop progression until growth ceases. PMMEs are even more influential after brace use stops. Any bracing naturally weakens an area, so core restoration at this time is essential to help maintain the client's gains from brace use.

Brace design

The following classifications, developed by scoliosis specialist Dr Rigo (see Fig. 5.7), are the 3-curve, 4-curve, and non-3 or non-4 types.

The main general differences among the types are, when observed from the rear:

- 3-curve: Pelvis shifted to the concave torso side, trunk imbalance on the convex side and noticeable rib hump (sic).

- 4-curve: Pelvis is shifted to the convex thoracic rib hump (sic) side and noticeable lumbar prominence.

- Non-3 or non-4 curve: The pelvis is neutral with a 'C' or 'S' curve above it.

Note that there is more than one variation under each basic heading, showing that each client needs an individualized exercise approach.

Other braces

Other bracing systems exist that, although not made specifically for scoliosis use, help posture affected by bone weakness and low muscle tone.

TheraTogs® and Spinomed® help certain people seeking brace alternatives for scoliosis.

A mentee contacted me and asked for a brace recommendation for an 80-year-old client with scoliosis. When reviewing her case, it became apparent that the issue was one of too much flexion in the woman's posture due to bone frailty. The Spinomed® did the trick for her.

The Nada-Chair and the XBack support

Parents and adults alike request recommendations for general postural help. Two other resources, the Nada-Chair and the XBack support, are resources to note.

One adult client with a 50° Cobb angle curve came for consultation and advice. Her only complaint was pain when playing the ukulele! This was hardly surprising since her sitting slump was impressive.

I suggested the use of the Nada-Chair, which has a low back sling with loops that loop around each knee, holding the lumbar spine in extension. Later the client explained that the Nada-Chair worked wonders to help have fun with her music group and encouraged her to find a better sitting posture (Nada-Chair, 2017).

XBack Braces is another resource that offers back braces for a variety of uses from strictly postural to use for acute spinal situations. Developed by an orthopedic surgeon and a physical therapist, these braces offer options especially for adults who need transient, episodic help or posture support. I used this one for low back support to prevent slumping during computer use (XBack Posture Correx Model T106, 2017).

Numerous clients and parents request recommendations for general posture aids. The PMME is wise to keep a running list of such resources.

Surgery

The last category is surgery. Clients may require surgery in youth especially with pre-adolescent Early Onset Scoliosis (EOS), to prevent further progression of the curves prognosed to dictate lifelong disability. Adult clients require surgery when the spine is failing, that is true instability, again prognosed toward full disability and loss of independence.

A1	A2	A3
Clinical criteria Pelvis translated to the concave thoracic side Trunk imbalance to the convex thoracic side Long thoracic rib hump going down into the lumbar region	**Clinical criteria** Pelvis translated to the concave thoracic side Trunk imbalance to the convex thoracic side Noticeable rib hump / no lumbar or minimal lumbar prominence	**Clinical criteria** Pelvis translated to the concave thoracic side Trunk imbalance to the convex thoracic side Noticeable rib hump / minor lumbar prominence
Radiological criteria Single long thoracic / fractioned lumbar TP imbalance to the convex thoracic side T1 imbalance to the convex thoracic side L4 horizontal or tilted to the convex thoracic side	**Radiological criteria** Single thoracic / no or minimal functional lumbar TP imbalance to the convex thoracic side T1 imbalance to the convex thoracic side L4 horizontal	**Radiological criteria** Single major thoracic / lumbar minor TP imbalance to the convex thoracic side T1 imbalance to the convex thoracic side L4 tilted to the concave thoracic side / negative L5–4 counter-tilting

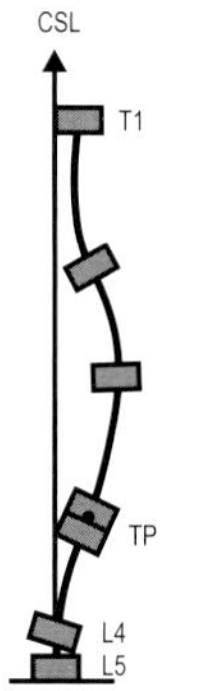 A1	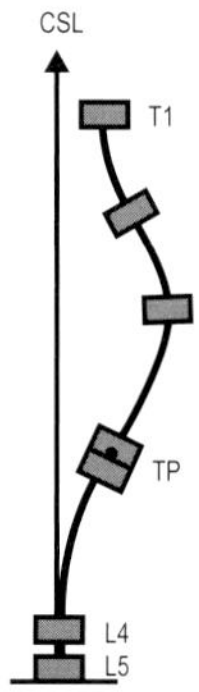 A2	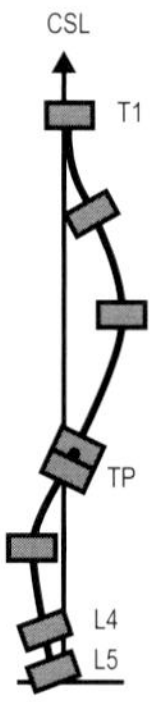 A3
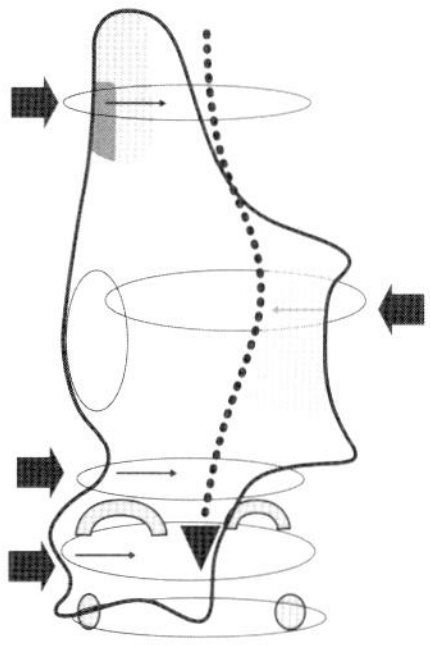 **Brace design** 3C 'Open pelvis on the convex thoracic side'	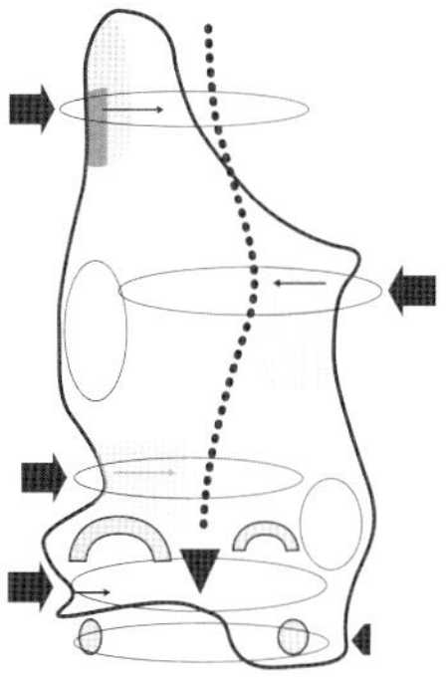 **Brace design** 3C 'Classical'	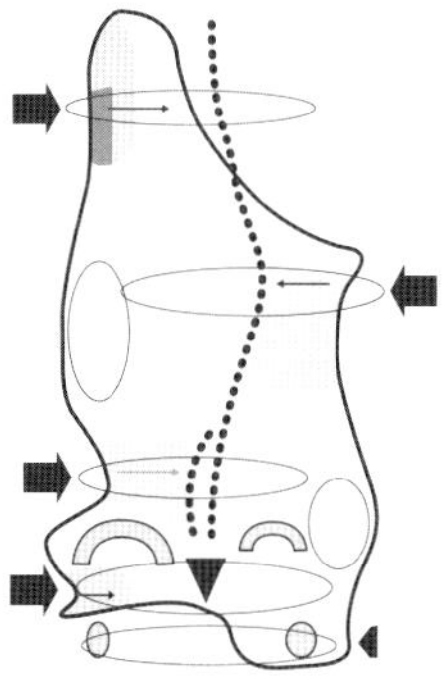 **Brace design** 3C 'Classical'

Figure 5.7

Dr Rigo's Brace Classifications. CSL = central sacral line. Open access. Rigo, M.D., Villagrasa, M., Gallo, D. (2010). A specific scoliosis classification correlating with brace treatment: description and reliability. Scoliosis, 5: 1. doi: 10.1186/1748-7161-5-1

B1	B2
Clinical criteria	**Clinical criteria**
Pelvis translated to the convex thoracic side	Pelvis translated to the convex thoracic side
Trunk imbalance to the concave thoracic side	Trunk imbalance to the concave thoracic side
Noticeable rib hump and lumbar or thoracolumbar prominence	Noticeable thoracolumbar prominence associated with a minor thoracic hump
Radiological criteria	**Radiological criteria**
Double thoracic and lumbar or thoracic and thoracolumbar	Major thoracolumbar combined with a minor thoracic curve
TP imbalance to the concave thoracic side	TP imbalance to the concave thoracic side
T1 imbalance to the concave thoracic side	T1 imbalance to the concave thoracic side
Positive L5–4 counter-tilting	Positive L5–4 counter-tilting (often, positive L4–3 counter-tilting

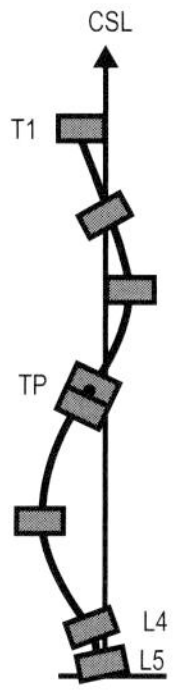 B1	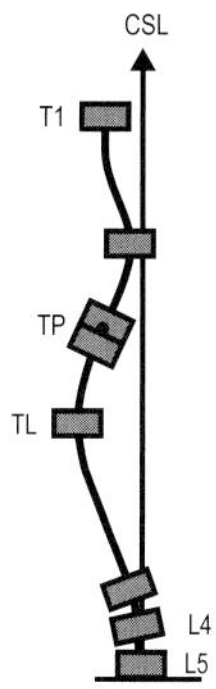 B2
Brace design	**Brace design**
4C 'Classical' eventually pelvis open at the concave thoracic side	4C 'Classical'

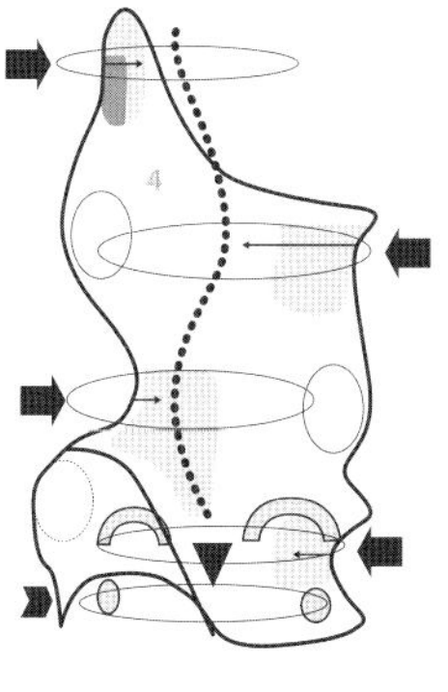

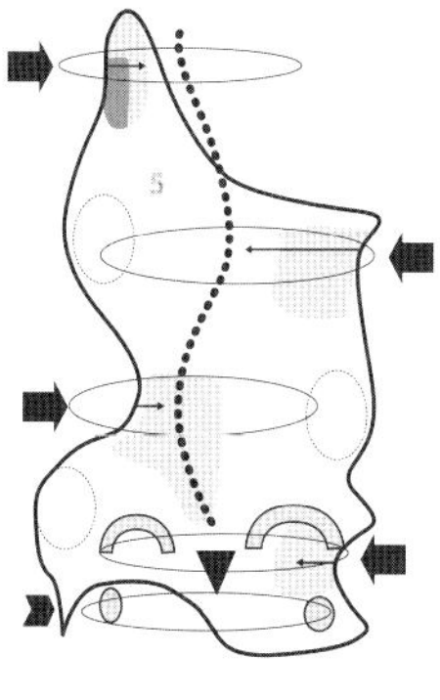

Figure 5.7
Continued

C1	C2
Clinical criteria Pelvis centered Trunk balanced Noticeable rib hump with lumbar spine rectilinear	**Clinical criteria** Pelvis centered Trunk balanced Noticeable rib hump combined with a noticeable lumbar prominence
Radiological criteria Single thoracic with no lumbar curve TP on the CSL T1 on the CSL	**Radiological criteria** Thoracic major and lumbar minor or double thoracic and lumbar (false double) TP on the CSL T1 on the CSL Negative L5–4 counter-tilting
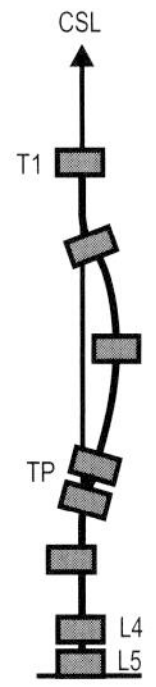 C1	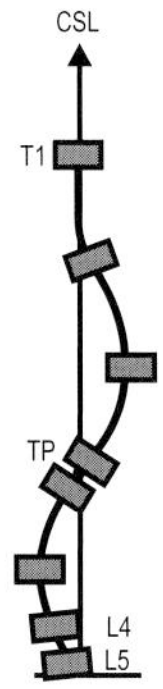 C2
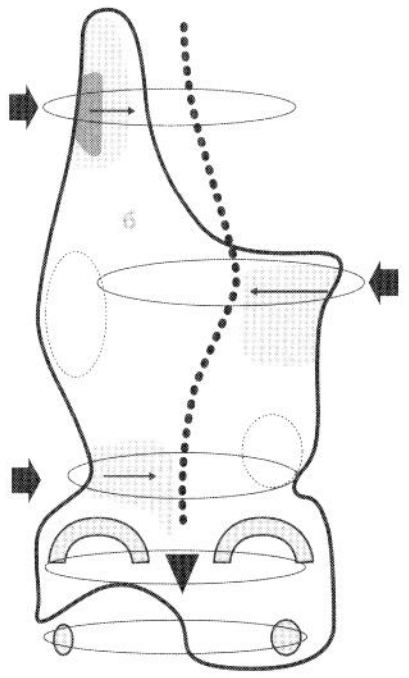 **Brace design** Neutral pelvis	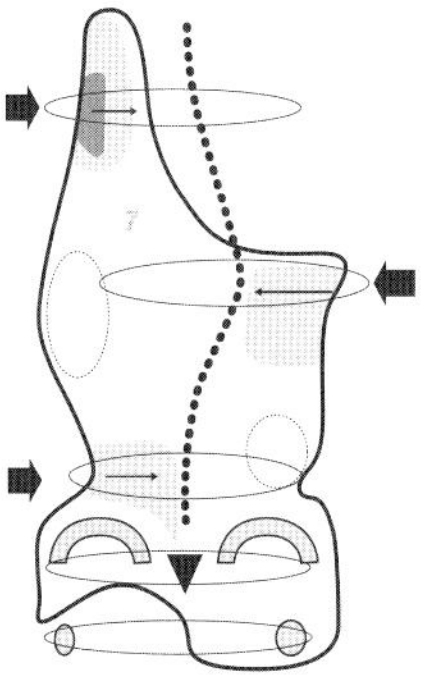 **Brace design** Neutral pelvis

Figure 5.7
Continued

PMMEs help enormously with the reacquisition of daily life and beyond for these surgical clients. Suggestions for helping this population appear in Chapter 12. Some further advice follows below.

Variations on surgical approaches depend upon the training and philosophy of the surgeon. I have seen many variations through the years. Rest assured that most surgeons desire the best functional outcome for their patients.

There are two basic approaches for fusion surgery, one from the anterior spine, and one from the posterior. Both involve chipping down the spine or pelvis, harvesting the chips and placing them along the desired correction area. A rod or cables, with or without pedical screws, as shown in Chapter 1, help to brace the healing repair until the bone chips fuse together to form a strong skeletal bond. I know someone who had hers removed later after the bond formed. Basically, the timeline is the same as fracture healing, about two months to bond and a full year to remodel (Abul-Kasim et al., 2011).

PMMEs need physician permission to work with these clients post-operatively. Little evidence exists on the exact expectations after such spinal surgery. It is unreasonable to expect a client to regain more range than they had previously, yet function improves with spinal stability.

Note that rotation decreases about 25% and full spinal articulation is not advised. Go slow. Be conservative to begin with. The scars and adhesions need to take hold to support first-line rehabilitation and are highly sensitive.

Youth recover quickly, within a couple of months. Adults recover more slowly. Encourage walking as much as possible in both cases. Concentrate on side waist equality, ribcage shift control, arm elevation range of motion, ankle use, and balance. Let the client know that the rod, or fixation is not a brace. One of my clients broke hers yet is still very functional. Caution them not to sag into the spine, but to find the core again, and lift up and out of the spine.

It is prudent for those with surgery to seek a lifetime support. One client's parents refused to allow fixation surgery when she was a teenager. In her 20s, after developing spinal instability, she opted for surgery while she was in medical school. Old videos showed a vibrant, happy young woman with lots of mobility. Now in her 50s, she developed pain, flexion collapse, difficulty standing up, and faced disability. After several years of collaboration, she improved with consistent programs to optimize long-term survivorship of spinal asymmetry and instability.

Conclusion

PMMEs benefit from knowledge of the experience, research and organization of classifications of the medical world to ground our practice with special populations. We are a part of the solution in both the allopathic world and the complementary world. This knowledge empowers and frees us to do what PMMEs do best ... medicine cures, yet Pilates heals.

Read on to find the framework to support our Method.

Bibliography

Abul-Kasim, K., Karlsson, M.K., Ohlin, A. (2011). Increased rod stiffness improves the degree of deformity correction by segmental pedicle screw fixation in adolescent idiopathic scoliosis. Scoliosis, 6: 13. doi:10.1186/1748-7161-6-13.

Chowanska, J., Kotwicki, T., Rosadzinski, K., Sliwinski, Z. (2012). School screening for scoliosis: can surface topography replace examination with scoliometer. Scoliosis, 7: 9. doi:10.1186/1748-7161-7-9

Doi T., Kido, S., Kuwashima, U., et al. (2011). A new method for measuring torsional deformity in scoliosis. Scoliosis, 6: 7. doi:10.1186/1748-7161-6-7

Grivas, T.B., Vasiliadis, E.S., Koufopoulos, G. et al. (2006). Study of trunk asymmetry in normal children and adolescents. Scoliosis, 1: 19. doi:10.1186/1748-7161-1-19

Heary, R. F., Albert, T.J. (2016). Spinal deformities: the essentials. Child's Nervous System 31(4), 631–632

Lam, G.C., Hill, D.L., Le, L.H., et al. (2008). Vertebral rotation measurement: a summary and comparison of common radiographic and CT methods. Scoliosis, 3: 16. doi:10.1186/1748-7161-3-16

Lenke, L.G., Betz, R.R., Harms, J., et al. (2001). Adolescent idiopathic scoliosis: a new classification to determine extent of spinal arthrodesis. Journal of Bone and Joint Surgery 83(8), 1169–1181

Levine B., Kaplanek, B., Jaffe, W.L. (2009). Pilates training for use in rehabilitation after total hip and knee arthroplasty: a preliminary report. Clinical Orthopaedics and Related Research, 467(6), 1468–1475

Magee, D. (2016). Orthopedic Physical Assessment, 6th edn. St Louis: Elsevier

Nada-Chair. (2017). Retrieved September 13, 2017, from Nada-Chair: http://www.nadachair.eu/

Osbourne, M. (2012). Why do females injure their knees four to six times more than men...and what can you do about it? Retrieved September 11, 2017, from University of Colorado Hospital Women's Integrated Services in Health: http://www.ucdenver.edu/academics/colleges/medicalschool/departments/Orthopaedics/clinicalservices/sportsmed/Documents/WISH_SPORTSMED_Female%20Knee%20Injuries%20and%20ACL.pdf

Rigo, M.D., Villagrasa, M. Gallo, D. (2010). A specific scoliosis classification correlating with brace treatment: description and reliability. Scoliosis, 5: 1. doi:10.1186/1748-7161-5-1

Saccucci, M., Tettamanti, L., Mummolo, S., et al. (2011). Scoliosis and dental occlusion: a review of the literature. Scoliosis, 6: 15. doi:10.1186/1748-7161-6-15

Scoliosis treatment. (2012). Retrieved August 14, 2018, from SpineCor®: http://www.spinecor.com/ForPatients/ScoliosisTreatments.aspx

Silva, F.E., Lenke, L.G. (2010). Adult degenerative scoliosis: evaluation and management. Neurosurgical Focus, 28(3), E1

Stokes, I.A., Bigelow, L.C., Moreland, M.S. (1986). Measurement of axial rotation of vertebrae in scoliosis. Spine (Phila Pa 1976), 11(3), 213–218

van Loon, P.J.M. (2012). Scoliosis idiopathic? The etiologic factors in scoliosis will affect preventive and conservative therapeutic strategies. In: Grivas, T. (ed.) Recent Advances in Scoliosis. InTech, pp. 211–234. Retrieved August 13, 2018, from: http://www.intechopen.com/books/recent-advances-inscoliosis/changes-in-conservative-treatment-of-spinal-deformities-based-on-increased-knowledge-on-etiology

Walston, J. D. (2012). Sarcopenia in older adults. Current Opinion in Rheumatology, 24(6), 623–627

Weinstein, S.L., Dolan, L. A., Wright, J.G., Dobbs, M.B. (2013). Effects of bracing in adolescents with idiopathic scoliosis. New England Journal of Medicine, 369(16), 1512–1521

XBack Posture Correx Model T106. (2017). Retrieved September 13, 2017, from Xback Braces: http://xbackbraces.com/products.html

Chief concepts: a framework of reference

The systems model

The PMME should adopt a systems model of the body, looking at the whole, rather than a reductionist model of simple leverage of one joint or motion segment at a time.

To describe the functional body, it is essential to start with the basics of musculoskeletal classical mechanics, separating each part for examination, recognizing that all subsystems work together where the parts become greater than the whole for ultimate natural motion.

The tension elements of the body in the soft tissues, muscles, ligaments and fascia contribute to the support system in essentially a truss model, where the basic unit is a triangle.

Three points mathematically define a plane. Planar triangles combine into structures of varying tension and compression, creating an efficient model of biologic structural support, tensegrity. Volumetric space in the body is a combination of these trusses forming more and more complex shapes, such as the icosahedron, offering a fourth dimension of structure encompassing multidirectional capability.

All natural structures possess these omnidirectional polyhedra allowing function in tension or compression. The bones are the compressive elements and the soft tissue (tendon/muscle, fascia, ligaments) are the tension elements, in an efficient, energy-conserving system. Evidence points to not only the existence, but also to the stability, versatility and efficiency of this system (Barnes, 1990; Schleip et al., 2012).

The body has approximately 206 bones and 602 muscles. Global control focuses on using all layers of muscle involvement, the deep and intermediate musculature allowing relative individual strength. Focusing only on the superficial 13 major muscle groups for body development, as in traditional fitness, does not achieve the relative strength desirable for an asymmetrical body.

While large muscle groups need to be exercised, many individuals with spinal asymmetry find limitation to accomplish significant absolute strength due to the disadvantage of the non-optimal mechanical joint leverages. For this reason, it is practical to focus on all muscle layers and incorporate the fascial sling system to achieve the best function available to the asymmetrical individual.

The three levels of organizing the spine

Three levels of whole-body organization exist, which add architectural assistance. It is possible to think of the body with asymmetry as a structure imploding upon itself where the outside pressures of gravity and atmospheric pressure overpower the internal structural elements.

The 3-E strategy

Three strategies help the client form full spinal connection and begin the process of the art of bodily control and awareness:

- Ergonomics
- Exercise
- Emotion.

Memorize the 3-E strategy. Ingrain it in your clients.

Ergonomics

Ergonomics extends into clothing, medical and non-medical braces, shoe wear, seating, mattresses,

Exercise

Level 1

There are four diaphragms within the body: cranial (horizontal eye level at the sphenoid bone); thoracic inlet (soft tissue ring where the shoulder girdle meets the neck); respiratory (at the ribcage base); and pelvic (underneath the pelvic floor musculature). These layers of fascia move with circulation. They are like parachutes that billow in relation to one another, creating circulation of air and fluids that drive homeostasis, the narrow range of bodily steady state regulating acid–base balance, hydration level, toxin elimination and cerebral spinal fluid distribution, among other functions.

Code 6.1 (free code)
The four diaphragms

Take the science of visceral biomechanics into art. Watch the video (Code 6.1). Then, stand. Imagine aligning these billowing parachutes vertically and acknowledging their relation for 6 breaths (Broomes, 2012).

Level 2

The Deep Frontal Fascial Line connects the internal asymmetrical body to impact spinal asymmetry. Discover the art of the science of asymmetrical management with this standing exercise.

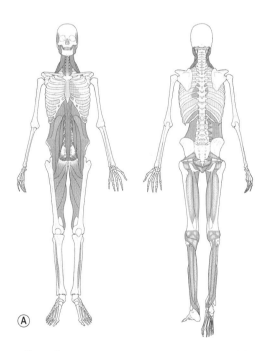

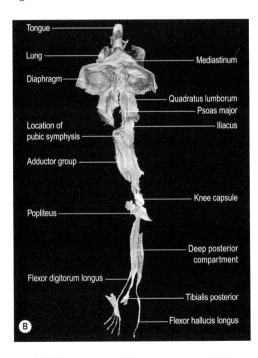

Figure 6.1
The course of the Deep Frontal Fascial Line runs inside the soft palate of the head down the posterior throat, dives deep into the ribcage back behind the heart and lungs, passes the diaphragm to continue back behind the intestines, along the front of the psoas into the inner thighs, travels down into the hamstrings and calves, where it finally ends in the soles of the feet.

Bring the feet about 3 inches (9 cm) apart. Now smile hard, lifting the cheeks and eyes, showing the teeth. Smile hard and breathe 4 breath cycles. Now frown, breathe 3 cycles. Repeat the smile cycle and the frown cycle. Notice the difference of feeling in your pelvis and soles of the feet. This whole-body connection is the Deep Frontal Line.

Level 3

Vertical elongation alone is not sufficient as a single corrective for an asymmetrical spine, yet is an essential element in anti-gravitational control. Used as a strategy when the body becomes tired or distracted, it is an invaluable tool for composing the entire body and decompressing vulnerable visceral and spinal structures. The phenomenon of the collapsing waist is best avoided before it becomes irreversible.

Bring art into the science of spinal decompression by imagining the spine as a deflated accordion. Next, use the breath to fill the torso from the bottom to the top, seeing the pleats of the accordion open up to give spinal height. Stay and breathe in, grow tall, exhale, grow taller for 3 breaths. The magic number of 3 helps to re-set the postural tone.

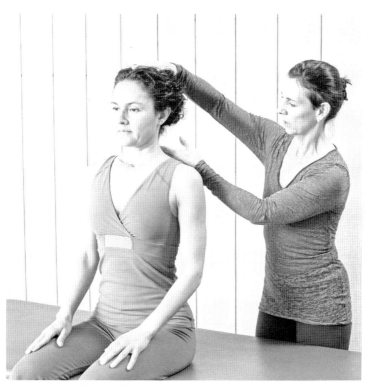

Figure 6.2
Use the Straw exercise, an elongation where it is as if the spine is being sucked up a straw, as a daily Body Skill for scoliosis management.

along with props and wedges to help daily comfort. Chapter 11 expands upon these strategic tools.

Exercise

Apply exercise in three fundamental aspects: somatic, corrective, and conditioning aspects of movement.

Somatic exercise: imagine, think, feel

Begin somatic exercise with the motto, *imagine, think and feel*, to move from the realm of ideas into the physical.

Somatic exercise begins with organization of the internal environment. People with spinal conditions benefit greatly by using inner focus and vision to access the inner regions of the body. Often an unfamiliar skill, this aspect takes training and time to develop. Evidence exists in sports, business and theatrical training that a physical effect takes place while using the imagination (Amasiatu, 2013).

Use descriptive imagery. Gentle humor aids retention. Use the art of imagery to enhance the science behind teaching. One such favorite image entails the back of the ribs having gills like a fish and then watching the bubbles emerge and float to the ceiling.

- *Imagine*. Explaining the expansion of the ribs posteriorly begins with metaphorical thought of bone motion.

- *Think*. Attaching an additional physical sensation to the image, such as self-touch and holding of the anterior rib cage while breathing encourages sensory input.

- *Feel*. Coupling mental rehearsal with gentle motions and physical sensation enhances the experience (Guillot et al., 2013).

Corrective exercise

Train clients when as well as how to use correctives. Start slow and add on as the client becomes more familiar with the program.

Move clients through and beyond remedial exercises by quickly establishing the individual's physical and behavioral scoliosis cues. The Client Profile, covered Chapter 7, formulates not only areas of need for core and structural embellishment, but also provides a template for monitoring both postural and behavioral tendencies in all other exercise using personalized scoliosis cues that serve as target goals beyond simple curve diminishment.

Personal cues follow the Client Profile and include monitoring vertical axis collapse, increasing non-dominant arm usage, gently contracting obliques along the protruding anterior ribs region, increasing inflation of concave lung lobes, and softening the convex ribs.

Adding lower body involvement is a boon. Attend to the less engaged gluteal side, the less used pelvic stabilizer (pelvic floor) side, imprinting weight into the foot, enhancing core to foot sequencing. Promote body skills such as aligning the head over the center of gravity and centralizing the pelvic arch, placing the feet 4 inches apart (10 cm).

Teach the use of the non-dominant eye and tongue position when appropriate. This method takes the science of analysis into artful exercise execution useful in both symmetrical and one-sided exercise.

Conditioning exercise

Guide and encourage clients toward conditioning.

The Pilates Method is a specific type of exercise integrating deep and intermediate layers of musculature with principles of potentiating movement using fascial slings, motor control and mental focus.

As a gateway to fitness, the Method makes conditioning using the 13 large muscle groups more effective and accessible. In *Return to Life*, Joseph Pilates says, "It would be a grave error to assume that even Contrology (the Pilates Method) exercises alone will remake a man or a woman into an entirely physically fit person."

He likens his Method to a lumberjack sharpening the saw to make the difficult task of bringing down a large tree faster, easier, and more effective (Pilates, 1945). The Pilates Method hones the body and is a gateway to fitness.

Emotion

Emotions offer a choice of reaction or response. Managing the ups and downs of progressing or non-progressing spinal curvatures requires a consistent strategy.

The 'fight or flight' sympathetic nerve chain lies directly on the bodies of the vertebrae, in this instance, skewed vertebrae, with a poorly understood effect upon the asymmetrical system. What is known is that this condition affects quality of life and self-esteem (Durmala et al., 2015).

Societal participation involving familial and inter-personal relationships, job ability, recreational pur-suits, along with a desire for plain, comfortable living receive heightened awareness.

Just as balancing pain management involves the dis-cipline of pulling focus toward pleasurable mental states and physical sensations, managing the highs and lows of asymmetrical body discovery and educa-tion takes special desire and effort.

Emotional management tools include the physical act of breath manipulation, the choice of exercise body positions, along with use of vocalization and focus on recognition of emotional state related to the body (interoception); all work to stimulate the parasympa-thetic feature of the nervous system, dominated by the vagal nerve. The astute PMME weaves these tools into the work (Porges et al., 1994; Shafir et al., 2016).

The motto of the parasympathetic system is rest, digest and heal:

- Rest

- Digest

- Heal.

Principles: the mantra

The mantra for functional management of asym-metry is to identify the pattern, break up the pat-tern, redirect the pattern, correct the pattern and go beyond the pattern.

- Identify the pattern

- Break up the pattern

- Redirect the pattern

- Correct the pattern

- Go beyond the pattern

Identify the pattern

The first principle, identify the pattern, starts with the creation of a Client Profile in Chapter 7. Awareness is necessary for the possibility of change but deliver the assessment findings in a kind and straightforward way. Clients are impressionable, especially youth. Youth need strength and guidance. Adults need infor-mation regarding time of life and a clear-cut plan.

The assessments in Chapter 7, SSPOT-1 and SSPOT-2 (Scoliosis Specific Physical Observation Test) and GPOA-1 and GPOA-2 (Global Profile Observational Assessments) serve two purposes: to give the PMME a place to start; and to educate the client on their indi-vidual asymmetry cues for the exercises, and all other exercise in which they participate.

Both groups need to re-examine strategies for study time, phone time, leisure time, home set-up and work spaces. Everyone needs management tools.

Breaking up the pattern

Soft tissue interventions

Tensile elongation in restricted and concave areas, and gentle compression of the convexities along with repetitive motions, change fascial restrictions and lat-erality biases.

Musculotendinous re-shaping along with fascial stretching and re-shaping are the logical tools for this principle.

The fascia

Asymmetrical bodies need specific fascial extensi-bility, loosening internal fascial strapping, as evi-denced in the conversation with Bonnie Thompson, as highlighted in Chapter 3. Fascia is not an inert, passive structure. It adapts and shapes its function-al importance, according to how you use it. It forms the inner scaffolding for the minute parts of the cell to give inner shape and to allow each part to work inde-pendently as well as to travel toward and away from each other. It gives cells shape and form.

Visceral organ tissues are all encapsulated with heavy fascial coverings to keep out unwanted invad-ers, such as viruses, bacteria, or cancers, as well as provide structure to keep organs located in a specific area in the body (Barnes, 1990). Asymmetry alters this all-important internal infrastructure. Opening shortened areas between and around the ribs, in the area supporting the waist and viscera, are part of the principles of the framework.

Nature is asymmetric. Chapter 1 notes two areas of structural asymmetry directly affecting functional asymmetry found in the respiratory diaphragm region and the pelvic sacral-to-hip relation. In addition, fascia reorganizes along lines of tension imposed upon the body (Figure 6.3), according to the less-known Davis's law, which is a corollary of Wolf's law of bone remodeling. Davis's law states that both overloading and insufficient challenge to soft tissue leads to loss of tissue strength, yet properly calibrated challenge induces tissue strength (Frost, 2003).

Osseous restrictions, such as spine asymmetry, physical accidents of life, leg length discrepancy (whether structural or functional) and biased pelvic rotation all contribute to more soft tissue alterations. By adding support, such as a back-pack load of books or an incorrect sitting posture, influencing gravitational loads to this misalignment, fascial strains intensify and spread like a pull in a sweater or stocking.

These powerful restrictions slowly tighten causing loss of mobility, and often pain, and interfere with normal muscle functioning (Barnes, 1990).

Muscular challenges

Special spinal muscle challenges await those with spinal asymmetry. Khosla examined the deep intercellular structure of postural muscles of the spine, the mutifidi, just before surgical insertion of a corrective spinal (Harrington) rod, showing how muscle cells alter by the stresses of an asymmetrical spine.

The issue is a weakness in the muscle to tendon unit. Especially on the concave side, both the muscle and tendon tissue fibers showed disorganization, along with scar tissue interwoven into the regular muscle tissue, as compared to the other side of the torso. Tendon fibers should organize along lines of force, implying that the muscle pull is impeded.

Tendon fibers literally mat up when they are not experiencing lines of pull from the muscles. The scar tissue within the muscle cell lessens the muscle's ability

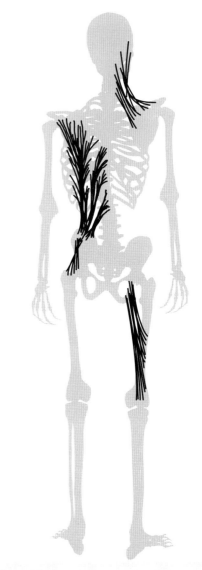

Figure 6.3
Fascia adhesions in asymmetry.

to contract. Muscles are bathed in nerve conduction. The scar tissue acts as an insulator against the nerve conduction in the muscle fibers. This information helps us to hypothesize that myofascial release therapy or fascial tensile engagement may normalize connective tissue, scar tissue and muscle in the region.

The study also found more arterial tributaries, meaning the muscle was struggling to find oxygen, just like a diseased heart develops extra blood routes in an attempt to supply oxygen and nutrients to the muscle (Khosla et al., 1980).

Breaking up the pattern means to fascially alter not only the curves, but all other patterns of asymmetry, to re-establish recruitment of the musculature and create new strategies different from the ingrained neurological habits such as dysfunctional breathing, task biases and unbalanced standing, sitting and walking. Tools to implement fascial changes include wedges, the Arc, the Magic Circle, rib motion mobilization and spinal shifting and rotary actions.

Using wedges and the Pilates Arc

Two types of wedging explain the importance for the need for options with the variations that walk into your studio door. Positional release is a relieving technique that helps the discomfort associated with the transitions between the curves.

The Activ-Wedge® works in opposition to the passive wedge technique. Use it during the active work of mat and apparatus exercises to challenge the shortening of the fascial lines in all the neurodevelopmental positions, described later in this chapter. Generally, place the wedges under the supine concave posterior rib region, the posterior elevated pelvis area. Other neuromuscular tools such as eye and tongue use help too.

The Activ-Wedge® also functions as a gluteal sit bone orthotic. For structural scoliosis, especially where there is spinal fixation surgery, place the wedge under the lighter sit bone to fill in the space. In a functional or more flexible scoliosis that does not contain hardware, place the wedge under the heavier sit bone to push the pelvis over to the lighter side.

Using the Pilates Arc is a great quick start for sessions. Take care with older adults who may have spinal degenerations. While on the Arc, one-lung breathing with the client draped over the Arc serves to restore accessory motion in the ribs and vertebra as able through breathing exercises.

Be sure to exert restraint in long duration or end-range rotation and side-bends in an effort to change the fascia. For this reason, delay introduction of the typical Mermaid on the Reformer until the client learns more about the control needed for true spinal rotation, a necessity for daily life.

Most importantly, be sure to note that the Activ-Wedge® in supine is not advised for those who have undergone spinal fixation. All other positions of sitting, kneeling, standing and inversions work well. Similarly, spinal extension, flexion or side-bending over any type of Pilates Arc is not advised for those with fixation. PMMEs are prudent to note these differences in use and concept between the operated versus non-operated individuals.

Redirecting the pattern

Chapter 10 introduces the concept of altering difficult movement patterns as much as the client is able, leading to a redirection of the scoliosis pattern.

Be sure to follow the sequence from Chapters 7–9 to prepare the client for a safe and effective approach to change: creating the profile to identify asymmetrical cues and tendencies, initiating education and foundational exercises, altering the fascia, and opening stuck or blocked movement patterns.

Redirecting the pattern becomes possible through small increments of what change is possible over time, ensuring safety. There will always be parts that cannot change, yet a good percentage can. Proceeding slowly, the unchangeable aspects, along with the manageable aspects, become more obvious. Programs that aim straightaway into assertive asymmetry change can be abrupt to the system and may not reveal a client's vulnerabilities. Patience is rewarded.

Several strategies become evident in this section. These include the use of the neurodevelopmental sequence positions and motions, the strategy of moving first into the direction or side of ease in asymmetrical, one-sided exercises such as Scooter, and then performing the movement into the direction or side that presents an obstacle.

Although it is tempting to only exercise one area, reasons exist to perform exercises on both sides of the body in such a chronic condition. The direction of ease serves as a reciprocal inhibition to help release the opposing side's resistance, serves as a level of 'overflow' in the spinal segments to help the second side receive some neurological input, and also serves as practice so that the second side has a sort of motor template to use as a guide on the more difficult side.

Avoid the tendency to never perform any symmetrical exercises. Instead, turn symmetrical exercises such as Footwork into asymmetric exercise with wedges, eye control, tongue position, and other asymmetry cues.

Eye control

Why does the use of the non-dominant eye matter? Adding the solo use of the non-dominant eye also aids rotation ease and range.

Chapter 4 discussed the implication of the vestibular balance system being affected in those with spinal asymmetry. Herman's model of asymmetry, see Table 1.2 and mentioned previously in Chapter 4, illustrates that the eyes are part of the spinal asymmetry puzzle although it is unclear whether it is the chicken or the egg. Interestingly, some people show an inability to close one or both eyes while merely performing the eye dominance test.

Chapter 4 described components of Herman's model showing the involvement of the oculomotor system, the brain area which controls the muscular motion of the eyes.

Taking this work and the work of scoliosis researchers in Chapter 4 that found differences in vestibular (balance brain area) function in those with scoliosis, one step farther, consider that eye use has a big impact on both the musculoskeletal and the neuromuscular systems.

The eye has six muscles for function control. Musculoskeletally, the six muscles then coordinate with the suboccipital muscles connecting C2 to the head at the back of the skull.

These muscles are felt when the index fingers are placed on the hairline at the back of the head. Then shift the eyes from side-to-side and feel the slight contractions of the suboccipitals. Due to the slight weight changes of the head, nuanced muscles counterbalance musculature all the way down the body.

If one eye does most of the work, the cerebellum on the same side as the eye dominance receives the most work. The cerebellum controls precision for head, hand and eye coordination. As a person performs biased motions, the side dominance gets stronger in that oppositional side of the brain that controls sensory input and muscle output.

Neuromuscularly, the eyes focus neurologically into both sides of the brain, which is different from the preceding explanation of how the musculoskeletal system works. The eyes receive the image upside down but then process the image, turning it erect in our vision to make sense of it.

Controlled by five nerve control systems, the six main eye muscles help keep the focus area of the retina on the object of interest by holding the head steady by way of the vestibular balance system, brain processing of images, or specific internal retinal systems to hold the object in focus.

The vestibular system of the semi-circular canals deep in the head, work on a three-dimensional basis since each canal is stimulated by head tilt in multiple planes. Focusing through one main eye then ingrains a pattern of repetition in the canals, then ingraining specific muscle and fascial sling patterns that react to this dominance. Eye physicians and technicians take this information into consideration when prescribing or correcting vision acuity (Goldberg et al., 2012).

The goal of the PMME is not to completely eradicate an asymmetrical person's habits or re-train a client to be ambidextrous. The idea is to simply use the non-dominant eye in chosen exercises or daily actions in order to allow the body to use formerly underused nerve pathways and muscle groups, thereby finding functional solutions to redirect the asymmetric spiral. Since PMME training focuses on postural and intermediate level muscle groups adding the ability to use the head and neck in a safe way is a bonus.

Tongue movement

The use of the tongue is another aspect to gain access and redirect the Deep Frontal Fascial Line as well as a safe method to engage the deep neck and thoracic outlet, the area of the ring of the shoulder girdle.

Chapter 7 assessments look at the level of the lower hand in arm elevation while standing. The client assessment generally, along with determining the side of the client's torso that gives into gravity the easiest, both help to establish which side needs elongating from an internal viewpoint.

Bringing the tongue up behind the top teeth away from the side that is falling into gravity, the side with the lowest hand in standing arm elevation or the side giving into gravity with gentle sitting shoulder compression, conceptually, and hopefully physically, lengthens the deep frontal fascial line.

Since spinal asymmetry and scoliosis impact the entire body, interventions need to reach the whole body. Functional solutions focusing on elongation and articulation of the spine, individual and group rib functional solutions, along with pelvic and leg interventions all need to be addressed on both the mat and on the apparatus.

Mat work promotes manipulation of the body weight and provides homework for in-between session maintenance. The apparatus is particularly effective in serving as a measure for side-to-side discrepancies, as an aid due to spring support, and a boon in establishing fascial glide and recoil attributes. The use of the Activ-Wedge®, choosing which side to start the exercise and adding the eye focus and tongue position all help to individualize each exercise without resorting to a global formula based on C, S or 2-, 3-, 4-curve protocols.

Neurodevelopmental sequencing

A recurrent theme throughout all the initial, corrective and progressing re-directive exercises is the use of the neurodevelopmental sequence (NS).

The NS is a normal progression of first year milestones for infants that hopefully culminate in the ability to walk. The positions start as a baby starts in life, in supine with head and neck control as its first priority. Then the baby finally begins to roll onto the tummy for prone. Prone is often difficult for most people in general.

It is actually best for asymmetric individuals to start with the legs below the horizon, by lying on a Long Box or starting with the Ice Cube Exercise so as to avoid overuse of the spinal erectors before the deep multifidi become engaged. Chapter 8 specifies the form needed for this population.

The Pilates Method typically uses sagittal plane rolling on a mat such as Seal and Rolling like a Ball. Initially, lateral rolling is preferable for the asymmetric spine.

The infant and child rolls side to side as a functional progression to attain sitting. Here, rolling accentuates spinal elongation, articulation and breaking up faulty or non-complete movement strategies, and serves as a gateway to spinal rotation.

Adults rarely use rolling as a movement strategy and their rolling is often deficient. Two options for rolling, the Baby Rolls and the X-rolls, are in Chapter 9. Breaking up the pattern: motion is lotion. Both work well as assessments in the SSPOT, and as fascial intervention and motor control techniques, coordinating upper and lower body.

Lateral rolling initiates from the legs or the arms. The core lies in between those kinetic and fascial chains to transmit force from one end to the other. Notice sticking points where the client simply cannot move any further without cheating or using momentum. Getting stuck usually does not indicate weak or inhibited muscles, but the presence of a broken pattern. Be sure to include some sort of lateral rolling.

Clients with scoliosis often have issues with sagittal rolling due to the ribcage and lumbar area prominences, perhaps causing discomfort at transition points. Short and long spine can be problematic for adults with any level of scoliosis until more pliability and control happens. Mermaid is also problematic in spinal asymmetric beginners to the Pilates Method.

Transition points for asymmetric individuals occur in two ways. Typical skeletal transition points occur at:

- The cervical to thoracic junction (neck to ribcage), thoracolumbar junction (where the ribcage meets the low back), and

- The lumbosacral junction (where the low back meets the pelvis) (see Fig. 4.6).

Transition points for asymmetric individuals occur in two ways. Spinal asymmetry has transition points above and below the lateral prominences, the curves:

- In a 'C' curve where there is one prominent long curve, the spinal transitions occur not only in the typical spinal junctions between regions but also above and below the asymmetric curve.

- In an 'S' curve style, often named the 3- and 4-curve pattern, where the head usually centralizes over the pelvis, there are even more transition points due to the multiple curve transitions above and below primary and secondary curves when added to the typical spinal junction transitions.

Notice in the client's Scoliometer® assessment the amount and direction changes of the degree readings for some interesting revelations.

For this reason, start with the lateral rolling suggested in Chapter 9 and proceed from there.

As a milestone, rolling serves to gain shoulder strength to push off from one shoulder and sit up, usually achieved around four months of life. Quadruped crawling soon follows.

In the Pilates Method, the long-sit position (hips flexed at 90° with a neutrally extended spine) helps to achieve hip dissociation, the ability to sit with an erect pelvis.

Although difficulty assuming this position is often misunderstood as a hamstring length issue, other tissue lengths are involved, such as the gluteals, the fascia between the gluteals and external rotators, along with deep and superficial back fascial lines.

Taking time to acquire the four-point Inner Unit foundational exercise in Chapter 8, where the extended toe position touches the floor instead of knee support, aids the development of the more difficult long-sit position.

The PMME is wise to use the variation of gently pulling the client backwards until full confidence of the quadruped position happens.

Most people assume they understand the basics of the knee and hand four-point position, simply hanging onto the bones. The quadruped position is

a gateway into mid-back and upper body strength, along with strengthening pelvic stabilizers for eventual walking.

Look closely at the nuances to make sure that the triceps and the serratus anterior are engaged as in the instructions in Chapter 8. This closed kinetic chain work forms an energetic ring within the deep and superficial fascial arm lines.

The serratus posterior, two chevron-shaped muscles at the top and bottom of the scapular areas, become activated, thereby helping the lung lobes to receive and exchange oxygen, helping the concavities to expand. Individuals with scoliosis often are weak in the upper body, from the waist up, a critical element in the adult collapsing waist phenomenon.

Older adults with a protruding belly confuse the accumulation of abdominal weight with the waist collapse, a similar issue of the protruding belly in osteoporosis. Attention here firms the belly, and optimizes the diaphragmatic breathing zone, the ZOA, explained in Chapter 7.

Quadruped on the Reformer, with No-spring Abs or reverse abdominals, often balances the asymmetric ribcage posteriorly. Experiment using the individual's scoliosis cues, engaging the external obliques along the anterior protruding rib area in combination with lengthening the waist side with the hip hike, adding in the eye and tongue cues. This example demonstrates transforming a symmetrical exercise into a personalized asymmetrical one.

The quadruped position transitions into crawling at around seven months. Reformer Jackrabbit exercises resemble this action. Full kneeling and half-kneeling bring an infant closer toward a standing position at around eight months (Cook, 2016). The astute addition of the Activ-Wedge® in these positions effectively balances out pelvic obliquity. I use the wedge in these positions for popular asymmetry consults at conferences to demonstrate quick correction results. Consistent use over time is even better.

Functional solutions in the pelvis involve educating the client as to the motions of the three bones of the pelvis and how their attached anatomy differs in influence between the spine and the legs. The Z-sit position for the Spinal Spiral and sidelying Pelvic Rotations on the Trapeze Table access Spiral Line fascial slings and musculature, enhancing pelvic mobility and balancing side-to-side uneven leg use. The NS final positions of plantigrade and retrograde involve inversions that progress to standing. Reformer Elephant modifications and Down Dog elongations on the Trapeze Table with the Activ-Wedge® allow even more fascial lengthening and hip dissociation, along with traction and decompression of the spine.

Foot to core sequencing using a wobble board aids full Deep Frontal Fascial Line engagement, coordinates deep pelvic stabilizers to foot and ankle use as well as addressing leg length global issues.

To sum, the NS is a positional and developmental template useful in organizing exercises individualized for the client by layering on the asymmetric client cues. Functional solution strategies for the spine, ribcage and pelvis become apparent and concrete as unconscious faulty and dysfunctional movement patterns redirect toward conscious improvement and ultimately unconscious improved functional movement strategies (Cook, 2011).

Correcting the pattern

Correcting the pattern is the glue that holds the improved strategies intact. It can be described as a de-rotation reinforcement program, where the 3 Es of ergonomics, exercise and emotion converge. Daily Body Skills emphasize the reduction of gravitational exposure of body parts out of a central vertical line, with the use of anti-gravitational correctives aiding muscle contractility and fascial recoil.

Encourage the client to accumulate simple home tools for ergonomic control and exercise enhancement such as a core pillow, Magic Circle, Foam Roller, Activ-Wedges®, Arc or therapy ball, Wobble board, tennis balls or foot rollers. A daily home program emphasizes the multi-directional systems needed to reinforce Pilates Method sessions, fostering a lifelong management system. Daily implementation of a management plan instills consistency and confidence for a fulfilling life.

Beyond the pattern, programming for the individual

Beyond the Pattern in Chapter 12 takes into consideration differing population spinal asymmetry needs and considerations. Gender differences, times of life differences and comorbidities help to set priorities for the PMME in Pilates Method training.

In general, youth seek to stem the progression of developing larger asymmetry, but also need training and guidance to pursue athletic, social, academic and artistic goals. In general, the adult also often has multiple reasons to seek help beyond the asymmetry.

A grave mistake is to overlook essential comorbidity needs such as pregnancy, hip replacement recovery, cancer restoration or body type conditions such as hypermobility training due to preoccupation with the spinal asymmetry. Use practical sense and wisdom in discerning what is most necessary, even if pressure exists from concerned loved ones.

Bringing art into the science of asymmetrical training regards the client's specific goals, a hook to guarantee engagement with the program along with the client's capabilities. Venturing into the Pilates Method world, learning the new language of imagery and the challenge of personal somatic intimacy, takes courage. PMMEs possess an enormous tool box from which to select the right tool for the right client. Through guidance and support from the PMME, the client moves into robust living.

Gender differences

Not all exercises are good for everyone. All exercises can be reframed for anyone. Select language and approach for each gender.

Males tend to be very direct, concrete and may appreciate a different approach than that applied to women clients. Remind the client that Pilates was indeed, a man. Adolescents comparing themselves to their peers need reassurance that many fitness role models besides Joseph Pilates overcame the weakness of undeveloped or weak bodies through focus, and devotion to a regular exercise regimen.

A man's pelvis shape is more funnel-like. In general, it does not possess the natural flexibility of a female pelvis. For this reason, finding true hip flexion without automatic flexion of the lumbar spine is often difficult for a man to embody.

The body skill of holding a neutral flat spine into a squat off a low seat is a simple tool to enter into pelvic floor work, and more accurate bending mechanics necessary to protect the lumbar spine. In addition, men often experience the task of heavy lifting, usually accomplished by use of the more dominant arm. A body skill of lifting more ambidextrously, along with the proper squatting technique is a valuable asset to any man with scoliosis.

Women are more used to detailed language involving body awareness than the typical gym anatomy. Females are usually introduced to the regular occurrence of pain at the time of menses which gives a different body experience than most men. Many are drawn to Pilates for its promise of a more flattering figure, an obstacle in drawing women into the deeper aspects of the work.

Although weight reduction or shape control is a by-product and not the main goal of the Pilates Method, these beneficial side effects might serve as the hook to keep a woman engaged in the process of attaining improved spinal health.

Times of life

Children aged less than 10 years old require a pediatric approach. Play is most important in this stage and a play-like approach may work better. Select different aspects of the SSPOT to start the conversation.

Adolescence is the most common time when the majority of those with idiopathic scoliosis seek help. This critical period is due to the asymmetry's potential for progression to a severe level. Disclose and educate in a spirit of optimism. Encourage coping skills. Proceed with graduated education since scoliosis is confusing even to scholars! Education in the Body Skills ensures concepts, exercises and habits that hopefully last for a lifetime of successful management. Allow time to support life dreams in terms of sport, artistry, education, career and rearing a family.

Child-bearing years are particularly tricky for women with scoliosis. The relaxin hormone creates global ligamentous laxity for about a year after childbirth possibly increasing the liability of scoliosis. Avoid heavy large muscle group activity postnatally. Although jogging eliminates extra pounds quickly, the impact potentiates likelihood of asymmetric exacerbations such as spine, pelvic and leg injuries.

Mid-life begins arthritis formation. Education in prevention and encouragement to condition the whole body helps since joints need movement to avoid stiffening with age, especially in the ribcage.

The abundance of youth may mask the real effects of asymmetry. By mid-life, if the larger muscle groups are allowed to dominate, the lateral curve pattern that may not have been of much significance in earlier life often increases.

Fall prevention starts at middle-age. Include balance activities. Include the wobble board use. Older clients with spinal asymmetry have a lot to lose. Keep encouraging single leg balance, and arm closed chain strength as able.

Menopause is transitional time for women. Changes in the pelvic area with pelvic floor muscle tone diminishment is a time to ensure a stable foundation for the spine. Moving to full Inner Envelope and diaphragmatic control and beyond simple sphincter use of the pelvic floor is critical.

70+ years is a time of bone thinning and muscle loss, the reality of aging (sarcopenia). Look at pictures of Pilates at age 60 and at age 80. Even for a fully developed individual, loss happens. At 70 years, both men and women experience bone loss. At 80 years, expect a muscle loss of about 40%. Look at a 40-year-old and an 80-year-old. See that they look different. At 80, one is different.

The spine with osteoporosis is recommended not to load in flexed positions due to the risk of compression fractures.

Everyone can improve. However, I recommend seeking a skilled practitioner for the fragile elderly. PMMEs need to keep in mind their own physicality as well as providing a safe environment for the fragile client. I advocate the use of an

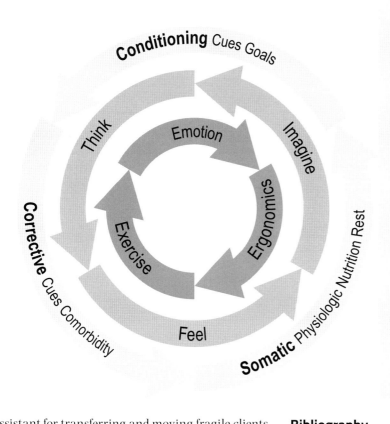

Figure 6.4
Strategies for spinal organization.

assistant for transferring and moving fragile clients around equipment.

Conclusion

Refer to Chapter 13 for a quick guide to the organization of the framework. Everyone needs to start somewhere yet avoid the temptation to 'cookbook' the classifications, especially when co-conditions and comorbidities exist. Fast-track youth into the play of SSPOT-2. Use the core corrective functional tests to begin the initial education with adults. Create the asymmetry cues exposing preferences and individual asymmetry characteristics. Use the NS positioning for more initial education and as a part of the functional solutions for the spine, ribcage and pelvis. Expose the client to the joys of fascial shaping and manipulation. Regard the 3 Es. Teach the body skills and enhance emotional stability through the training of functional breathing.

Go slowly to begin. Have fun with youth. Encourage adults. Be joyful. You have a lot to give.

Bibliography

Amasiatu, D. A. (2013). Mental imagery reharsal [sic] as a psychological. Educational Research International, 1(2), 69–77. Retrieved October 6, 2017, from http://www.erint.savap.org.pk/PDF/Vol.1(2)/ERInt.2013(1.2-07).pdf

Barnes, J.F. (1990). What is myofascial release? In: Barnes, J.F., P.T. Myofascial Release: The Search for Excellence. A Comprehensive Evaluatory and Treatment Approach. pp. 17–19. Paoli, Pennsylvania: Rehabilitative Services Inc.

Broomes, G. (2012). The 4 diaphragms. Retrieved November 3, 2017, from The fascia therapy blog: https://thescienceofphysicalrehabilitation.blogspot.com/2012/07/the-4-diaphragms.html

Cook, G. (2011). Movement: Functional Movement Systems. Screening—Assessment—Corrective Strategies. Aptos, California: On Target Publications

Cook, G. (2016). Why is the neurodevelopmental sequence important to trainers? Retrieved August 14, 2018, from: On Target Publications: https://www.otpbooks.com/neurodevelopmental-sequence-for-trainers/

Davis's law. Retrieved November 3, 2017, from https://update.revolvy.com/topic/Davis%27%20law&item_type=topic

Durmala, J., Blicharska, I., Drosdzol-Cop, A., Skrzypulec-Plinta, V. (2015). The level of self-esteem and sexual functioning in women with idiopathic scoliosis: a preliminary study. International Journal of Environmental Research and Public Health, 12(8), 9444–9453

Frost, H. (2003). New targets for fascial, ligament and tendon research: a perspective from the Utah paradigm of skeletal physiology. Journal of Musculoskeletal and Neuronal Interactions, 3(3), 201–209

Goldberg, M.E., Eggers, H.M., Gouras, P. (2012). The ocular motor system. In: Kandel, S. J., Schwartz, J.H., Jessell, T.H., et al., eds. Principles of Neural Science, New York: Elsevier, pp. 660–677

Guillot, A, Moschberger, K., Collet, C. (2013). Coupling movement with imagery as a new perspective for motor imagery practice. Behavioral and Brain Functions, 9(8), 1–12

Khosla, S., Tredwell, S.J., Day, B., et al. (1980). An ultrastructural study of multifidus muscle in progressive idiopathic scoliosis. Changes resulting from a sarcolemmal defect at the myotendinous junction. Journal of Neurological Science, 46(1), 13–31. Retrieved November 3, 2017, from https://www.ncbi.nlm.nih.gov/pubmed/7373342

Pilates, J. H. (1945) [2010]. Return to Life Through Contrology. Miami: Pilates Method Alliance.

Porges, S.W., Doussard-Roosevelt, J.A., Maiti, A.K. (1994). Vagal tone and the physiological regulation of emotion. Monographs of the Society for Research in Child Development, 59(2–3), 167. Retrieved August 14, 2018, from ResearchGate: https://www.researchgate.net/publication/15215400_Vagal_Tone_and_the_Physiological_Regulation_of_Emotion

Schleip, R., Findley, T. W., Chaitow, L., Huijing, P. A. eds. (2012). Fascia: The Tensional Network of the Human Body. Edinburgh, UK: Churchill Livingstone

Shafir, T., Tsachor, R.P., Welsch, K.B. (2016). Emotion regulation through movement; unique sets of movement characteristics are associated with and enhance basic emotions. Frontiers in Psychology, 6: 2030. doi:10.3389/fpsyg.2015.02030

Stokes, I.A.F. (2007). Analysis and simulation of progressive adolescent scoliosis by biomechanical growth modulation. European Spine Journal 16(10), 1621–1628

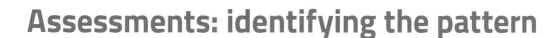

Assessments: identifying the pattern

"We must look globally, act locally, and then act globally to integrate our local remedies in the whole person's structure."

Thomas W. Myers: *Anatomy Trains*

Identifying the pattern creates a flexible profile. Flexibility allows for the composite client profile to differ in motion, in standing versus horizontal, and over time.

The focus of this book is to create functional solutions. We begin with general postural observations and then proceed to the functional tests such as core and leg use, postural sway, vertical compression, eye dominance effect upon spinal rotation, ribcage excursion and breathing analysis.

Observation assessments and tests

This chapter is part of a program summarized in Chapter 13 and is designed for the PMME to create profiles for both youth and adult clients.

Global posture observation assessments Parts 1 and 2 (GPOA-1, GPOA-2) are suitable for everyone. Adults proceed to the Scoliosis Specific Physical Observational Test Parts 1 and 2 (SSPOT-1, SSPOT-2). SSPOT-2 is most helpful to begin with when assessing youth along with GPOA-1 and -2, the initial postural observations. The definition for youth is age 5–20.

Identify the pattern

Specific observational tests identify the surface anatomy and motions to aid the non-radiological

positioning of bones and lines of force. Radiographs analyze mostly the rib, spinal and pelvic elements of the body in two dimensions. The Cobb angle is measured in two dimensions and extrapolated into three.

Other imaging confirms the detailed twists such as MRI, which describes volume. The three-dimensional x-, y- and z-axes are mathematical concepts from the Cartesian coordinate system that define how an object is organized in space. The same system defines the basic corkscrew of the asymmetry pattern.

Note the difference between planes and axes (Figure 7.1). Axes define motion. The x-axis is a horizontal axis parallel to the floor, defining flexion and extension. The y-axis is a vertical axis that runs from the middle of the tip of the head down between the legs, defining rotary action. The z-axis impales the body in a front-to-back line, defining side-bending action.

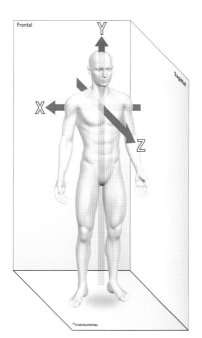

Figure 7.1
X, Y, Z axes
of the body.

Table 7.1

Adults	Youth
GPOA-1 and -2	GPOA-1
SSPOT-1: Parts A and B	SSPOT-2

Although knowing the three dimensions in the coronal and sagittal planes when looking at the block system of twists is critical, the PMME requires more information regarding muscle tone and direction of fascial pull, acknowledging the fourth dimension of functional use. Greater insight comes not only with observing skeletal twists and turns, but also soft tissue formations, shadows and textures. Imagine the body underneath the surface bringing art into the science of analysis. Keep in mind the highlighted image of the body with its fascial restrictions in Chapter 6 (Fig. 6.3).

Beginning words

Be kind with yourself and the client. No one is perfect. Therefore, preface your observations with the statement, 'I say everything to you with love.' Being playful with youth has its benefits and takes pressure off the nit-picky details pronounced by adults. Keeping youth engaged so that they want to participate is primary.

Train your eye yet suspend judgment. The eye develops observation skill with spaced repetition of practice. Having a starting reference point is invaluable. It serves as a place to engender encouragement and inspire you both on your journey. This is the road map for a successful ride.

Observations can go wrong even with a developed analysis skill set. Bias from emotion, upbringing, environment and experience impede a detached observational eye, and willingness to learn. Strive for neutrality.

The overall purpose:

- to record the client's initial postural observations, functional measurements and bony landmarks in order to create a roadmap for change

- to create markers to gauge improvement over time.

GPOA-1 and GPOA-2

The GPOAs begin with general impressions from the posterior coronal view and the side sagittal view (Figure 7.2).

Suspend judgment and collect data. Explanations of why certain shapes happen come to light with progress through the entire postural and functional assessments process. GPOA-1 and -2 break the body into general blocks of head, shoulders, ribcage, waist, pelvis, legs and feet. Observe the contours of these blocks of the body from the posterior for overall effect.

Next, GPOA-2 views the central plumb lines from the posterior and the side. The posterior view plumb line is a vertical gravity line, a y-axis, not a plane, separating the body from right to left by a sagittal mid-line plane. The side-view plumb y-axis separates the body from the anterior to the posterior cut by a coronal plane.

Examine how the body weight starting at the top affects the body parts below (Magee, 2016; Kendall et al., 1993; Barnes, 1990).

GPOA-1: from the posterior coronal plane view

Plumb line from the posterior view

Under the surface

- The plumb line from the posterior is the central vertical spinal line (CVSL), which is either a normal straight line or a lateral curvature of the spine.

- The posterior line falls from the middle of the head and lands between the two feet (Figure 7.3). Standing reveals both functional and structural components of asymmetry. Notice what stands out the most.

- Start at the top and work downwards. The right to left waist indentations, shoulder height tilt and orientation of arm hang reveal asymmetries. In average posture, the shoulder on the side of the dominant hand is lower. Notice the body weight distribution between the legs. The muscular distance between the thighs, calves and legs normally falls equidistant from the plumb line. When the plumb falls closer to one leg, it means that the heaviest part of the body weight, the center of gravity, dominates to that side.

Head alignment

- Is the head more or less centered (called compensated) over the spine? Or is it not (called non-compensated)?

- Is one ear closer to the shoulder, indicating tilt? In which direction?

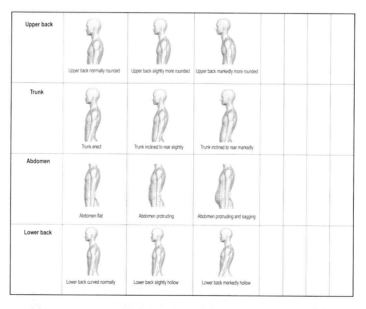

Figure 7.2

GPOA-1 and GPOA-2: general observations from the posterior and the side.

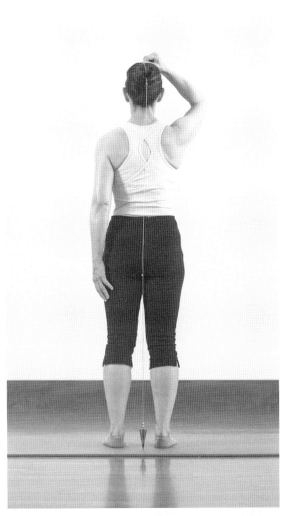

Figure 7.3

- Are both ears visible or is one more fully seen than the other, indicating a rotation?

Shoulder angle

- Is the horizontal shoulder line fairly level?

- Is one shoulder higher than the other? A right-handed person usually has a lower right shoulder and the left is lower in left-handedness.

Lateral thoracic prominence or rib convexity

- Does the spine and/or ribs protrude sideways? To the right? To the left?

- If there is more than one prominence, which one is larger or more eye-catching? Does it spread into the waist?

Lateral vertical waist indentations

Look at just the soft tissue of the vertical sides of the waist, the area between the ribs and the pelvis.

- Is one side of the vertical waist more indented than the other? The right? The left?

- Is there a skin or fat crease that is larger or tilted on one side?

Lateral lumbar prominence or (lumbar hypertrophy)

- Does the spine between ribcage and the pelvis protrude outwards or sideways? To the right? To the left?

- Can you see a difference in the muscle tone on one side of the back than the other?

Usually the ribcage prominence is called the convexity and the lumbar area prominence is lumbar hypertrophy as there are no ribs here.

Pelvic/pant waist level

Check just the line and avoid pelvic specifics at this point.

Note: Be sure to not to change the clothing alignment by smoothing it out beforehand. Creases in the clothing help to detect asymmetries when clients are not disrobed.

- Does the client's pant waist line appear more or less horizontal?

- Is there more space between the forearm and the side of the pelvis on one side?

- Is one gluteal fold, the smile line where the buttocks meet the back of the thigh, higher than the other?

Achilles/heel line

- How far apart are the feet?
- Are the angles of the feet pointed outwards? Inwards?
- Is one side different than the other?
- Is each Achilles line vertical or at an angle toward the mid-line or away from the mid-line of the body?

GPOA 2: from the side sagittal plane view

Side observation (Figure 7.4) reveals deviations from the expected gravitational curves, usually due to poor posture. Improving general gravitational curve issues often improves asymmetric spinal conditions. In fact, start here to reveal the real lateral curve issues:

- Observe:
  - The lateral, side-view line optimally runs from the earhole (auditory meatus) down through the shoulder past the side of the pelvis and ends at the heel of the foot.
  - Line up the plumb with the ear. Use a dowel for best view.

Head alignment

The cervical spine normally is in extension (lordosis), with concavity between the head and the shoulders. Head position guides the lower spine. Imagine it is a bowling ball sitting on a small tree trunk.

- Is the middle of the ear in line with the middle of the head and the middle of the shoulder? Is it forward or behind the line?
- Is there a noticeable crease behind the neck?
- Does the chin jut forward?
- Does the head sag downwards?

Upper back

The upper back (thorax) is normally convex, in flexion (kyphosis), with the apex at T8. Is there a long, smooth slope of a convex curve to the roundness of the ribcage? Clients with scoliosis are often flat here.

- Is the middle of the arm at the shoulder in line with the ear?

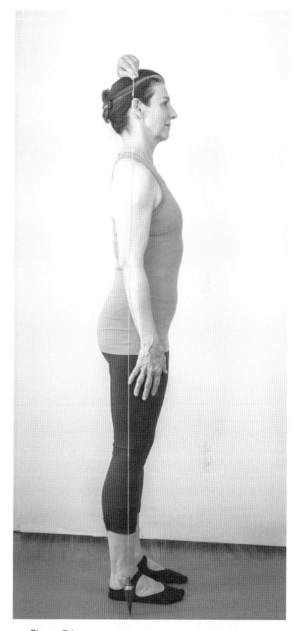

Figure 7.4

- Is the head behind the upper back?
- Does the upper back appear so rounded that the eye is drawn to the roundness of the upper back?

○ Does the upper back seem so round that the client appears to be stooped forward?

Upper trunk to lower trunk alignment

Look at the angle from the apex of the waist up along the back of the thorax toward the head to decipher a sway back posture.

- Is the middle of the shoulders in line with the middle of the pelvis?

- Does the thorax appear to be leaning backwards?

Abdomen

Focus on the line from the pubis up toward the navel. Suspend judgment about whether the area is fat or not. A protruding abdomen: Is it a sign of osteoporosis, fatigue, or a spine condition like scoliosis? A collapsing waist also protrudes the belly.

- Does the abdomen appear flat, protruding or sagging?

- Does the abdomen appear a normal bulk for the body type?

- Does the client report constipation?

Lower back

Lumbar spine lordosis is a normal concavity between the ribcage and the gluteus maximus. The apex of the curve is roughly just above the waist line at L3. The lumbar area is particularly vulnerable to collapse and side shifting due to lack of bony support at the waist. The middle of the side of the thorax should line up with the middle of the side of the pelvis, optimally creating a vertical line.

Be careful about confusion between an anterior pelvis and a hyperlordotic lumbar spine. Sway back people often appear hyperlordotic. Yet when the thorax is upright, the lumbar area is often undeveloped.

- Does one side of the buttocks appear full while the other is recessed (flat)?

- Does the thorax appear to be pulling forward of the pelvis?

- Does the apex of the low back appear unusually curvy?

SSPOT-1: Part 1

Functional solutions for asymmetry require more than static standing posture assessments so use your three-dimensional sense to ferret out what is happening underneath the surface of the skin (Barnes, 1990; Kendall, 1993; Lee, 1999; Mitchell, 2002).

Standardize the test

Place your foot in between the client's feet to standardize the width between the legs with the feet parallel to each other, even if this position is not the client's normal or comfortable stance.

The SSPOT-1 observational tests are:

- Beighton Hypermobility Score

- Higher hand in elevation

- Clavicle position

- Anterior rib crest angle

- Chin to sternal notch vertical line

- Anterior plumb vertical mid-line

- Level anterior superior iliac spine (ASIS) position

- Scoliometer® use

- Forward-bend book convexity observation

- Knee 'Q-angle' marker without the use of a goniometer

- Ankle pronation/supination.

Beighton Hypermobility Score

This assessment is not a diagnosis. The score generally identifies those with loose joints or connective tissue. It uses many classifications in the spectrum from benign to severe (see Figure 7.5). Chapter 12 highlights some important aspects of training the hypermobile population.

The 9-point Beighton Scoring System for Joint Hypermobility Scale

- Score one point on each side:

  ○ Passive dorsiflexion of the fifth metacarpophalangeal joint to 90°

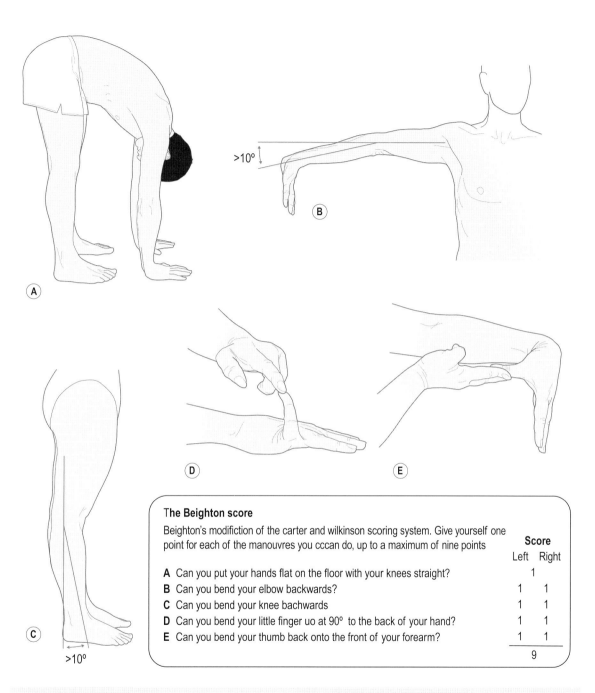

The Beighton score

Beighton's modifiction of the carter and wilkinson scoring system. Give yourself one point for each of the manouvres you cccan do, up to a maximum of nine points

	Score	
	Left	Right
A Can you put your hands flat on the floor with your knees straight?		1
B Can you bend your elbow backwards?	1	1
C Can you bend your knee bachwards	1	1
D Can you bend your little finger uo at 90° to the back of your hand?	1	1
E Can you bend your thumb back onto the front of your forearm?	1	1
		9

Figure 7.5
The Beighton Hypermobility Score.

○ Touching the thumb to the flexor aspect of the forearm

○ Hyperextension of the elbow beyond 10°

○ Hyperextension of the knee beyond 10°

○ Plus one point: forward trunk flexion placing hands flat on the floor with knees extended.

A score of 4/9 = general hypermobility. A score of 9 indicates more hypermobility. The higher the score, the greater the concern for injury with activity (Knight et al., 2012).

Higher hand in elevation

Which hand is higher in elevation? Match the third fingers. Note each side. How far is the upper arm from the head? See Figure 7.6 on page 94.

Under the surface

Notice how the shoulder blades sit on the ribcage, and which way the armpits face. A lower or tighter arm could be pulled from the waist, an internal shortening of the trunk or pelvis. Think shortened deep hip flexor, inner envelope, or unnecessary habit as arms elevate. This tests the z-axis side-bend asymmetry.

Clavicle position

- Note each side. Are the clavicle positions symmetrical from the mid-line? Is one is higher than the other? See Figure 7.7 on page 95.

- Is one at an angle? If so, what is the tilt angle (horizontal, outer edge higher, middle edge higher)?

- Is one more forward in space than the other?

- Look at the shadow underneath the collar bones. Is one area of soft tissue more concave under one side?

- Note the protrusion of ribs just under the collar bones. Does one side of the ribs look more prominent than the other?

- Notice the muscle girth of the upper trapezius on each side.

Under the surface

The shoulder girdle literally spins around the ribcage and twists with asymmetry. A shadow underneath

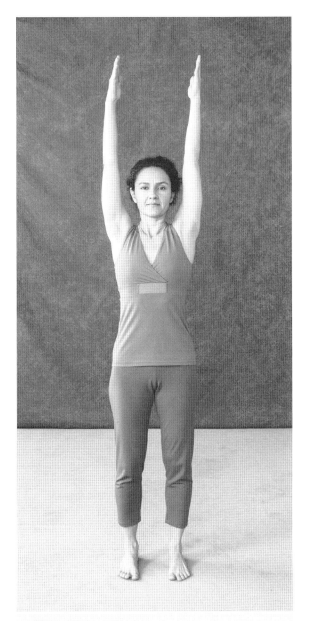

Figure 7.6

the clavicle usually indicates a tight pectoral minor, a winged scapula and ribs rotating to the posterior.

The bones need free movement to glide up and down to protect the cervical nerves that dive between the collar bones and the first rib. A difficult and often fragile

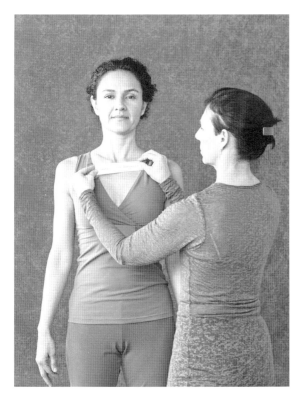

Figure 7.7

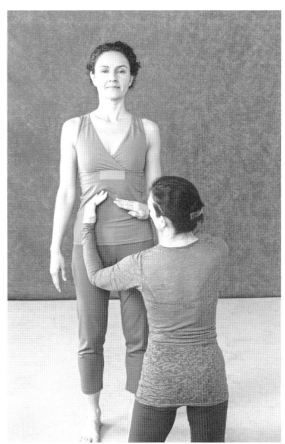

Figure 7.8

area for direct exercise, use of the eyes, tongue, awareness and imagery tools combined with spine articulation and arm exercises balance the neck, shoulders, arms and hands. Each rib pair creates a functional ring around the spine. A revelation for most is that the upper trapezius musculature needs strengthening; it functions to hold the shoulder girdle up.

Anterior rib crest angle

- Note each side. Are the anterior (front) rib crease angles symmetrical? Is one higher than the other? See Figure 7.8 on page 95.

- What is the tilt angle? Horizontal? Outer edge higher? Mid-line edge higher?

- Does one side of the anterior ribcage protrude forward?

Under the surface

Giving clues as to orientation of the internal and external ribcage in relation to the pelvis, this test reveals the asymmetrical impact upon the internal fascia and diaphragmatic, intercostal and upper oblique abdominal tightness. The protruding side is important in scoliosis cue correctives indicating the internal obliques there are tight and weak. If the upside down 'V' of the angle is tilted, consider that the internal pleural fascial area of the mediastinum, the fascia hollow between the lungs and heart, is essentially twisted or restricted.

Chin to sternal notch vertical line

The *sternal notch* lies between the clavicles in the center of the chest:

- Is the chin in a vertical line with the sternal notch? See Figure 7.9.

- Is the chin to the right, left or in line with the notch? A ruler, pencil, or straight line identifies positioning.

- Do the neck muscle lines of the sternocleidomastoid (SCM) form a symmetrical 'V' shape?

- Is the 'V' angle of the chin pointing to the right shoulder, center or left shoulder?

Under the surface

The sternal notch observation reveals head placement and orientation upon the neck. Asymmetry of a 15 lb

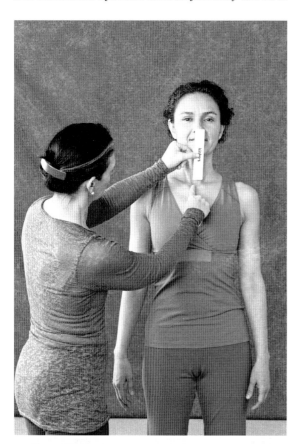

Figure 7.9

head (6.5 kilos) impacts large orientation muscles and fascia. The gravitational drop down into the body impacts the symmetry of the central plumb line. This measure helps to show clients where the head needs optimal positioning to affect all other structures.

Anterior plumb vertical mid-line

Take a dowel, place it on the chin and line it up with the mid-pubis region and let it touch the floor (Figure 7.10):

- Where does the plumb line fall?

- Is the navel at the center or to the right or left of the dowel?

- Which way is the 'V' of the groin area pointing? The 'V' at the groin is formed by the two hip creases, the pant lines.

The anterior line reveals and confirms the asymmetric distortions. A great home program strategy is an exercise using a mirror to optimize a near-perfect central lineup of the chin, navel and pubis.

Level of ASIS positions

Slide your thumbs up and under the bony prominences, not on top, for accuracy (Figure 7.11):

- Are the thumbs horizontally level, or is there one higher than the other?

- Are the thumbs equidistant from the anterior plumb line and also the hip joints at mid-way on the pant line?

Under the surface

The positioning of the pelvic bones detects pelvic obliquity, a common condition with an asymmetric spine. An ASIS side lower than the other indicates a hemi-pelvic (one side of the pelvis) rotation (anterior innominate) toward the floor, creating a longer leg and more heaviness into the ground. The distance of the thumbs from the mid-line indicates a presence of a hemi-pelvic flare, with one side being closer to the mid-line than the other. See the video for an illustration of pelvic motions (Code 7.1).

The sacrum rotates about six axes and creates a figure-of-eight motion in walking. See Functional solutions for the pelvis in Chapter 10 for more.

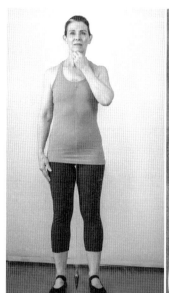
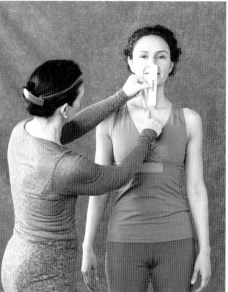

Figure 7.10

Code 7.1 (free code)
Pelvic bone motions

Code 7.2 (free code)
Scoliometer assessment

Scoliometer® assessment

Observe. With the client's hands in the swimmer's dive position and with feet hip-width apart, the client slowly bends over toward the floor (see Figure 7.12 and Code 7.2). Simultaneously slide the indentation side of the Scoliometer® down the line of the spinous processes. Feel for the spinous processes as they wander from central line of the torso. Keep the sides of the Scoliometer® in contact with the ribs.

- At which part of the spine does the Scoliometer® tilt to either side?
- What is the degree of tilt? Is it equal to or more than 7°?

Under the surface

On-line Scoliometer® apps are available and provide color zones that denote severity.

The Scoliometer® strictly measures axial trunk rotation, a functional measure (Figure 7.13). It correlates with yet is not the same as the Cobb angle. Used primarily in school screening to determine if a youth should be referred to a medical service, it has value for the PMME to better understand the twists and bulk of the asymmetry. It is a validated instrument through stringent research.

If the Scoliometer® measurement is equal to or more than 7°, and the client is an adolescent, it is recommended that the client seek medical attention. Avoid disappointment by not relying only on changes in the Scoliometer® reading for improvement. Spinal asymmetry has both structural and functional components. In one of my courses, I demonstrated the difference between the readings when I rolled down and up with controlled experience compared with when I completely released the control. The class was astounded!

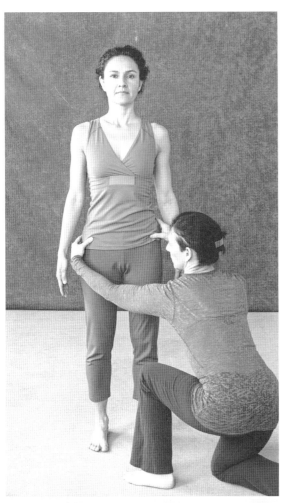

Figure 7.11

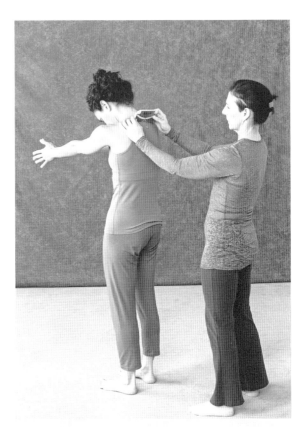

Figure 7.12

Do not be fooled that the Scoliometer® shows only structural changes. Also, do not promise clients or families that a certain degree will change. You will both be disappointed. The true value of its use is in repeated readings, so as to alert the client to any true progressive worsening of the curves.

When observing the tilts of the Scoliometer®, the raised side indicates a thoracic convexity, in slang, a rib hump. The bodies of the vertebrae here are twisting toward the rib convexity. The raised side in the posterior waist often indicates overbuilt erectors, called lumbar hypertrophy. Touch the spinous

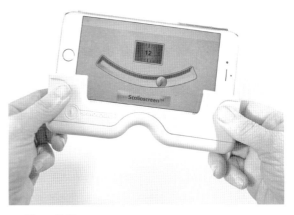

Figure 7.13

processes to note direction of the twist. Accurate values for spinal, rib and pelvic rotation and ribcage are only accomplished with X-ray, MRI, and CT scan (Beauséjour et al., 2013; Bunnel, 1993).

Forward-bend book convexity

At which part of the spine does the book tilt to either side? To which direction? (See Figure 7.14.)

Take the book away and observe once again. The area with the higher level of ribs, or the higher level of muscle tone is the sign of asymmetry.

Under the surface

Using this validated visual forward-bend test to detect presence or progression avoids harmful effects of repeat radiograph exposure for youth. However, refer to the Scoliometer® for accurate degree referral to the medical system (Chowanska et al., 2012).

Q-angle approximation

Approximate the Q (quadriceps) angle by comparing one side to the other with a line drawn with a cord from the mid-patella to the tibial tuberosity (TT) (Figure 7.15). Generally, the line should be vertical.

- Is there a vertical line or it is an angle?
- Compare sides: are the lines fairly symmetrical?

Under the surface

Technically, the Q-angle (quadriceps) occurs from two lines intersecting at the mid-patella from the ASIS to the patella and from the patella to the TT, the prominent bony landmark at the top and front of the tibia. Measured with a goniometer, it is significant

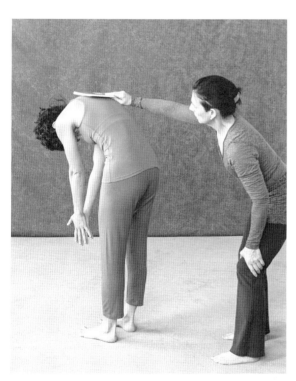

Figure 7.14

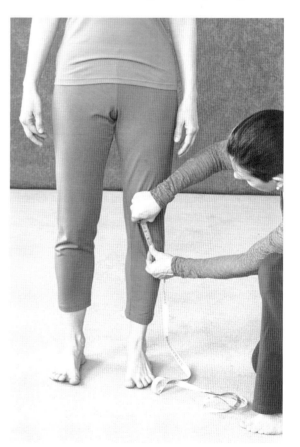

Figure 7.15

for knee pain if it is greater than 17°. Approximation observation from the patella to tibia tuberosity gives good insight into leg imbalances. The greater that the line veers from vertical indicates the greater the twist between the femur and the tibia. Strengthening and aligning the fascia and musculature of the legs has a profound effect upon balancing the pelvis and stabilizing the spine.

Ankle pronation/supination

View the ankles and feet from the front. Note the client standing still, then rolling the ankles in and then outwards (Figure 7.16).

- Are the ankles fairly symmetrical in terms of the rolling in or out of the ankles?
- Does the client stand on the outside of the feet? On the inside?
- Are the toes lying on the floor, or are some lifted?
- Are any toes crossed over the others?
- Are the great toes pointing toward the little toes (bunions)?

Under the surface

Equalizing the weight between the feet is a useful body skill for anyone. In spinal asymmetry, one leg hits the ground more than the other. Think of a cow standing sideways on a hillside where the lower set of hooves are in supination and the higher set is in pronation. Generally, the leg with the greatest Q-angle is a shorter leg with a supinated ankle. The longer leg with generally an anterior hemi-pelvic rotation is the longer leg, with a slightly flexed knee to equalize the sides.

SSPOT-1: Part 2

Preferential movement biases and directions

Identifying preferential tendencies serves two purposes. First, it is informative to reveal a usual strategy or preference. One image is of the internal alien, where asymmetrical people feel a constant internal twist. Identifying the elements that comprise the internal twisting gives hope to make peace with it.

The second purpose is to decide which side to begin an asymmetrical exercise. Asymmetrical exercise is critical in the treatment of scoliosis. Do include both directions and sides of exercise instead of focusing on one side versus the other. Each side of every part of the whole body, not just the trunk, works in an oppositional way with and against each other.

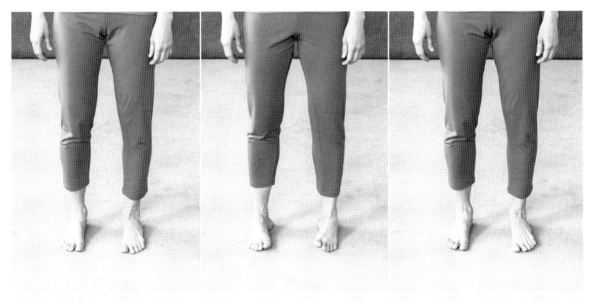

Figure 7.16

Asymmetrical imbalances, by virtue of the spiraling nature of the condition, cause a DNA-like helical three-dimensional imbalance pattern that is difficult, at best, to fully analyze. Functional assessments ferret out various directional and lateral biases to address the need for whole body, multidirectional intervention.

The functional tests listed here are:

- Handedness
- Seated pelvic rotation
- Eye dominance test
- Vertical compression test
- Seated spinal rotation test
- Core muscle straight leg raise
- Tensor fascia lata (TFL) dominance (Figure 7.17)
- Rib excursion
- Breathing count, pattern and style.

The overall purpose:

- To observe the client's initial intuitive strategy when given the request to perform the motion.
- To determine individual preferences in directions of motion to break up habitual motor patterns that may be exacerbating the scoliosis.

Handedness

Ask the client to sit and write something on a piece of paper. Notice if the client sits straight forward or twists to write on the paper. Record whether the client is right- or left-handed. One strategy to break up this dominance is to have the client color in a color book with the non-dominant hand (DeNooijer, et al. 2016).

Seated pelvic rotation

This test determines the pattern of transverse rotation restriction due to laterality preference of handedness as described by Boyle. It is related to breathing dysfunctions and correlates with imbalances in functional leg length and stride length (Boyle, 2013). Watch the video for a demonstration of this test (Code 7.3).

Code 7.3 (free code)
Beta study: laterality interventions

Test

The client sits on a stool or chair toward the edge of the seat with the feet on the floor, about hip-width apart. Place a book or stiff paper in front of the knees. Hold the upper body fairly steady as the lower body rotates, bringing one knee ahead in space than the other. Observe the differences from side to side in range of motion. Note which one goes farther.

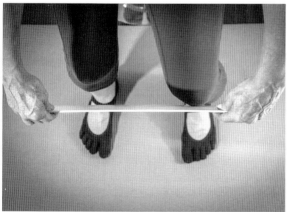
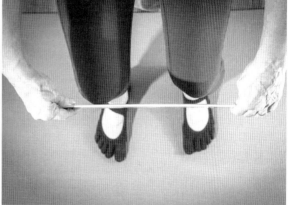

Figure 7.17

Eye dominance test

The dominant eye use relates to sub-occipital muscle use due to C1–2 positioning along with the semi-circular canal positioning for balance (see Ch. 6) in functional communication of reading, speaking, and electronic device use, among others. Variations in the exercises to include eye use foster integration and coordination of the head and hand use (Carey & Hutchinson, 2013).

Test

Make a diamond with your hands by touching the thumbs together and the index fingers together (Figure 7.18). Look at an object across the room through the diamond with both eyes. Then close each eye. Which opened eye keeps the object in the same location as when both eyes are open? This eye is the more dominant eye.

Vertical compression test

The side that falls more, or is perceived to fall more, is probably the more flexible side, the concave side, giving into gravity. This is an indication of dysfunctional side-bending on the z-axis combined with an x-axis flexion, indicating need for elongation on that side. Understanding which side gives into gravity the most specifies the tongue position for exercise. When used in exercise, the tongue is placed behind the opposite side's top teeth to pull and elongate the Deep Fascial Frontal Line on the concave side (Barnes, 1990).

Test

The client sits on the Trapeze Table, preferably with feet dangling to isolate the seated torso or on a chair without leaning back into it. Place one hand with flat, open fingers, on each superior shoulder closer to the neck on the soft tissue, not on the bony shoulder girdle as much as possible. Gently press downwards on the shoulders at the same time. Hold about 10 seconds and observe (Figure 7.19).

Which side seems to feel as if it is falling toward the table, or collapsing slightly? Which side feels like it cannot hold up against the pressure?

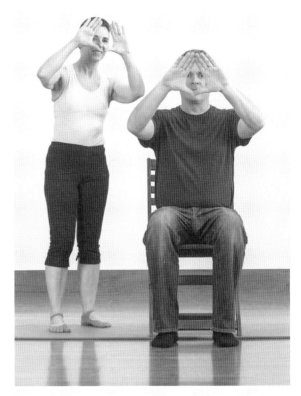

Figure 7.18

Seated spinal rotation test

This test observes strategy for ease of movement and detects rotation compensatory motion. Do not push the client. It is a functional y-axis observation. Part 1 is the simple test. Part 2 adds closing the dominant eye to determine if the range changes (Barnes, 1990; Mitchell, 2002; Carey & Hutchinson, 2013).

Test

The client sits on the Trapeze Table, preferably with feet dangling or on a chair.

Cue the client to gently twist to one side and then the other. Do not indicate which direction. Note which direction the client turns. Ask the client's impression of which way seems easier to turn or has a larger range of rotation. Observe whether there is any lateral translation (side shifting as a compensation) to make the motion go farther or easier (Figure 7.20).

If a lateral shift occurs during the rotation, gently hold the rib cage in alignment with the pelvis and repeat. Is the result different? One strategy is to include a side shift, making the direction range feel larger or easier. Record the direction of ease with the correction. If there was a lateral translation (a shift, or cheating) to make one direction easier, then gently hold the ribcage to prevent the compensation and try again.

Which way is easier to the client now? If unsure, choose the direction of ease.

Lateral pelvic sway test

Lateral sway indicates how much the pelvis moves from one side to the other in gait and determines the leg the client prefers to stand on. Again, it is a combination of z-axis side bend and x-axis flexion. Standing and walking more centrally between the legs prevents leg overuse and injuries such as bursitis among other knee and ankle problems. The side with weaker hip abductors, responsible for strength in standing on one leg, indicates the easier direction (Kinikli et al., 2011).

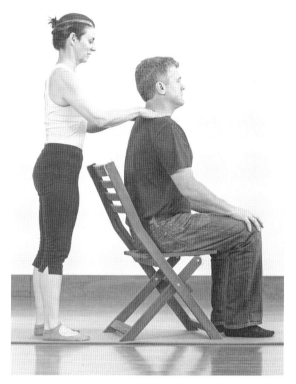

Figure 7.19

Figure 7.20

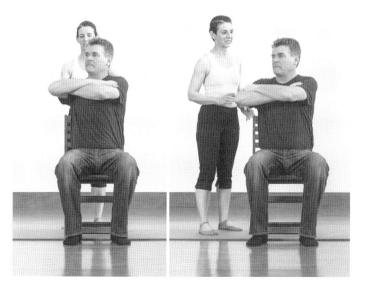

Test

The client stands in the *1st parallel*. This term will mean, throughout the entire text, that the legs are placed into a vertical line drawn from the second toe, the one next to the Great Toe, in line with the center of the kneecaps and mid-way on the pant line, where the femur head flexes the hip joint.

Find the greater trochanter (GT) of the femur. Locate the GT by sliding the hand gently from the top of the side of the pelvis to the top of the side of the thigh. Gently push horizontally at the GT level, side to side. Guide more than push (Figure 7.21).

Which way does the pelvis move more, according to the client? According to you? Which way moves easier? Watch the video from Chapter 1 (Code 7.4) to see a demonstration of the seated rotational test and the pelvic sway test.

Code 7.4 (free code)
Beta study: laterality interventions

Test

Part 2: TA ASLR test

TA: ASLR with anteriorly compressed ilia

The purpose of the TA ASLR test is to imitate the shortening contraction use of the TA to see if the designated heavier or more difficult leg to lift improves in ease, less pelvic rotation or lightness.

Place cupped hands around the ilia at the ASIS and simultaneously press the hands toward each other. Focus on pulling the fascia from the posterior pelvic sides toward each other following the curved nature of the bones. Then cue elevation of the 'more difficult' leg. Repeat this action several times to determine consistency of the finding and record the result.

Three functional core muscle group tests: straight leg raise

This specialized, supine (backlying) straight leg raise test helps to identify which of the lumbar spine stabilizing muscles are most imbalanced with leg use. The lumbar spine stabilizing muscles are known as a group as 'the inner unit.' They are the *transverse abdominals* (TA), the *multifidi* (MF) of the lumbar spine, the *pelvic floor* (PF) as a group, and the *respiratory diaphragm*.

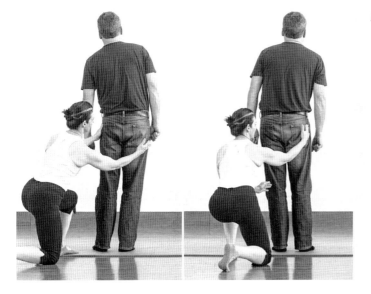

Figure 7.21

Test

Part 1: test reference – ASLR

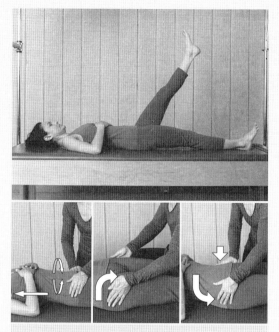

Figure 7.22

The client lies in supine with no instruction given except to lie as heavily as possible on the table. Cue the client to raise a leg about 45° from the horizon of the table or mat, one at a time. Do not indicate which side in order to see which one the client prefers. Ask which is harder to lift. Note whether the chosen leg is accompanied by a pelvic rotation when the leg lifts. If so, hold the pelvis stable, repeat the test. Does the selection change? Pelvic rotation often is a compensation. If the leg selected as being harder to lift is accompanied by a pelvic rotation toward that side as the leg was lifted, repeat the test for a second time. On the second trial, hold the pelvis firm to correct the pelvic rotation, yet light enough to allow movement. At times, when the pelvic rotation is corrected, the opposite leg is then determined to be harder to lift. The pelvic rotation may be a compensatory motion hiding the real results. Which leg-lifting appeared more difficult or uncoordinated, or heavy to perform the action to you? To the client? Did it cause pelvic rotation as it lifted?

Determine between you and the client which leg will be the test leg for the next variations of the ASLR.

Test

Part 3: MF ASLR test

MF: ASLR with posteriorly compressed ilia

The MF ASLR test imitates the shortening contraction of the MF to determine if lifting the more 'difficult' leg produces less pelvic rotation, a greater feeling of ease or greater sense of coordination with the handhold maneuver from the PMME. Places the hands on the sides of the client's pelvis. Place the hands on the sides of the ASIS region, and not on top of the bones. Cup the palm (duck hand) around the sides of the large iliac bones. Gently tug the fascia of the bones back toward the spine. Motion down toward the table and follow the curved nature of the pelvic bones to the back of the body. Upon request, the client then elevates the 'more difficult' leg. Repeat this action several times to determine consistency of the finding and record the result.

Test

Part 4: PF ASLR test

The PF ASLR test imitates the use of the pelvic floor musculature in the stabilization of the movement of the legs. The PF is like a parachute with muscles, tendons and fascia. It forms a flexible sling, pulling from the base of the bowl up and inside the bowl of the pelvis toward the spine. This action connects the legs into the pelvis.

Again, the test aims to find if lifting the more 'difficult' leg produces less rotation, a greater feeling of ease or greater sense of coordination with the handhold maneuver from the PMME. Place flattened hands on the sides of the client's thigh at the GT. The hands are now lower onto the bony mound of the GT, and not on top or side of the iliac bones. The fingers are pointing down toward the mat.

Gently press the GTs of the femurs toward the midline of the body, along with a slight lift toward the head. Think about trying to move the skin and fascia rather than attempting to drive the bones in a certain direction. Upon request, the client then elevates the more 'difficult' leg while this pressure is maintained by the PMME. Repeat this action several times to determine consistency of the finding and record the result.

Test

Part 1: Parallel Position

Part 1 starts with the client supine upon the mat. First, observe hip flexion without touching the area of interest, pointed out in the photograph (Figure 7.23, left and middle images). Note if one of the hips seems to hike up toward the ribcage with the action. Next, gently cup the finger pads where the hip creases on the lateral portion where the thigh meets the pelvis. The TFL is a small muscle right at the crease. Larger muscle girth occurs on the more dominant side.

Cue the client to flex each hip. Repeat the action a second time, using tactile aid to determine the timing of muscle use. Often the more dominant side contracts first. Repeat this action several times to determine consistency of the finding and record the results.

Begin with an active straight leg raise (ASLR) to use as a test reference (Lee, 1999). The goal is to reveal core muscle weakness of coordination and strength of the lumbar spine against leg weight. However, if pain with leg lifting or pain with the compression tests occurs, refer the client to a medical service.

Which tests helped to increase the ease of the ASLR of the more difficult leg to move? Match up the results with the correctives in Chapter 8, forming a foundation to start the Asymmetry Program. If a certain test made the client's response worse, creating more rotation or a heavier or less coordinated action, then do not focus on that test's corrective exercises. Avoid confusion by attempting to ascertain why a test made the response worse. The tests are not meant for this purpose.

Part 2: Walk Position

Part 2 of the test uses the 'walk' position with the knees bent and opened in an easy 'frog' position (Figure 7.23, right image). Do not allow the thighs to merely flop open. Maintain some muscle tone. Place the foot weight onto the metatarsals and pads of the toes. Perform the same knee-folding motion, first observing for any click and then repeat with tactile aid to determine the motor control. Repeat this action several times to determine consistency of the finding and record the results.

The TFL dominance test (Sahrman, 2002)

The TFL dominance test investigates the compensatory use of the TFL instead of the deep hip flexors, the iliopsoas complex. The hiking hip indicates a slight difference in how and when the feet are hitting the ground in normal walking, creating a functional if not structural leg length difference. Often accompanied by a clicking or snapping hip, the two assessment positions reveal subtle differences in strategy. The frog position especially highlights whether the joint needs help coordinating motion and strength to eradicate, or lessen, the clicking. Chapter 8 provides detailed correctives for both test positions.

Parallel Position with knees straight up for Part 1 of the test (Figure 7.23).

Identifying breath excursion, pattern and style

Functional breathing patterns are important. Breathing is a function of both the autonomic nervous system as well as the sensory-motor nervous system. We breathe automatically, but we can also consciously change our breath.

The shape of the female ribcage is narrower from the front to the back in general than the male ribcage. Men have a more barrel shape, perhaps allowing more leverage for stronger muscular connections from the arms to the scapula, vertebra, ribs and pelvis (Bellemare et al., 2003). Scoliosis is associated with a flat thoracic curve region, and other unusual sternum shapes. Be ready to observe more than the typical rib and lumbar area prominences. Support the

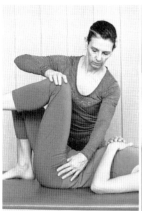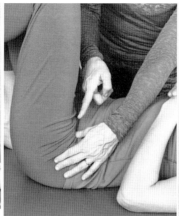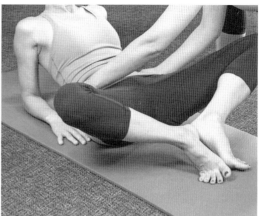

Figure 7.23

client and the family as they seek the care they need. Functional solutions are always within reach. A big help is to focus on the breathing pattern (Jaroszewski et al., 2010).

Breathing pattern disorders (BPDs) and scoliosis are most common in women. Be reassured that true lung failure occurs most commonly at the extreme of measured spinal curves of 90°. These clients know who they are and are likely under medical care. However, it is prudent to measure the chest excursion to achieve more activity in the thorax, optimize the ZOA and Inner Envelope fascial stocking, and promote emotional stability through vagal nerve stimulation.

Chest excursion

Chest excursion is the distance the ribcage expands between each inhalation and exhalation. Take a simple tape measure. Place it around the ribs about 1–1.5 in (2–3 cm) below the breasts, or about where the xiphoid ends (Figure 7.24). Take three trials. Place the tape, then instruct the client to exhale out. This is the first measure. Then ask them to breathe in, in, in, in ...take the second measure; do not move the tape. Exhale. Repeat to inhale for 4 counts, slide the tape if it moves, exhale, then at the end of the third inhalation instruction, hold the tape where the last inhalation ended and that is your measure. Take three trials to give a good reading. If the excursion measure is less than 1.55 in (35 cm), be

prudent and refer the client to their family physician or a pulmonologist (Weinstein et al., 2003).

Breath pattern

Observations of accessory breathing, location of breath origin, and direction of breath flow along with qualitative factors determine functional breathing. Symptoms of BPD include shortness of breath; however, true fainting and dizziness need medical attention. Qualitative symptoms include labored or quick breathing although the excursion measured as normal, chest tightness, chest pain, breathlessness with Pilates or easy exercise exertion, frequent yawning, and hyperventilation (Thomas et al., 2001). Other reported symptoms are fatigue, pain at the back and neck, anxiety, brain fog, tingling in the shoulders or arms and cold hands (Schleifer et al., 2002).

Check for diaphragmatic breathing. In a *supine hookline position* (lying on the back with knees bent and soles of the feet on the floor), place the hands on the abdomen. Bring the thumbs together at the bottom of the sternum and index fingers together at about the navel. Check to see if the fingers at the navel move before the ribs. Inquire where the feeling of the breath originates (Chaitow, 2012.) The breath should originate at the navel. Imagine two cones with the bases at the waist and the apices up above the clavicles. Imagine the cones filling from the bases up to and beyond the clavicles.

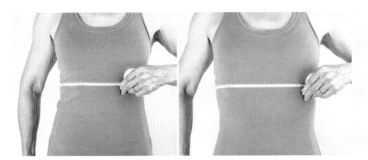

Figure 7.24

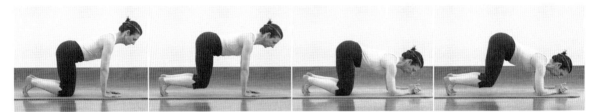

Figure 7.25

Breathing style

Assess the client's breath style. BPDs include chest breathing, mouth breathing, and hyperventilation or over-breathing. Check the number of breaths in a minute. Many people do not recognize over-breathing. Program your timer for one minute. Cue the client to count breaths. One breath is an inhalation and an exhalation. The PMME counts as well. Then compare the two. An ideal rate is 3–4 breaths per minute. Average is 12–16. A daily habit of counting to 15 on exhalation is a good way to begin progress toward functional breathing.

SSPOT-2

SSPOT Progressions are both assessments, goals and session movement progressions directed toward, yet not limited, to youth. SSPOT-2 is not intended for those who have had any spinal surgery.

Rate them as levels from poor to fair to good to excellent.

Planks: three variations

Observe planks in all three orientations of closed mechanical chain positions, from the front, the side, and the back. Start from the beginning of each section to determine the level at which the progression begins. No one probably starts at 'excellent' in order to allow time to improve form.

The front plank

The front plank functional use balances leg length difference and optimizes functional overhead reach. Beginning in a half-plank, the progression proceeds toward inversions.

Inner Unit (half-plank, see Figure 8.22)

The High Axis version is with the elbows extended in quadruped. Cue the client to lift the knees 1.5 in (3 cm) and breathe (Figure 7.25).

Rate:

- Good if the abdomen does not droop, the client needs no help to elevate the knees with a duration of 3 breaths and with no complaint of wrist irritation.

- Fair if the client cannot hold the knees elevated for 2 breaths. Then substitute the Low Axis version with the forearms on the mat to begin.

- Poor if the client cannot elevate at all.

Full plank

Full plank position begins in the quadruped and walks out to extended legs. Check here for side shifts, shoulder and head droop, pelvic rotation and Achilles tendon girth, texture and length.

Rate:

- Good if a high axis version lasts 5 breaths, the thorax is in line with the pelvis, little pelvic rotation, with neutral hip extension and the distance between the legs is 1.5 in (3 cm) with the toes in extension.

- Fair if there is an evident shift laterally, the legs are disorganized, the shoulder girdle and/or head is sagging.

- Poor if the plank lasts only 1–2 seconds.

Leg Pull Front

Progressions begin with the classic PM mat exercise performed with audible 2-count sniff inhalations through the nose and audible 2-count ha-ha exhalation with each leg exchange (sniff-sniff/ha-ha).

Check here for uneven shifts of weight, uneven leg lift heights, externally rotating legs, drifting leg lifts to either side.

See the photo progression (Figure 7.26) from full plank to leg kicks to the Down Dog variations in the next section.

Rate:

- Good if the plank height is maintained through 5 sets (one set equals one alternation of right and left leg kick) with good form.

- Fair if the plank begins to sag and form is lost after 4 sets.

- Poor if the plank sags with only 2 sets.

Down Dog: three variations

These versions are the most advanced, yet offer most benefit, moving repeatedly into a plank on one leg with the shoulders moving in and out of shoulder flexion range as in an inversion.

Rate:

- Good if the plank occurs on one leg and moves between a horizontal plank and a Down Dog position with the elevated leg maintaining the torso line.

- Fair if the plank occurs with only one support leg but the motion between the plank and

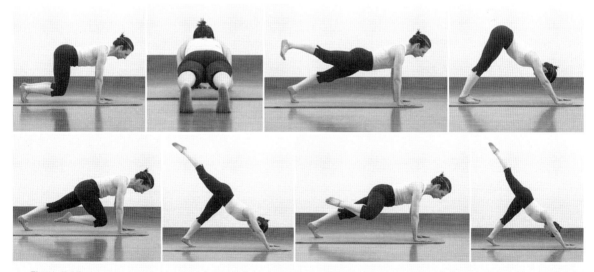

Figure 7.26

inversion is limited or the lifting leg is not above the horizon.

- Poor if the plank occurs with one support leg but the elevated leg touches back down to the floor quickly or the body quickly disorganizes without double leg support.

Side plank

Side plank finds its functional use in diminishing waddle from side to side in gait and evening pelvic listing in stance. Five versions progress through more advanced levels.

Double Z hip lift with Rainbow Arm

Sit upon one side of the pelvis with knees flexed, hips flexed and the tibias stacked upon each other. Lean onto one hand with a slight elbow bent. Exhale, then inhale and reach up onto a high axis arm, elevate the pelvis, and with a rainbow reach up to the ceiling, touch the mat farther past the support hand, keeping the spine flexed (Figure 7.27).

Rate:

- Good if the full rainbow sweep of the arm is achieved with the pelvic elevation.

- Fair if the top hand of the gesturing arm must assist the pelvic elevation.

- Poor if the client must rock onto the top hand and barely lift the pelvis up.

Side hip lift variations (Figure 7.28)

Full side hip lift: low axis

The low axis begins on the forearm. Lie on the easier side to lift first. Experiment to see which one. Place the elbow below the level of the shoulder toward the feet to protect the rotator cuff. Dorsiflex the ankles strongly. Line up the pelvis so that one side of the pelvis is over the other. Exhale, press down upon the fifth metatarsal and forearm. Elevate the pelvis until the lower hip is at least in neutral abduction. Slowly lower for 4 counts, stop before allowing all the body weight to contact the mat, then begin again for

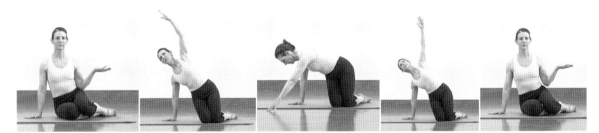

Figure 7.27

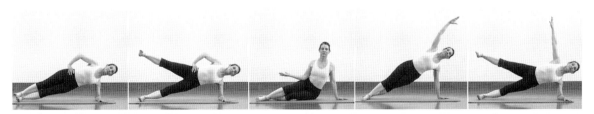

Figure 7.28

3 more repetitions. Check for the form points of: Hip Abduction Ability, Pelvic and Thoracic Rotation, and Shoulder Girdle Neutral (not protracted).

Rate:

- Good if the pelvis elevates up to a neutral body line with the top hand upon the pelvis for at least 2 repetitions.

- Fair if the client must lean forward onto the top hand to elevate the pelvis.

- Poor if the client must bend the knees and lean forward to lift the pelvis.

Full side hip lift: high axis in parens (side bend)

The high axis version with weight on the hand starts with one ankle crossed over the other. The support arm is now with weight upon the hand. Exhale. Straighten the legs. Come up onto the hand, placed underneath the ribcage. Elevate the pelvis, making an arc shape with the body. Hold for 3 breaths and lower. Check for the form points of: Hip Abduction Ability, Pelvic and Thoracic Rotation, and Shoulder Girdle Neutral (not protracted).

Rate:

- Good if the pelvis elevates and the feet do not slide away from the hand.

- Fair if the pelvis elevates slightly but the form points show rotation, and the pose cannot be held for one breath.

- Poor if the client attempts but then falls immediately before attaining the pose.

Static Star: low axis

The Static Star is an optimal goal. Go onto the easier side to lift. Fully dorsiflex the ankles. Exhale, press down upon the fifth metatarsal. Elevate the pelvis. Abduct the top shoulder. Check for the form points of: Hip Abduction Ability, Pelvic and Thoracic Rotation, and Shoulder Girdle Neutral (not protracted), ability to hold the ankle into dorsiflexion and eversion.

- Good if the form points are achieved for 4 breaths.

- Fair if the ankle lacks full dorsiflexion.

- Poor if balance is lost or if the top arm is abducted in a non-vertical position.

Shooting Star: low axis

Exhale. Elevate the pelvis and abduct the arm simultaneously for 4 counts, and lower back to the mat and return the arm to neutral for 4 counts.

Check for the form points of: Hip Abduction Ability, Pelvic and Thoracic Rotation, and Shoulder Girdle Neutral (not protracted), ability to hold the ankle into dorsiflexion and eversion.

Rate:

- Good if all the form points are met and the transition from down to up and down again are smooth.

- Fair if the form points are generally met, but the elevation is abrupt in an attempt to achieve the top position only.

- Poor if elevating and lowering appears too difficult on the shoulder.

Back plank

The back plank has two versions. It reveals pelvis rotational issues and shoulder girdle weakness and chest range issues. The dynamic version aids equality of stride in gait. Form points to observe are the distance between the feet, emphasis on pelvic elevation instead of back extension, the ability to hold a tricep dip position, and minimal pelvic shift off the center line in both static and dynamic versions.

Static back plank

Start in supine. Place the hands behind the torso. Roll the shoulders up and back. Lean back slightly. Bend the elbows with the fingers pointing toward the feet. Feel like an imaginary hand is holding the sacrum. Exhale. Posteriorly rotate the pelvis to elevate it. Breathe in and out for 10 breath cycles with the sniffy breaths (sniff-sniff/ha-ha). Check the form points of hips in neutral rotation, and that the pelvis is central between the legs and lined up with the thorax (Figure 7.29, left and center).

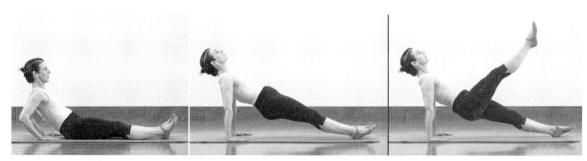

Figure 7.29

Rate:

- Good if the tricep dip pose, the pelvic elevation and the 10 breath cycles are achieved.

- Fair if the shoulders have trouble with the arm position and/or the pelvis is elevated very briefly for 4 breaths.

- Poor if the pelvis is unable to elevate. In this case, keep the pelvis on the mat and perform the breath cycles.

Leg Pull: a dynamic backwards plank

This exercise is the classic mat exercise. It is an excellent test of rotational stability and lateral sway. The emphasis in the dynamic version is not the height of the leg kick. Instead emphasize the bottom leg pushing into the mat and opening the legs away from one another. Check for width of leg excursion with movement.

Begin the same way as previously. After pelvic elevation, begin to alternate leg lifts using the sniffy breaths for 10 leg alternation sets, with right and left equaling one set (Figure 7.29).

Rate:

- Good if 10 alternation sets are completed with the breaths and pelvic elevation.

- Fair if only 5 sets are completed.

- Poor if the pelvis remains on the mat. Do complete the 10 breath cycles of sniffy breaths in this case as a modification.

Long sit with overhead dowel reach

The Long Sit is one of the most difficult positions for anyone to achieve. Its functional use is to develop a good pelvic foundation for sitting. It promotes both spine extension and hip dissociation. It reveals not only shoulder flexion range and hamstring length but also gluteal and back line fascial tightness. It is a great opportunity to experiment to see if a wedge sitting orthotic is appropriate for the client. Monitor if the client is leaning backwards and if the pelvis is upright. Observe any shift or list of the ribcage from the back. Inquire which hemi-pelvis seems lighter and then place a wedge diagonally between the ischial tuberosity and the GT to see if the client is more comfortable or appears more centered. This section may not be suitable for those with spinal fixation with hardware or disc herniation.

Sit on the mat with the hips flexed and knees as extended as possible. Reach up with a dowel. Stay sitting tall for 5 breath cycles (Figure 7.30).

Rate:

- Good if the knees are reasonably extended and the dowel is mostly vertical.

- Fair if the torso is overly flexed or the client is leaning backwards.

- Poor if the knees are very bent and the dowel is not upright.

Balancing 'O'

This exercise was inspired by hippotherapy, the use of therapeutic horseback riding for those with

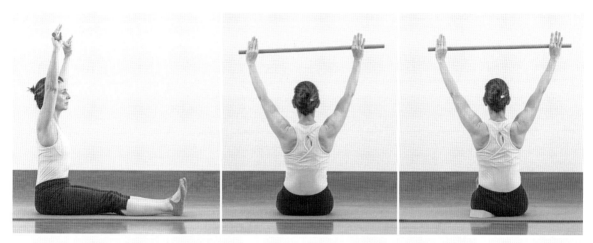

Figure 7.30

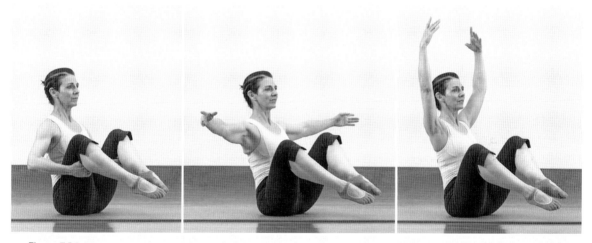

Figure 7.31

neurological issues. It uses spinal reflexes to stimulate the righting reflex. It dovetails with Pilates' notion of the balance point, activating multifidi as well as the psoas due to its leg position. This is one of the most beneficial exercises to promote functional sitting endurance, strength and spinal extension. It has two versions, one static and the other dynamic.

Sit on the mat. Flex the hips and knees and bring the great toes close to one another. Place the hands underneath the thighs and slide the hands along the backs

of the thighs toward the knees. Pull the elbows toward the back wall to help support the back and achieve more spine extension. Then slowly drag the toes toward the pelvis. Gently lean back. Elevate the feet off the floor and balance. Try to abduct the arms, then elevate the arms to a high 'O' position. Cue the client to breathe in, get tall and exhale, get taller for 3 breath cycles. Check to see if the head height lowers with the exhalation, if there is wobbling, a lack of confidence, a difference in arm height or any stiffness in the hips (Figure 7.31).

Rate:

- Good if the balance is achieved and 3 breath cycles are accomplished with the arms in a high 'O' position.

- Fair if the client is unable to balance in the high 'O'.

- Poor if the client must lean back upon the hands and assume only part of the leg position.

Dynamic balancing 'O'

This version promotes spinal extension endurance and the ability to counterbalance against the arm weight. The same exercise is performed as previously (Figure 7.31), then add the arms circling from the knees, upwards toward the high 'O' and then opening sidewards for each breath cycle. Coordinate the breath with breath in, lift from the front, exhale and circle out to the side. Monitor once again the ability to not drop the torso as the arms open sidewards and down.

Rate:

- Good if all 3 arm cycles are achieved with good spinal form.

- Fair if the cycles are mostly completed yet the spine still wobbles.

- Poor if there is a loss of balance out of the position.

Lateral rolling

Lateral rolling breaks up directional bias and promotes spinal articulation. There are two versions, the Baby Roll and the X-rolls. Lateral rolling replaces the sagittal rolling typical of traditional Pilates mat exercises.

Baby Rolls

Baby Rolls are a safe variation that most people can perform. Use a pillow or towel underneath the head if necessary; however, most youth do not require such assistance. The neck rotation is a critical element. Lie on one side. Flex the hips and hold onto each knee with the same-side hand. Begin to roll onto the back, opening one thigh, then the other. Delay the head movement as long as possible in the original position (Figure 7.32). Watch a demonstration of this exercise (Code 7.5).

Rate:

- Good if the hand remains on the knees throughout the exercise, the head delays and a smooth motion occurs.

- Fair if the hands lose grip on the knees and the spine stiffness is apparent creating a choppy motion.

- Poor if momentum is abrupt and the spine is unable to imprint.

X-rolls

X-rolls (Code 7.6) require more coordination and reveal greater discrepancies in regions of the spine making smooth transitions with one another. They show organizational difficulties across the body integrating top with bottom, establishing diagonal pathways

Code 7.5 (free code)
Baby Rolls exercise

Code 7.6 (free code)
X-rolls exercise

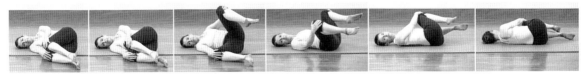

Figure 7.32

through the body. They promote internal fascial resiliency. Intended for youth, adults will benefit if the spine is deemed safe for such mobility. It may take time to acquire. The Arc fascial stretches in Chapter 9 (see Figure 9.2) facilitate the lateral rolling action with the position with the side of the pelvis at the height of the Arc.

- Lie in supine in an X position with the legs past hip width and arms behind the head on the mat past shoulder width. Use the right leg as a leader leg. Begin to lift the right leg across the left. Feel the reach between the right foot and the right hand as is crosses the body (Figure 7.33, top row).

- Continue pulling with the right leg until rolling over onto the front of the body. Reverse the action. Reach the right foot across and behind the left on the mat. Feel the pull of the right foot against the right hand that remains on the mat. Allow the right foot and leg to drag the torso back to the X supine position, rippling the spine smoothly back to the position. Repeat with the left leg leading.

- Now begin the upper body, leading with the right hand (Figure 7.33, bottom row). Touch the right hand to the sternum, then reach to the left hand. Stay and feel the reach between the right hand and right foot that has remained in the X position. Then allow the right arm and shoulder to continue reaching the body onto the front.

- Settle the body into a comfortable X. Reverse the action by reaching the right hand back toward the right pelvis, then move the whole right shoulder behind the torso, and trace the right hand back to the upward position of the supine

X. Repeat with the left hand leading, moving from the chest to the other hand, pulling over to the abdomen.

- Then reverse by reaching the hand back, then the shoulder and re-trace the path up to the X. Check the forms points for stiffness, choppiness, especially with the arms leading into the backwards motion. This is an awkward moment. Allow the client to move slowly until this motion is more familiar.

Rate:

- Good if able to smoothly perform the X-rolls with either the legs or the arms leading the exercise.

- Fair if able to perform the X-rolls with the legs but the rolls with the arms leading are difficult or the foot pushes the body over instead of allowing the arms to pull the body into the cross action.

- Poor if the arms feel too stiff or the spine feels too uncomfortable to perform the action. In this case, refer to Chapter 9 and perform Arc fascial stretching instead (see Figure 9.2).

Lunges

Lunges help functional gait. Systematically assessing the ease of holding one hip in deep flexion, the ability to keep a uniform distance of 1st parallel (2.5 in/5 cm between the legs), keeping the legs in neutral rotation, the ankles in comparable dorsiflexion, and progressing to rotational range in the lunge are valuable form points.

Start in quadruped to standardize the distance between the legs, observe the difficulty to posteriorly

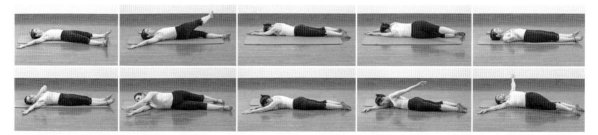

Figure 7.33

rotate the pelvis to flex the hip and proceed to the lunge with upper body rotation (Figure 7.34). Use a mirror for good feedback for the client's form.

- Step 1. Establish the quadruped position of the 2.5-in (5-cm) distance between the legs in a neutral pelvic 90° hip flexion. Position the shoulders so that the face is in front of a line made from hand to hand.

- Step 2. Right hip flexion with the left knee remaining on the mat. Notice the difficulty of the posterior pelvic rotation to accomplish the move.

- Step 3. Extend the back leg into hip and knee extension. Check the ability of both. Note the stiff one. Does the leg rotate or cross the mid-line to reach backwards?

- Step 4. Bend the right elbow, imagine pulling a thread toward the ceiling and try to straighten the arm. Note the verticality.

- Step 5. Bend the left elbow, point it toward the ceiling and try to straighten the arm. Note the verticality. Which side is more limited?

Rate each step:

- Step 1:

  ○ Good if the distance between the knees is equal about 5 cm apart, the pelvis is neutral and the head is forward in front of the hands. Other traditional form points apply here.

  ○ Fair if the pelvis remains in posterior rotation and the legs, torso or shoulders are disorganized.

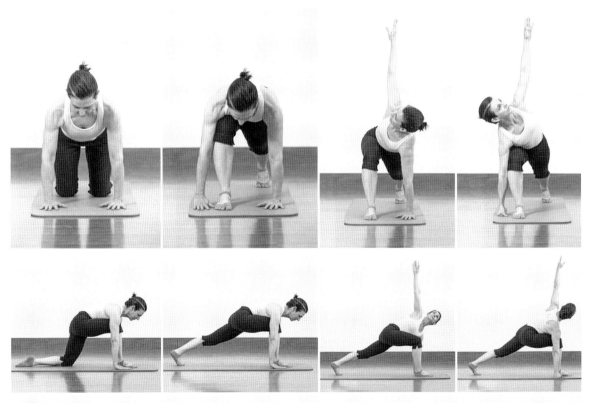

Figure 7.34

○ Poor if the above applies even after correction of position.

- Step 2:

  ○ Good if the hip flexion was smooth and the distance between the legs remained steady.

  ○ Fair if the hip flexion was abrupt or the foot had to swing out to the side to move forward.

  ○ Poor if the hands had to leave the floor and the torso reach up into a kneeling position to move the leg.

- Step 3:

  ○ Good if the back leg is not rotated, the hip is extended, fairly level with the other hip, with the knee fully extended.

  ○ Fair if the hip and knee are slightly bent.

  ○ Poor if the hip and knee cannot extend and the back leg must rotate to accommodate the position.

- Step 4:

  ○ Good if balance is mostly maintained with no substantial pelvic lateral shift, and the arm is more or less vertical.

  ○ Fair if balance is challenged perceived by a pelvic shift or bracing of the supporting hand on the front leg.

  ○ Poor if a full loss of balance occurs, or the arm is only slightly beyond the horizon.

- Step 5:

  ○ Good if the left elbow is about ten o'clock, the shoulders are rotated so that most of the chest is facing the side wall and the opposite hand can reach the mat.

  ○ Fair if the left elbow is more horizontal than vertical, the chest is more halfway between facing down and to the side wall and the opposite hand needs a block for support.

  ○ Poor if the left elbow is almost horizontal, the chest is facing mostly down and the hand needs a chair for support.

Squat to inversion to roll up

This series promotes discovery of the hollow above the pubic bone, that is, to pull up and create a deep lower abdominal connection to the center of gravity in the pelvis (Figure 7.35, Code 7.7). Functionally, its use is a connection to the ability to balance with the head down, move from supine to standing, promoting a balanced plumb line stance as well as balance in functional reach to lift and lower objects, such as out of a high cabinet. In a simpler

Code 7.7 (free code)
Squat to roll up training

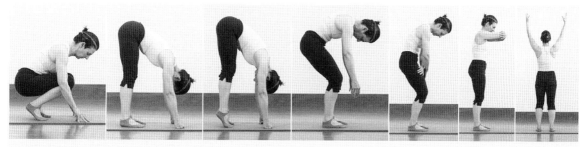

Figure 7.35

explanation, mortality correlates to the lifelong ability to get up from the floor to a standing position (Klima et al., 2016). If possible, train adults in this skill. Chapter 12 uses the Trapeze Table for a similar version.

- Step 1. Start standing in the 1st parallel position. Flex the spine and reach the hands to the floor as the hips and knees flex. If the hamstrings are too short to reach the hands to the floor, modify the reach to the floor with a Box.

- Step 2. Squat. Flex the hips and knees with the coccyx coming down toward the heels – the coccyx to heel connection. Note any discrepancy in heel height. The heel higher from the floor indicates a tight Achilles tendon.

- Step 3. Invert the position by straightening the legs as much as possible. Spot the client for balance by holding the pelvis with duck hands. Cue the client to elevate the heels. Note if the upper body or lower body are in line with each other. Note shifts from the sagittal line, such as the pelvis being to the right of the ribcage.

- Step 4. Cue the hollow above the pubic bone to elevate toward the ceiling. Hold the hollow as the heels lower. Note if one side of the abdominals is bulging toward the floor, and if both heels elevate at the same height.

- Step 5. Cue the head to be heavy, tailbone heavy. Then guide the client to roll up the spine smoothly, one vertebra at a time. Note if the coccyx points down in between the ankles at the mid-foot or toward the heels. Check for loss of balance.

- Step 6. Cross the hands across the thighs and end with the arms elevated. Note if the mid-ribcage lines up with the mid-pelvis from the side.

Rate each step. Rate this sequence for more motion ability rather than side-to-side discrepancies. The asymmetry cues will train out the sides.

- Step 1:
  - Good if the spine is able to move sequentially with abdominal support, and the hands are within several inches (cm) from the floor.
  - Fair if the motion is initiated from the pelvis with no spinal motion.
  - Poor if reaching to the floor is with more gravitational momentum than control, with little pelvic motion, or the hands only reach to the height of the Long Box.

- Step 2:
  - Good if the coccyx is reasonably close to the heels and the heels are within several inches (cm) from the floor.
  - Fair if the fingertips only touch the floor, the back is flat, and the heels are elevated.
  - Poor if the hips do not flex, the trunk is more vertical, and the heels are substantially high from the ground.

- Step 3:
  - Good if inversion balance is achieved, and the face plane is parallel to the floor. Moderately bent knees are allowed.
  - Fair if the balance is shifted to one side, leaning and with one knee bending more than the other.
  - Poor if the head attempts to remain vertical, the fingers are on the Box and only the heels lift, not the pelvis.

- Step 4:
  - Good if comfortable in this position.
  - Fair if there is a loss of balance forward.
  - Poor if there is a request to get out of the position.

- Step 5:
  - Good if a smooth transition through the flexing spine occurs.
  - Fair if an initial spine extension occurs but can change to a flexion when guided.
  - Poor if there is an attempt to extend the spine and initiate becoming vertical by extending the spine instead of rolling up through the flexion.

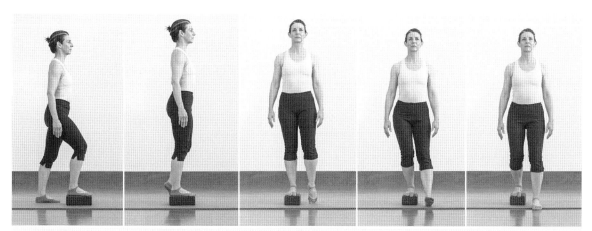

Figure 7.36

- Step 6:

  - Good if the final position has the mid-ribcage lined up with the pelvis.

  - Fair if the ribcage ends in front of the pelvis.

  - Poor if the ribcage ends up behind the pelvis at the end.

Step Down

The Step Down (Figure 7.36) gives good information about directional bias overuse due to pelvic sway and hip hike in walking, running and jumping. Improved function here helps correct leg malalignment, which often leads to athletic injuries.

- Step 1. The client stands with one foot on a yoga block or tall book. The other foot is placed to the side in back.

- Step 2. Cue the client to step onto the block and then keeping the support foot on the block, step down in front with the free leg. Do this several times.

Note the shift of the pelvis with the reach down from the block for knee to mid-pant line alignment, and for hip hike.

Rate the step-down portion:

- Good if there is little pelvic sway, the ribcage remains fairly vertical and the second toe,

patella and mid-pant line are lined up vertically. Some lateral excursion is expected.

- Fair if the hip elevates on the step down, the knee drifts toward the mid-line or the chest tilts forward.

- Poor if there is significant hip hike with the knee moving toward or past the mid-line or the chest tilt is excessive.

Bibliography

Barnes, J. F. (1990). Visual standing analysis, body language. In: Barnes, J.F., P.T. Myofascial Release: The Search for Excellence. A Comprehensive Evaluatory and Treatment Approach. Paoli, Pennsylvania: Rehabilitation Services, Inc., pp. 37–50

Beauséjour, M., Goulet, L. Parent, S. et al. (2013). The effectiveness of scoliosis screening programs: methods for systematic review and expert panel recommendations formulation. Scoliosis, 8: 12. doi:10.1186/1748-7161-8-12

Bellemare, F., Jeanneret, A., Couture, J. (2003). Sex differences in thoracic dimensions and configuration. American Journal of Respiratory and Critical Care Medicine, 168: 3. doi:10.1164/rccm.200208-876OC

Boyle, K.L. (2013). Clinical application of the right sidelying respiratory left adductor pull back exercise. International Journal of Sports Physical Therapy, 8(3), 349–358

Bunnel, W. P. (1993). Outcome of spinal screening. Spine, 18(12), 1572–1580

Carey, D.P., Hutchinson, C.V. (2013). Looking at eye dominance from a different angle: is sighting strength related to hand preference? Cortex, 49(9), 2542–2552

Chaitow, L. (2012). Breathing pattern disorders and lumbopelvic pain and dysfunction: an update. Retrieved

August 14, 2018, from leonchaitow.com: http://leonchaitow.com/2012/01/23/breathing-pattern-disorders-and-lumbopelvic-pain-and-dysfunction-an-update/

Chowanska, J., Kotwicki, T., Rosadzinski, K., Sliwinski, Z. (2012). School screening for scoliosis: can surface topography replace examination with scoliometer? Scoliosis, 7: 9. doi:10.1186/1748-7161-7-9

DeNooijer, J.A., Willems, R.M. (2016). What can we learn about cognition from studying handedness? Insights from cognitive science. In: Loffing, F., Hagemann, N., Strauss, B., MacMahon, C. eds. Laterality in Sports. London: Elsevier, pp. 135–150

Jaroszewski, D., Notrica, D., McMahon, L., et al. (2010). Current management of pectus excavatum: a review and update of therapy and treatment recommendations. Journal Board of American Family Medicine, 23(2), 230–239

Kendall, F.P., McCreary, E.K., Provance, P. G. eds. (1993). Muscles: Testing and Function, 4th edn. Baltimore: Williams and Wilkins

Kinikli, G.I., Yuksel, I., Yakut, Y., et al.(2011). Of postural sway in adolescent idiopathic scoliosis. Fizyoterapi Rehabilitasyon, 22(1), 17–22. Retrieved November 16, 2017, from https://www.researchgate.net/publication/287321981_Alterations_of_postural_sway_in_adolescent_idiopathic_scoliosis

Klima, D.W., Anderson, C., Sarah, D., et al. (2016). Standing from the floor in community-dwelling older adults. Human Kinetics Journal, 24(2), 207–213

Knight, I., MacCormick, M., Bird, H. (2012). Managing Joint Hypermobility – A Guide for Dance Teachers. London: Southwest Music School

Lee, D. (1999). The Pelvic Girdle, Vol. 1. Toronto: Churchill Livingstone

Magee, D. (2016). Orthopedic Physical Assessment, 6th edn. St Louis: Elsevier

Mitchell, F. (2002). Relevant gross anatomy of the trunk, evaluation and treatment of the thorax and lumbar spine. In: Mitchell, F., Mitchell, P. K., eds. The Muscle Energy Manual, Vol. 2. Lansing: MET Press, pp. 2–12, 173–217

O'Sullivan P.B., Beales, D.J. (2007). Diagnosis and classification of pelvic girdle pain disorders –Part 1: A mechanism based approach within a biopsychosocial framework. Manual Therapy, 12(2), 86–97

Rakhimov, A. (2018). Ideal breathing pattern: 3 breaths/min for maximum body oxygen. Retrieved August 14, 2018, from: www.normalbreathing.com: http://www.normalbreathing.com/patterns-ideal-breathing.php

Sahrman, S. (2002). Diagnosis and Treatment of Movement Impairment Syndromes. St Louis: Mosby

Schleifer, L.M., Ley, R., Spalding, T.W. (2002). A hyperventilation theory of job stress and musculoskeletal disorders. American Journal of Industrial Medicine, 41(5): 420–432

Thomas, M., McKinley, R.K., Freeman, E., Foy, C. (2001). Prevalence of dysfunctional breathing in patients treated for asthma in primary care: cross sectional survey. British Medical Journal, 322, 1098–2102

Weinstein, S.L., Dolan, L.A. Spratt, K.F. (2003). Health and function of patients with untreated idiopathic scoliosis. A 50-year natural history study. JAMA, 289(5), 559–567

Laying the foundation: initial education, organization, coordination

Initial education: somatics

Be sure your client is ready to begin an exercise program. Not all clients are in distress, yet some will be. Many young clients do not necessarily experience pain outside of brace use.

Be prudent. Use the entire Scoliosis Team to coordinate proper care. Clients who wear a brace to stem progression are best to not wear the brace during exercise such as the Pilates Method. Consult the medical team if there are questions.

Start by teaching breathing and the basic neurodevelopmental sequence (NS, introduced in Ch. 6) to position internal organization. Next, implement the individual asymmetry cues in the NS positions using the wedge. Then train the client in their profile functional correctives from the SSPOT-1 or -2. See Chapter 12 on more programming for individuals.

Controversy exists about the safety of 'core' exercises. It is the responsibility, and liability, of all PMMEs to ensure the safety and efficacy of all exercises. Beginning in a strong sense of neutral and expanding from there ensures a positive experience.

Lay the foundation to foster body awareness, and begin acquisition of life skills of asymmetry, the Body Skills necessary for the lifelong management of spinal asymmetry.

Note

The following chapters contain symbols to guide appropriateness according to Cobb angle severity and for those who have undergone internal spinal fixation. The exercises and methods in this chapter are intended for all clients who are at least four months' postoperative or who have not had any surgery, with a few exceptions.

Degree guidelines for severity of the Cobb angle

A = 0–10° Normal expected degree of spinal asymmetry

B = 10–20° Mild

C = 21–40° Moderate

D = >40° Severe

E = >70° Severe with possible medical breathing issues.

Use extra precaution with any operative clients that either have or do not have spinal or other hardware due to joint replacements.

☑ indicates the exercise is appropriate for either those with spinal fixation or who have not had any surgery. ⚠ indicates the exercise is not appropriate for those with spinal fixation.

Initial body organization

Functional breathing

Initiate total body organization with the art of breathing. Breathing is especially important in the management of spinal asymmetry due to its impact upon intrathoracic and intra-abdominal pressure, along with deep fascial structures.

Joseph Pilates identified breathing as the key to heart control and recommended the recumbent, lying down position of the mat environment as beneficial to reduce strain in visceral organs.

Physiologically, below a Cobb angle of 70°, scoliosis produces no signs and symptoms of respiratory problems. Ninety degrees is associated with lung failure. Larger Cobb angles, greater than 40°, are associated with the development of restrictive lung disease, yet the most significant issue is one of breathing dysfunctions and subsequent muscular deconditioning in even mild to moderate levels of scoliosis.

Torsion of the diaphragm makes the work of breathing more difficult. The intrathoracic pressure increases due to the inefficiency of the diaphragm around T8, which affects the Zone of Apposition (ZOA).

The ZOA is the functional area of respiratory diaphragm excursion from T8–L1. Whether the primary is on the right or the left does not make a difference.

The key to laying the initial foundation lies in the understanding of the fascial anatomy of the deep trunk, the ZOA and the Inner Envelope, and its biomechanical use in functional breathing.

Fascial anatomy of the ZOA and Inner Envelope

The ZOA is the cylindrical aspect of the diaphragm that touches the lower mediastinal wall, the floor of the space between the lungs that houses the heart. It accounts for most of the surface area of the ribcage. The mediastinal organs are encapsulated with a double layer of fascia. Their fascial aspects connect, called communication, with the respiratory diaphragm. The region of the ZOA extends from the lower end of the diaphragm insertion at the costal (rib) margin and extends toward the head to the costophrenic angle, the area of the diaphragm which meets the ribcage and connects to the phrenic nerve to drive breathing. Here the diaphragmatic fibers break away from the rib cage to create the diaphragm dome. The ZOA depends upon the orientation of the ribcage rather than the height of the dome: this is why scoliosis in the thoracic region has a big effect on breathing and the function of the ZOA. The top of the ZOA is generally located near T8, usually at the apex of a normal thoracic kyphosis.

The abdominal and oblique muscles control the ZOA as they direct the diaphragm tension. Diaphragm tension dysfunctions, such as accessory muscle overuse, the use of the scalenes and neck ring of the thoracic outlet and shoulders as the primary breath driver instead of giving a greater role to the respiratory diaphragm, are not desirable.

Chest wall stiffness including rib mobility issues associated with scoliosis, and lung hyperinflation (not exhaling fully), are diaphragmatic functions that affect the normal rest position of the ZOA, which occurs at the end of exhalation. Pilates advocated squeezing out every atom of air!

Optimizing the ZOA and spinal asymmetry

Optimization of the ZOA (Figure 8.1), the Upper Core, works in conjunction with the Inner Envelope, a part of the Pelvic Core. Connect the two into one comprehensive teaching. The ZOA is compromised in multiple ways due to sustained sitting in slumped or flexed spinal postures. Mechanical effects include lessening of rib mobility and thoracic mobility, and continue down into the pelvis through the fascial Inner Envelope, along with unfavorably altered breathing patterns. The Inner Envelope describes a web of support, the myofascial 'inner stocking' that encases the prevertebral (in front of the vertebra) and intrapelvic myofascial connections. These connections communicate, connecting the pelvic floor with the diaphragm (see Figure 8.2).

The medial arcuate ligament proceeds from the superior psoas fascia. This is the upper scaffolding of the quadratus lumborum where the diaphragm also connects.

Notice the right and left *crurae* (plural Latin for singular *crus*) of the diaphragm that attaches to the spine. See how they form a loop over the openings of the esophagus and aorta. Notice how the crurae are asymmetrical. This asymmetry accounts for the rotary breathing action described by van Loon (van Loon, 2012). The crurae along with their fascia overlap the psoas, blend into the psoas musculature and then finally blend with the anterior longitudinal ligament running on the front of the vertebrae.

Notice how the descending psoas has lower medial fascia that thickens at its lowest portion and blends into the pelvic floor. The conjoint tendon is where the medial fibers of the internal oblique aponeurosis, the large sheet of fascia, unite with the deeper fibers of

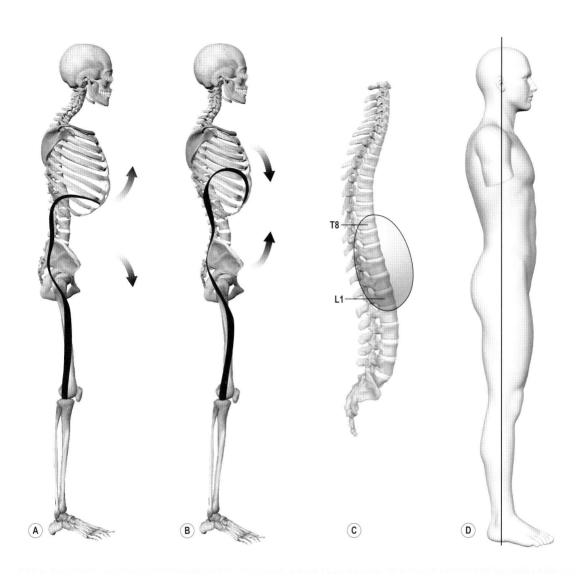

Figure 8.1
Optimal and non-optimal ZOA.

the transversus abdominis aponeurosis. The fascia of the posterior fibers of the psoas attach firmly to the pelvic brim as they pass over the brim to finally insert into the lesser trochanter of the femur, where the iliopsoas complex inserts. As the muscle fibers of the psoas and associated fascial fibers move over the pelvic brim, they connect into the intricate structure of the pelvic floor, especially in the pubococcygeus region (pubic symphysis to tailbone) (Chaitow, 2012). The posterior portion of the psoas is innervated by ventral (front) connections (rami) to spinal nerves T12–L4 supplying the waist, yet the anterior muscle fibers are innervated by branches of the femoral nerve (L2–4), giving a nerve connection to the hip adductors (Gibbons et al., 2002). This means the psoas exerts influence on both the spine and the legs.

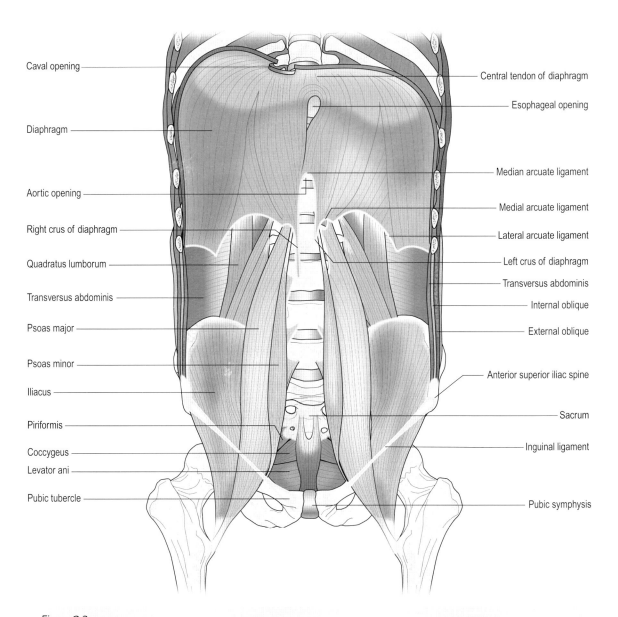

Figure 8.2
The Inner Envelope is made up of the deep fascia extending from the respiratory diaphragm and extending throughout the pelvic diaphragm.

The positive and negative biomechanical effects of the combined postural anatomy of the Upper Core of the ZOA coordinate with the Pelvic Core of the Inner Envelope.

Combining the Upper Core and Inner Envelope theme of torso malalignment is Janda's description of dysfunctional posture, the inability of a structure or physiological system to perform its job, often manifesting in the body through reflexive compensations. These compensations result in disorganization and imbalances of the body called 'upper and lower crossed syndromes' depicted in the sagittal plane (see Figure 8.1B and refer to Figure 4.8).

Simply stated, Janda's Upper Crossed Syndrome reflects the sunken chest issue of tight pectorals interacting with tight upper trapezius and levator scapula creating a pull down on the lower anterior chest, specifically impeding the efficiency of the ZOA. The cross pattern then continues into a forward head pattern where the deep neck flexors on the anterior cervical area are weakened along with the lower trapezius and serratus anterior in the posterior ribcage area.

Janda's Lower Crossed Syndrome reflects either a forward dumping pelvis or a posteriorly rotated, 'tucked,' pelvis. The first pelvic model, the Anterior Pelvic Crossed Syndrome, reflects an issue of tight iliopsoas use interacting with tight erector spinae, specifically impairing the delicate fascial structure of the Inner Envelope. This pattern relays a compressive force in the lumbar spine region and in turn weakens the gluteus maximus along with the anterior abdominal wall.

The Posterior Pelvic Crossed Syndrome is characterized by imbalanced coactivation of the trunk muscles with the more dominant work observed in the extensors, coactivation increased activity in the upper abdominal wall, piriformis and hamstrings combined with lower activity of the lower abdominals, deep hip flexors and low back extensors (Page, 2011; Williams, 2011).

An extrapolation of Janda's crossed syndromes is a subset of the Lower Crossed Syndrome, the Lower Pelvic Unit (LPU), considered a subgroup of crossed pelvic syndromes exerting influence on the functioning of the deep Inner Envelope.

The pelvic ring, the three bones, the three joints, and the four layers of the pelvic floor along with the fascial slings comprise the all-important connection of the spine to the legs. The sacrum–coccyx complex has the double role of serving the spine as well as the two side bones, the ilia.

Inclusion of obturators, iliacus, psoas, and all their interconnecting fascial sheaths provides structure and many functional roles by means of a fascial stocking, the Inner Envelope. Among its roles is to provide deep anterior support to the lower half of the spinal column, and along with the spinal intrinsics, such as multifidi, intertransversarii and rotatores, it contributes to lumbopelvic control. In addition, it contributes to generation of intra-abdominal pressure (IAP), necessary for unloading spinal elements.

The IAP unloads the spine in two ways: directly by pressing upwards on the rib cage via the diaphragm and indirectly by generating an extensor moment on the lumbar spine that decreases the back-muscle activities that compress spinal elements. In this way, the influence of the LPU promotes maintenance of continence, and optimal respiration (Key, 2010; Arjmand & Shirazi-Adl, 2006).

Summary

Evidence shows the ZOA and Inner Envelope are important in spinal and pelvic health and function. Attention to the sagittal postural imbalances of the spine are just as important as attending to the lateral curvature patterns in optimizing internal fascial organization. Connecting the Upper and Pelvic Core/Inner Envelope areas is beneficial in optimizing functional breathing. Address the basic sagittal issues of the client in general, such as sway back or pelvic weakness, while still attending to the lateral curves prominent in asymmetrical spines. Your correctives and education here optimize the client's breathing and can influence leg length, back pain, and spine stability in functional activities.

Turn science into art

Turning science into art uses a teaching method of *thinking* rather than *doing* to produce measurable and consistent changes in the relative position of skeletal parts. The theme of imagine, think and feel helps to find the connection between the upper core and the pelvic core once described by dance alignment expert Professor Lulu Sweigard as, "the most important for balance of the central skeletal structures and for freedom of movement of the lower extremities" (Sweigard, 1974).

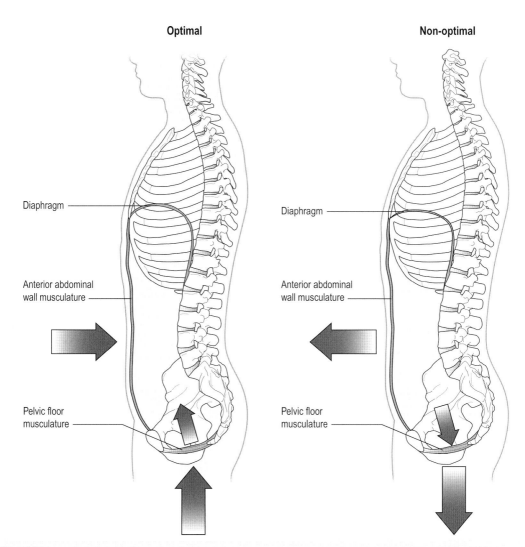

Figure 8.3
Optimizing the ZOA allows optimization of intra-abdominal pressure, which then allows the pelvic diaphragm, part of the Inner Envelope, to assume optimal function.

Aligning the ZOA and Inner Envelope

Exercise

☑ *Standing ZOA cues: A–E*

- Stand with your feet about 3–4 in (8–10 cm) apart. Point the toes forward. Let the arms hang freely downward.

- Imagine an X inside the body in the mid-line sagittal plane. One line extends from the lower end of the sternum to the front edge of the sacral promontory, the flat part of the top of the sacrum. The other line extends deep within the body underneath viscera from the front of the 12th vertebra to the inside of the pubic symphysis.

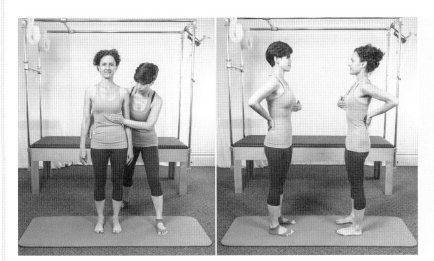

Figure 8.4

- Imagine the 4 diaphragms (horizontal cranial at the eye level, thoracic ring inside of the clavicles, respiratory diaphragm ring, and pelvic floor diaphragm) as parachutes floating and billowing with every breath.

- Think of these lines closing from an X-shape to one vertical line that lines up with the imaginary central axis of the trunk.

- Feel the breath and motion of the diaphragms within the shape. Breathe in for 4 counts and out for 4 counts a number of times. Shake out. Relax and then repeat the exercise twice more.

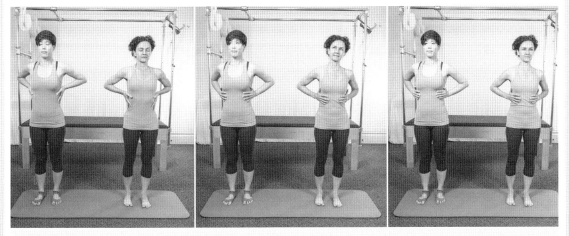

Figure 8.5
Use the movement acquisition strategy of imagine, think, feel (left to right): imagining the lines, thinking about the anatomy, to feel the ZOA.

Exercise

☑ *The Pelvic Spool: A–E*

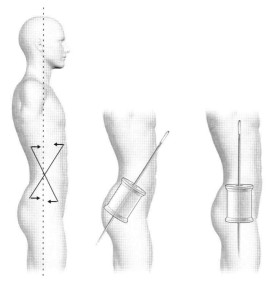

Figure 8.6
The Pelvic Spool. Use the image of a needle inside of a spool to align the ribcage with the pelvis.

- While still standing in the neutral stance, imagine the pelvis is a large spool of thread with a needle through the central opening.

- Imagine the spool is tipped so that the top of the needle is forward and in front of the body while the bottom of the needle is back behind and below the level of the pelvis, outside of the body.

- Think of the needle moving so that the needle now aligns with the imaginary central axis of the trunk.

- Imagine the 4 diaphragms (horizontal cranial at the eye level, thoracic ring inside of the clavicles, respiratory diaphragm ring, and pelvic floor diaphragm) as parachutes floating and billowing with every breath.

- Feel the breath and motion of the diaphragms within the shape. Breathe in for 4 counts and out for 4 counts a number of times. Shake out. Relax and then repeat the exercise twice more.

Exercise

☑ *Breath of Fire: A–E*

Watch the video via Code 8.1 for a demonstration.

- Sit on a chair with the sit bones toward the front of the seat.

- Inhale into the sides of the ribs for 4 counts. Exhale for 4 counts.

- Perform one percussive exhalation, a strong outward breath through the nostrils with closed lips. Hold for 4 counts. Feel like the area between the navel and pubis are wringing out a wet washcloth.

- Then exhale from this region repeatedly, and strongly for 20 more repetitions. Keep the lips closed throughout the exercise.
- Repeat twice more

Code 8.1 (free code)
Breath of Fire exercise

Exercise

☑ *Balloon Breathing into the torso: A–E*

Code 8.2 (free code)
Balloon Breathing exercise

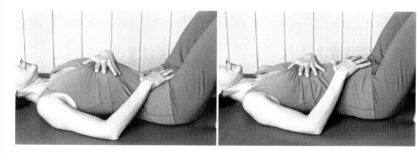

Figure 8.7

This exercise is not only an internal fascial influencer, increasing breath excursion, it is also a pain reliever. In addition, it stimulates the parasympathetic system, the opposite of the fight or flight response to distress. Think of the mantra: rest, digest, and heal.

- Lie on your back with your feet about hip-width apart. Knees are bent with the soles of the feet on the mat.
- Place one hand upon your breastbone with the thumb between the breasts; place the other hand on the abdomen with the thumb upon the navel.
- Inhale slowly and smoothly through your nose. Allow your nostrils to gently flare out. Inflate the ribcage and let the air move up and into the jaw and eyes. Expand the ribs sideways, allowing the breastbone to elevate for a slow luxuriant breath.
- Exhale through your mouth. Make a gentle 'ha' sound at the back of your throat.

Continued

- Allow the abdomen to fill, and gently distend, rising toward the ceiling to allow the pelvic floor to relax.

- Keep the low back touching the floor or mat.

- This action completes one cycle. Perform at least 5 cycles of this exercise. More cycles are beneficial and provide a meditative experience.

Bring art into science by imagining that your spine is a flexible old-fashioned mercury thermometer. As you inhale and inflate the ribcage, see the metallic silver move up toward the base of the skull at your hairline and then flow all the way down to your tailbone as you exhale to distend the abdomen.

- Imagine also that the vertebrae are making little ripples as the mercury moves up and down the spine.

- Imagine the pull and traction along the back of your body. As you inhale and move the mercury up the spine, feel like your hair could almost slide along the floor, elongating the top of the spine. As the mercury flows down the spine, gently rippling the vertebrae down toward your legs, feel as if there's almost a gentle tug of your pants toward your heels.

Exercise

☑ *Counting to 15 during exhalation: A–E*

After strengthening the diaphragm and increasing fascial excursion in the ZOA, focus on longer and deeper exhalations. Dysfunctional breathing, such as hyperventilation, focuses on many inhalations. Counting the exhalations in 1 minute, then attempting to lower the number of exhalations in 1 minute takes practice. Aim for 9 respiration cycles in 1 minute.

Neurodevelopmental positions

The acquisition of the neurodevelopmental positions, an initial Body Skill, is critical training for this population. The ultimate goal is for the client to learn how to position themselves in any exercise model, not just the Pilates Method, and also to better understand how to find a neutral (strong) back in any position.

Once the client is familiar, adding the Activ-Wedge® then begins the use of the scoliosis cues for the individual. Begin the positions without the wedge first, then add the wedge according to the client's needs in that position.

Watch the video to view the Activ-Wedge® (Code 8.3).

Code 8.3 (free code)
Activ-Wedge® use

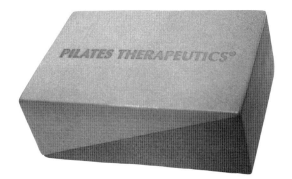

Figure 8.8

Exercise

⚡ *Supine: A–D*

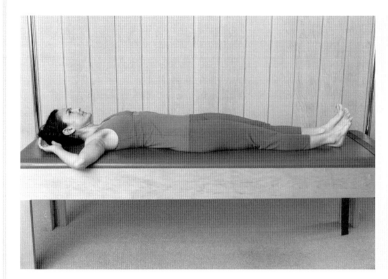

Figure 8.9

A main characteristic of the asymmetrical spine is lack of spinal erectness.

Although seemingly simple, Supine trains optimal erect standing posture. The back of the head, the back of the rib-cage, the back of the pelvis, the back of the thighs and the calves should all lie heavily into the mat. There is a small low back curve, yet not very pronounced.

The front of the neck is too tight if the chin juts upwards, or the top back neck is too tight (either in fascia or muscles). If the ribcage is accentuated off the mat, the lower posterior ribcage is too tight (either in fascia or muscles). If the posterior thighs lift and tilt toward the torso, the anterior hips are too tight (either in fascia or hip flexors muscles).

Note

When using the Activ-Wedge®, place one perpendicularly underneath the ribcage concavity. Place another perpendicularly underneath the side of the pelvis that is lighter on the mat between the levels of the greater trochanter and ischial tuberosities. Please note the Activ-Wedge® is not intended for general use in the Supine position with clients after spinal fixation surgery.

Exercise

⚡ Sidelying: A–D

When lying on the side, brace with the lower arm to lift the upper ribs at the chest level away from the mat. Point the lower elbow to the front. Create ample space between the waist and the mat. Attempt to get the high ribs at chest level off the mat. The pelvis is neutral, with strong hip extension. The bottom leg floats off the ground just a bit to emulate the legs in stance. If there is discomfort on the side of the bottom pelvis, use padding.

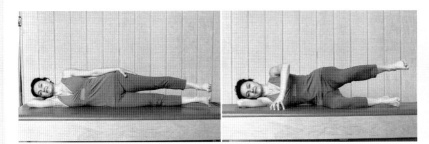

Figure 8.10

Do not endure pain here. If there is neck discomfort, usually due to weakness, bend the bottom elbow, and point it forward, using the hand to actually hold the head weight.

This position benefits the deep abdominal wall musculature. The transverse abdominals (TA) are the most length-ened in the sidelying position due to the orientation of the fibers. This position reveals rotary imbalance and is also very informative for the participant to note discrepancies in the waist lines.

Note

When using the Activ-Wedge®, place one underneath the convex side first to help the client learn how to move away from it. Then go to the next side to show how the sides differ.

Exercise

✓ Sitting: A–E

The model in the lower photograph (Fig. 8.11) shows how a lateral curvature can be straightened out with an Activ-Wedge® or small prop like a small book. Place it under the heavier side as perceived by the client.

The prop is placed on a diagonal between the ischial tuberosity (IT) and the greater trochanter. However, clients that have spinal fixation rods and fusions often find placing the prop underneath the lighter side is more comfortable on the back. The arm of this model is touching the shoulder on the convex side of the lateral curving spine. Her curve is very slight.

The neutral sitting position is with the pelvis slightly tipped forward on the ITs in order to create a closed sacral position, a firm sitting foundation from which the spine elongates.

In asymmetry re-training, it is critical to attempt a straight sitting position so that the pelvic foundation aids the elongation reflex of the spine. Functionally, scoliosis can be thought of as a condition of fatigue, causing a sitting slump.

When using the Activ-Wedge®, place one diagonally between the IT and the greater trochanter on the lighter sitting-side if the client has no hardware. Place it underneath the lighter pelvic sitting-side for a client that does have hardware.

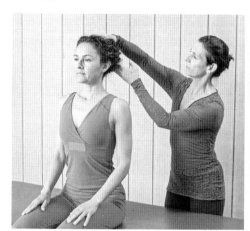

Figure 8.11

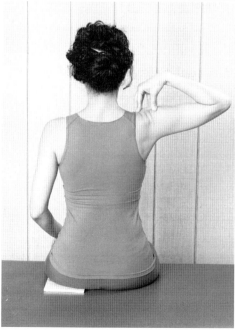

Exercise

Prone

Assume a Prone position. Imagine an ice cube under the waist so that the abdominals slightly elevate toward the ceiling.

Gently press down on the forehead and slightly elevate the Adam's apple (throat) toward the ceiling in order to activate the neck and upper back. Lengthen the coccyx toward the heels. Plant the pelvis onto the mat. Make 'smile lines' between the gluteus maximus and the hamstrings.

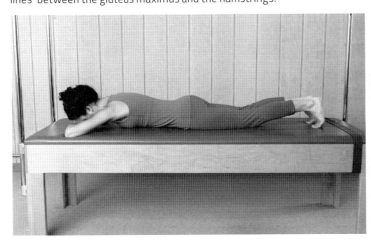

Figure 8.12

If the position is uncomfortable, place a small towel under the forehead, or underneath the waist to elongate the low back.

This position performs direct back work since any limb or head elevation places an anti-gravitational load on the muscles. In this work, the primary goal is to recruit the deep back muscles first before using orientation muscles that create large positions like a full Swan where the back bows into extreme arches. Being able to assume this position, with its emphasis on engaging the appropriate images and muscles, is a main skill in strengthening the back against the pull of the curves.

When using the Activ-Wedge®, place one or more perpendicularly underneath the ribs falling more heavily into the mat and have the client reach away from the wedge. Place another perpendicularly underneath the pelvic side that is lighter on the mat, cueing the client to press down into the wedge.

Exercise

☑ *Quadruped: A–E*

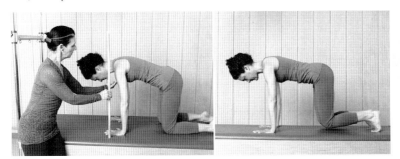

Figure 8.13

The client goes on their hands and knees. The hands are underneath the shoulder line and not in front of the shoulders. The breastbone should have a little lift. The head comes straight out of the neck, not hanging or lifted toward the ceiling. Cue the voice box to gently lift toward the ceiling to activate the anti-gravitational use of the cervical flexors, the longus colli muscles. The back of the pelvis, the back of the ribcage and the back of the head are all assuming a fairly straight line. The knees are underneath the pelvis. Avoid locking the elbows. Cue the inside of the elbows to face one another, not toward the front of the room with some elbow flexion.

This is called the Push-up Plus or Bulldog. A powerful teaching position, it is the foundation of planks and push-ups. Coordinating the deep psoas muscle on the front of the body with the deep back muscles, it engages the abdominal corset of the oblique abdominals, while training in the use of IAP to take load off the lumbar spine. It is the beginning of coordinated back work with the limbs.

When using the Activ-Wedge®, place one underneath the knee that is lighter on the mat. Ask which is heaviest, and then use the other.

Exercise

☑ *Kneeling: A–E*

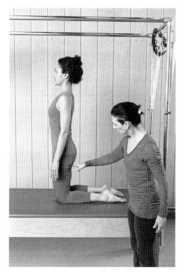

Figure 8.14

Go onto both knees. Bring the pelvis forward into the knees so that a 'smile line' is created between the thighs and the gluteals. The ribcage should line up directly over the pelvis. The back of the neck is elongated.

Avoid knee irritation with kneeling pads if necessary. Still try even if the client cannot assume a precise position. Encourage the client to use the position as a goal. If a comorbidity such as knee replacement exists, do not force the position on them. However, the kneeling position stretches the quadriceps, and promotes neutral hip extension, allowing the gluteals to fully engage without gripping. It engages the posterior pelvic floor, which is advantageous in protecting the position of the spine. Attaining this position greatly improves standing neutral alignment. Asymmetrical spines tend to shorten one side of the pelvis.

When using the Activ-Wedge®, place one underneath the knee that is lighter on the mat. Ask which is heaviest, and then use the other.

Exercise

☑ *Half-kneeling: A–E*

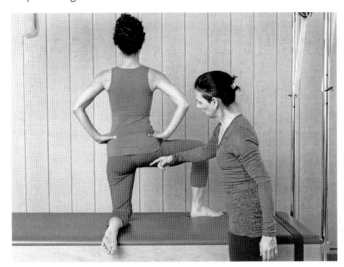

Figure 8.15

Go onto the left knee in this example. Place the other foot on the floor to the side and quite a bit ahead of the horizontal line of the support knee. Adopt the Pilates 'V' in slight external hip rotation. Find the smile line on the back of the support hip. Feel the stretch along the front of the thigh. Drop the right sitting bone toward the floor and pull it toward the left IT, which is the use of the ischiococcygeus of the deep pelvic stabilizers. Attempt to keep the support thigh vertical. Assist balance with a dowel or a chair.

Shortening of the smallest hip adductor at the highest part of the groin, the pectineus, causes obliquity. The position helps to balance the adductors and engage imbalanced or low-performing deep pelvic muscle stabilizers. Their strength greatly benefits overall body endurance for a weak spine.

When using the Activ-Wedge®, place the narrow end straight underneath the sole of the forefoot in line with the foot, then apply pressure on it.

Exercise

⚡ *Imprinting Compressions: A–D*

This exercise is a basic skill that underlies every movement preparation, stabilizing the spine before any larger motion. It promotes body awareness of the parts and full length of the line of the spine, even if the spine is asymmetric. Isometric activity through the central line of the trunk co-contracts and coordinates anterior and posterior trunk musculature and fascial slings. It also develops awareness of the neutral pelvis and pelvic floor in embracing the center of gravity in the pelvis at S2.

Place a small towel underneath the low back for individuals with pain. When using the Activ-Wedge®, follow the directions described previously in the Supine section.

- Lie on your back in a 'neutral' spine. Feel your head, shoulders, rib cage and pelvis are all heavy against the mat. Bend the knees and place the soles of the feet about 4 in (2 cm) apart. There is a small space behind your low back and the mat as well as a small space between your neck and the mat. Feel the backs of your thighs are very heavy. Your shoulder blades are like warm sponges softening into the mat.

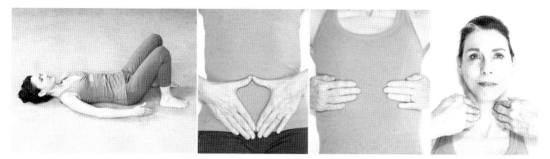

Figure 8.16

Code 8.4 (free code)
2-Diamond pelvic setup

- Bring the thumbs together and index fingers together. Place the thumbs on the navel and the index fingers on the pubic bone. Imagine that the pelvis is a bowl of water. Gently rock the bowl of water until the water spills behind the navel to the floor. Then rock the bowl so that the water spills between the legs to the floor. Rock back and forth several times and let the pelvis come to a balance in between the two points.

- Now think of the diamond at the bottom of the body made by four bony points, the pubis the coccyx, and the two ITs. Think of this area as a billowing parachute floating toward the head from the front, urinal area, and the back, rectal area. This is almost just a thought and not a forceful pelvic contraction. Now 'imprint' or 'hollow' the area above your pubic bone toward the mat. Imagine pressing a pearl into sand. Press two times with the breath, exhaling and hollowing more deeply each time.

- Next, proceed up to the navel area. Feel like the area between the 'hollow' and the navel are being pressed into the mat as if a flat iron is making an impression of the middle bone of the pelvis, the sacrum, into the mat. Press gently with the breath for 2 breaths and relax.

- Then imprint your ribcage, 'the solar plexus' area, by squeezing your ribs together in the front. Below the sternum, the ribs create an upside down 'V' shape. Try to exhale, squeeze the ribs together in the front and at the same time make the lines of the 'V' come together. Inhale. Feel the breath move the fingertips apart. Exhale gently and compress the ribs to bring the fingertips closer together. This is the solar plexus cue.

- Proceed up to the neck. Feel the area on the sides of your Adam's apple or Eve's apple (the larynx or voice box). Feel the weight of the fingers giving heaviness to the front of the cervical spine. These are your deep neck flexors, the colli muscles that are important for neck health. Inhale, exhale, gently feel the weight for 2 breath cycles.

Continued

- Now perform the whole exercise. Imprint the hollow, navel, solar plexus, then the apple and hold for 4 counts (saying 1-alligator, 2-alligator, etc.), and then release.
- Perform this about 5–6 times for full benefit.

Avoid holding the breath. Watch the video demonstration for the setup and exercise (Code 8.4).

Chapter 9 details variations of this basic exercise using the Activ-Wedge®.

Exercise

☑ *Isometric Body Setting: A–E*

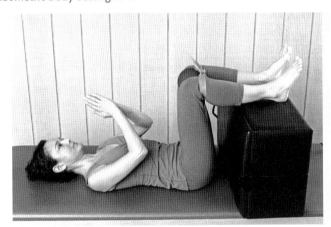

Figure 8.17

This exercise benefits those with low back pain, sacral instability and pelvic pain in general. It helps to organize the pelvis for sitting since it is essentially a seated position while on the back, lying down. It begins to neutralize the asymmetric fascial spiral line.

- Place the calves upon the long box or other similar height surface. Place a ball or a pillow to hold the thighs about 5 in (3 cm) apart. Place a non-stretchy strap around the thighs, tightened so that there is no motion when pressure is exerted upon it from either side.
- Float the pelvic diaphragm parachute toward the head. Feel that the ribcage is widening as you breathe. Imagine as if you have the gills of a fish on the back of your ribs.

Now alternate these two isometric (non-moving) exercises:

- Gently press the hands and thighs toward each other. The intensity should be reasonably firm but not gripping. Meet the boundary; don't try to beat the boundary. Hold this intensity and breathe through the nose and out through the open lips for 30 seconds. It helps to place the tip of the tongue behind the top teeth and gently gap the lips.
- After the 30 seconds, interlock the fingers and gently attempt to pull the hands apart. The interlocked fingers prevent the hands from coming apart. At the same time, gently press the thighs outwards (without externally rotating the legs or moving the feet) against the belt. Hold this intensity and breathe through the nose and out through the open lips for 30 seconds. After this 30-second set, one cycle is completed. Perform 3 cycles of this exercise for best effect.

Exercise

☑ *Prone sacral stabilizer: A–E*

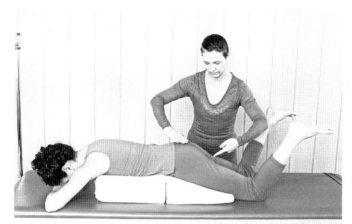

Figure 8.18

Not everyone needs this exercise; however, it is useful for those with sacral instability. An especially esoteric exercise, it utilizes deep pelvic musculature.

Often more difficult to access, engage this posterior pelvic musculature with gentleness rather than with a heavy force. The exercise uses the deep hip rotators to help stabilize the sacrum and increase pelvic muscle coordination and motor control with the legs. Postpartum women should wait a month after birth to assume this maneuver if they are at risk for infection.

- Imagine there is an ice cube underneath the abdomen and gently retract the abdomen up toward the spine, creating a small curve. Gently press the elbows into the mat. Gently elevate the breastbone toward the ceiling as if someone has a finger gently giving pressure upwards the ceiling. Open the legs apart just past hip width and bend the knees.

- Anchor the tailbone down, making 'smile lines.' Before the feet move, feel as if the back of the pelvis at the inner gluteal/anal area is gently drawing together and moving up into the front of the sacrum (rectal area).

- Now move the feet toward each other (externally rotate the hips); try to hold onto the muscle tone. Then using the same technique of drawing the inner sacrum up and into the spine, move the feet away from each other (internally rotate), while not moving the thighs apart; this completes one cycle.

Perform approximately 6–10 cycles while focusing on the coordination of the back of the pelvis with the leg motions.

Exercise

☑ *Lower body toner: A–D*

This exercise addresses imbalances of the pelvis and legs, rectifying the right to the left side of the body. Performed with concentration, it is an essential part of successfully managing the pelvic imbalances associated with scoliosis, by identifying unbalanced motor recruitment between the sides of the ITs and hip musculature.

- In supine, let your arms rest comfortably. Anchor the line of the spine as in the Imprinting Compressions. Lift your feet up, first one and then the other, while holding the spine and pelvic connection. Then flex your

Continued

knees below the horizontal level, and actively press them together. Bring the knees a little closer to the head than usual to avoid back strain. Use your hands to feel the indentations, 'dimples', around the glute area as in the picture.

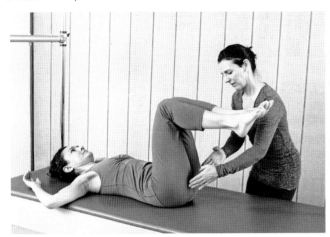

Figure 8.19

Code 8.5 (free code)
Lower body toner

- Slowly reach the feet up toward the ceiling. Stop just before straightening the knees all the way. Pause for one breath. Then slowly begin to lower the tibias, intensifying the 'dimple' and leg contractions. The therapist monitors the side that is having trouble engaging and taps it gently for a tactile cue. This is one set. Work up to doing 3 sets while not losing the engagement of the ITs to come together. Another helpful cue is to place two fingers between the adductors and ask the client to continually squeeze them. This reveals the weaker pelvic side.

- Do not overdo this exercise. Perform only one set per day. Watch the video (Code 8.5).

Exercise

☑ *Pelvic Floor: A–E*

This exercise also reveals one-sided pelvic weakness during leg motion. It recruits deep internal pelvic musculature coordination of leg motions with pelvic and low back stabilization. Avoid breath-holding.

Lie on your back. Flex the hips and knees into the 90/90 position (90° hip flexion with 90° knee flexion). Open the legs apart in neutral leg rotation, not external rotation. Place your hands just inside your knees. Find and contract your checklist:

- Imagine you have a dog's tail that is coming up between your legs and attaching just above the pubic bones.
- Engage your anal area with a 'wink'; then complete the action by elevating the pelvic floor parachute toward your head.
- Engage your urinal area, again elevating it rather than just squeezing it.
- Engage the gluteals with a gentle contraction.
- Now engage the inner thighs, pressing your thighs against your hands while also pressing the hands against the thighs.
- Then slowly move to a count of 4, bringing your legs together to 1.5 inches (3 cm) apart. Intensify the contractions for 10 counts, thinking of all the checkpoints. Then completely relax into the original position, while gently rocking the thighs. This is one cycle.
- Repeat 2 more times. On the last time, imagine that the ITs are moving away from each other.

Due to the intensity of the exercise, perform this one only once per day. Watch the video (Code 8.6).

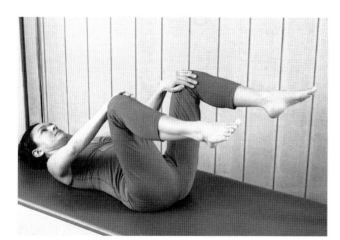

Figure 8.20

Code 8.6 (free code)
Pelvic floor exercise

Exercise

☑ *Straw exercise: A–E*

This Body Skill staves off fatigue in the afternoon, fatigue experienced while out at dinner with friends, or fatigue from standing while waiting in lines or visiting a museum. With practice, the entire maneuver becomes strictly an internal exercise, imperceptible to others.

A postural setting exercise, it greatly aids recruitment of vertebral segments that are difficult to engage and elongate. It is a decompression tool increasing sitting endurance, and for standing to decrease back discomfort. It is also a perfect exercise for sitting in traffic, with the shoulders back against the back rest, and the back of the head touching the head rest. Muscles recruited include the multifidi, paraspinals, psoas, pelvic floor, deep abdominals and respiratory diaphragm, along with elongation of the fascial Inner Envelope.

- The client sits toward the edge of the seat, preferably with the feet not touching the floor and the legs not crossed at the ankles.

- The PMME places one hand, flattened, to rest gently yet firmly upon the top of the client's head. The client slightly slumps like a deflated accordion, with minor spinal flexion. The PMME supplies gentle downward pressure with the flat of the hand (not a cup upon the skull) upon the top of the head. This pressure enables the client to feel the polarity of the downward reach into the pelvis with the simultaneous reach up against gravity.

- Begin to bring the sit bones together as if they are two magnets pulling the sit bones together. Roll slightly forward onto your rocker bones, the sit bones.

- Keep applying consistent, gentle pressure against the top of the client's head, try to not to push the head off center.

- Stroke the client's back traveling from the pelvis upwards toward the spine, with lifting up of the skin of the low back.

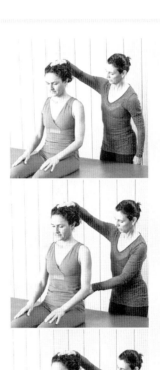

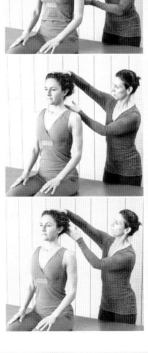

Figure 8.21

- Continue to stroke upwards to cue the ribcage upwards, off the pelvis, while cueing the client to continuing press firmly down into the ITs.
- Cue the client to imagine the ribcage is a lampshade and try to push up through it.
- Give extra tactile aid to any concavities along the sides of the spine.
- Continue to push the spine up through the yoke of the shoulder girdle.
- Cue the client to continue reaching up through the low neck and high neck pressing toward the PMME's hand.
- Cue the client to grow up taller through the spine to this command: "Breathe in, get tall, exhale get taller." Repeat this saying 3 times. Cue the client to relax yet stay floating in the upright position.

This is one cycle. A great home exercise, repeat it throughout the day; morning, noon and night until it becomes automatic.

Code 8.7 (free code)
Straw exercise

Exercise

☑ *Inner Unit exercise: A–E*

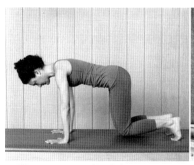 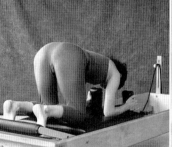 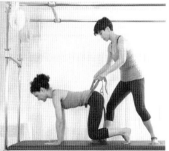

Figure 8.22

This exercise automatically recruits muscles known to aid lumbar spine stability. It is an excellent first exercise for anyone including those with recent spinal disc strain or herniation. Add the scoliosis asymmetry cues for intensity to promote serratus anterior strength, engage the oblique imbalance of the anterior protruding ribs, and identify and rectify hip hike using guidance from the PMME. It is a mainstay in my mat classes and one of

Continued

my favorites. An alternate area for this exercise is upon the reformer for those who are unable to go onto the mat or Trapeze Table. It is shown here on the Trapeze Table for a better view. If wrist tenderness is an issue, try using the fists.

- Go onto the hands and knees. First move the shoulders forward placing the shoulders into the frame of the arms and hands so that the face looks down in front of the hands in the Bulldog. Then walk the knees forward to come underneath the pelvis. Flex the hips in a 90° angle. Try to achieve a 'flat back', where the back of the head, the back of the shoulders and the back of the pelvis are in one long line, like an ironing board. Tuck your toes under (extend) in order to prepare to stand on the metatarsals (balls of the feet).

- Mat: exhale and elevate the knees 2.5 in (5 cm). Stay there and breathe 2–3 times, then lower the knees. Perform about 2–3 repetitions of this exercise.

- Reformer: use 2–4 springs to anchor the carriage as needed. Place the forearms on the mat and allow the hands to hug the shoulder pads. Exhale and elevate the knees 1 inch (2 cm). Stay there and breathe 2–3 times, then lower the knees. Perform about 2–3 repetitions of this exercise.

To advance this exercise on the Reformer, remove all springs or merely lighten the load to promote more core activation.

Imagine the torso is floating up toward the ceiling in order to lighten the load.

Initial body coordination

Pelvic imbalance solutions (from the SSPOT in Chapter 7), Part 1

Three functional core muscle group test correctives from the straight leg raise tests

Choose from a repertoire of exercises for each need. Make them homework. Although listed here as correctives, they are appropriate for any part of a mat regime or class.

TA correctives

Exercise

☑ *Sacral stabilizer: A–E*

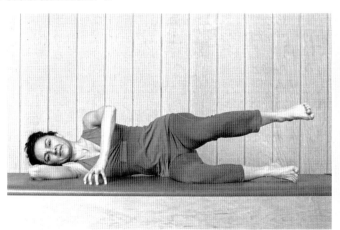

Figure 8.23

An essential element to create TA strength is the sidelying position due to the anti-gravitational load on the orientation of the muscle fibers running from one side of the abdomen to the other, aided by the tightening of the thoracolumbar fascia.

Named the *sacral stabilizer,* it activates each piriformis, which crosses the sacroiliac joint in an isometric (non-moving) act in a lengthened position on either side.

- Go onto the side of the waist concavity first. Roll the bottom shoulder back and point the bottom elbow forward. For comfort, use the lower hand to hold the head weight up.

- Press down onto the bottom shoulder and pelvis to assist with the waist lift. This detail is a critical detail.

- Bend both knees to a sidelying 'sitting' position at a 90° hip flexion with a 90° knee angle. Use a 'lizard hand' with the top arm in order to help assist stabilization of the trunk. Use the sidelying alignment cues. Start with the tibias on top of each other. Then exhale and very slowly 'levitate' the top leg just to the level of the top part of the pelvis. Hold and breathe 3 times and then lower. Repeat this action at least 4 times.

Exercise

⚡ *Articulating Bridging (not suitable for those with spinal fixation): A–E*

Bridging exercises are prone to improper execution for effectiveness. Engage the coccyx curl and smile lines to prevent this error.

- Lie on your back, with knees bent about hip-width apart. Imprint the pelvis into the mat. Start to gently flex the coccyx, beginning the tail curl as low toward the heels as possible. Elongate the low back. Imagine a dog's tail curling through your legs and threading it just above your pubic bone.

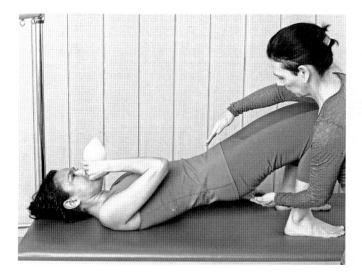

Figure 8.24

- Then start to elevate the pelvis several inches. Feel the engagement of the 'smile lines,' the creases between your gluteals and the hamstrings. Keep the sternum breastbone heavily implanted toward the mat, so that the pelvis level remains higher than the sternal level. Breathe twice and then slowly lower

Continued

through the spine to the pelvis, beginning at the breastbone, navel, waist, low back, pelvis and then finally the tailbone coming down at last to a neutral pelvis.

- Perform this action several more times for effectiveness.

Modify this exercise for those with spinal fixation by removing the spinal articulation and substitute neutral spine pelvic elevation. Levitate the pelvis from the hip extensors only.

The use of a balloon increases the effectiveness of the bridge. See Chapter 9 for more insight into balloon use.

Multifidi (MF) correctives

☑ **Multifidi training: A–E**

Multifidi training is an important Body Skill, described in Chapter 11.

Inner Unit exercise

Listed previously, this exercise is excellent for any back problem, but a special favorite for post-spinal disc bulging or herniation problems, as well as for clients with recent spinal surgery.

Exercise

☑ *Ice Cube exercise: A–E*

This exercise sets up all exercise work performed while lying on the front of the body. It allows the smaller muscle groups of the back, the multifidi, to turn on before the larger and heavier back-muscle activity.

- In the Prone position, place your hands underneath your forehead. Let your knees touch the mat. Tuck your toes under (extend) in order to prepare to stand on the metatarsals (balls of the feet).

- Gently press your elbows into the mat. Feel like a finger is gently pressing your breastbone toward the ceiling. Imagine that there is an ice cube underneath your navel and you are slightly lifting up your abdomen to get away from the cold. Feel an imaginary hand gently tugging the sacrum toward the feet to lengthen the low back. Anchor the smile lines into the mat.

- Holding all those points, begin to slowly extend the hip, straightening the knees, while also lengthening the coccyx toward the heels away from and not toward the ceiling.

- Feel the back of the gluteals and the hamstrings engage. Think of elevating the posterior pelvic fascial slings between the ITs and the coccyx toward the head. Stay and breathe 3 times and lower the knees. Repeat this exercise twice more.

Watch the demonstration (Code 8.8).

Code 8.8 (free code)
Ice Cube exercise

Pelvic floor (PF) correctives

☑ **Lower body toner: A–E**

Listed previously, this exercise is excellent for equalizing the engagement of the pelvic stabilizers of the PF musculature. It helps correct pelvic obliquity.

☑ **PF exercise: A–E**

Listed previously, this exercise is excellent for equalizing the engagement of the pelvic stabilizers in coordination with leg motion. It helps to create the pelvic foundation of the Pelvic Core.

☑ **Prone sacral stabilizer: A–E**

Listed previously, this exercise is excellent for accessing balance in the deep posterior pelvic region, an area particularly helpful for stabilizing the sacral to spine connection.

Functional group correctives (from the SSPOT in Chapter 7), Part 2

Tensor fascia lata (TFL) dominance correctives

The TFL dominance reflects a faulty movement strategy for the flexion of the hip, causing a hip hike, the elevated side of a pelvic obliquity. A compensation for the lack of psoas to flex the thigh, the TFL, a small muscle on the outer pelvis, tries to do the work of the larger psoas muscle group.

These exercises activate the psoas, and the quadratus lumborum, between the ribs and pelvis. The half-kneeling exercises on the mat or equipment work as a corrective as well.

Lower body toner

Listed previously, this exercise is excellent for equalizing the engagement of the pelvic stabilizers of the PF musculature. It helps correct pelvic obliquity.

Psoas trainers and Toe Touches

Two versions of psoas training help. The first trainer is more technical. The second Toe Touch version is simpler for most clients. The psoas originates about T11–12.

Version 1. ⚠ Psoas Trainer: A–E (Figure 8.25)

- In Supine, gently flex the trunk and imprint the spine with a forearm brace. Use an exception to neutral with a true posterior rotation of the pelvis, concentrically activating the psoas with hip flexion.

- Slowly lowering the leg uses the anti-gravitational, eccentric muscle use. Stabilizing strongly with the opposite waist and ribs against the weight of the moving leg corrects pelvic rotation, and hip clicking. The slow descent timing allows the hip capsule to clear in the joint through psoas contraction promoting posterior and inferior femur head glide.

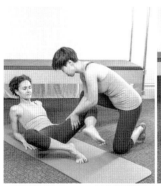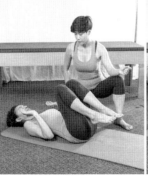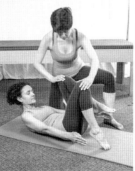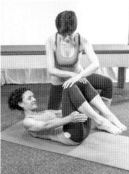

Figure 8.25

• The feet are in the 'walk' position, with weight upon the metatarsal heads of toes 3–5. First imagine that the psoas muscle contracts up toward the imprinted ribcage, then begin the hip flexion. Attempt to lift the leg starting with the heel, not the knee. Repeat 6 times on each leg.

Training joint congruency, this exercise helps to avoid labral tears and promote optimal pelvis to leg coordination. It also creates awareness of the insertion of the psoas on the lesser trochanter, an often-elusive connection for most people. This is a very technical exercise, yet the reward is a truly trained hip.

Version 2. ☑ Toe Touches: A–E

Toe Touches are simpler to teach and are more directly imitate the use of the moving thighs in a reciprocal fashion, a rhythmic one-then-the-other oppositional motion, while stabilizing the trunk.

A brisker exercise, it promotes equal use of the legs in walking. A TFL dominance indicates a slight, or not-so-slight, hip hike while walking, and pelvic sway to that direction, a common issue with spinal asymmetry. Resetting the body coordination improves a more balanced gait pattern.

• Imprint the spine in Supine. Elevate the legs one at a time to table top (tibias parallel to the floor). Be sure to touch the flesh of the calf against the hamstrings.

• Bring the backs of the hands to the shoulders and levitate the elbows off the floor in a preparatory position, the puppy dog.

• Touch the great toe of one foot then the other in a regular rhythmic cadence for 16 alternations of the legs with arms surrounding, but not touching, the legs. Do not waddle with the leg motion. Also cue the pelvic hip hike side to lengthen.

☑ Half-kneeling cueing: A–E

Half-kneeling is a particularly effective position during a corrective session to cue the TFL dominance pattern, whether as a stand-alone exercise or with Reformer or Chair exercises in a half-kneeling position. It was covered previously under Neurodevelopmental positions. Versions of half-kneeling exercises are in Chapter 10, under heading Functional solutions for the pelvis.

Functional group correctives (from the SSPOT-1 in Chapter 7), Part 3

☑ Sidelying handedness correctives: A–E

Break up the continual lateral patterning due to handedness with the two parts of this corrective. ZOA alignment and handedness have a combined effect upon the patterning of leg use.

This exercise is an exception to the general rule of exercising on both sides of the body. The overriding theme of the framework is to exercise in both directions. Interestingly, experimentation with this exercise occurred in several settings with seated observers in lecture halls as well as in a studio setting. It is surprising that this corrective along with the ZOA and eye dominance rotary correctives significantly altered a good percentage of asymmetric

---

Exercise

Go onto the side of handedness close to a wall. For example, I am right-handed so I will go onto the right side of my body and firmly press the right foot into the wall. Place the spine in a gentle flexion. Flex both the hips and knees at a 90° angle. Place a pillow between the legs (Figure 8.26).

• Part A. The client exerts pressure from the front of the top knee to the back of the pelvis as if the PMME is gently pressing the client's top knee backwards, exhaling for 6 counts. Maintain the slight spinal flexion. Then release. Repeat this motion 4 more times.

• Part B. Next, the client internally rotates the top leg, pressing the top knee against the bottom knee, exhaling for 6 counts. Release. Repeat this motion 4 more times.

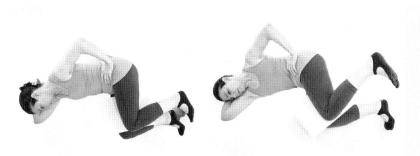

Figure 8.26

Code 8.9 (free code)

Beta study: laterality interventions

patterning for a pilot sample of approximately 200 people. More research will define its role for those with spinal asymmetry.

The video below (Code 8.9) briefly illustrates the technique originally discussed in Chapter 1.

Chapter 9 continues the theme of breaking up fascial and directional preferences.

Bibliography

Arjmand N, Shirazi-Adl, A. (2006). Role of intra-abdominal pressure in the unloading and stabilization of the human spine during static lifting tasks. European Spine Journal 15(8), 265–275

Bialek, M., Pawlak, P., Kotwicki, T. (2009). Foot loading asymmetry in patients with scoliosis. Scoliosis, 4(Suppl. 1): 019

Boyle, K.L. (2013). Clinical application of the right sidelying respiratory left adductor pull back exercise. The International Journal of Physical Therapy, 8(3), 349–358

Boynton, B.R., Barnas, G.M., Dadmun, J.T., Fredberg, J.J. (1991). Mechanical coupling of the rib cage, abdomen and diaphragm through their area of apposition. Journal of Applied Physiology, 70(3), 1235–1254

Chaitow, L. (2012). Breathing pattern disorders and lumbopelvic pain and dysfunction: an update. Retrieved August 20, 2018, from: http://leonchaitow.com/2012/01/23/breathing-pattern-disorders-and-lumbopelvic-pain-and-dysfunction-an-update/

de Mauroy, J.C., Lecante, C., Barral, F., Pourret, S. (2014). Prospective study and new concepts based on scoliosis detorsion of the first 225 early in-brace radiological results with the new Lyon brace: ARTbrace. Scoliosis, 9: 19. doi:10.1186/1748-7161-9-19

Gibbons, S., Comerford, M.J., Emerson, P.L. (2002). Rehabilitation of the stability function of psoas major. Orthopaedic Division Review, January/February, 9–16. Retrieved July 31, 2017, from https://www.researchgate.net/publication/262912731_Rehabilitation_of_the_stability_function_of_psoas_major

Kendall, F.P., McCreary, E.K., Provance, P.G., eds. (1993). Muscles: Testing and Function, 4th edn. Baltimore: Williams and Wilkins

Key, J. (2010). The pelvic crossed syndromes: a reflection of imbalanced function in the myofascial envelope; a further exploration of Janda's work. Journal of Bodywork and Movement Therapies, 14(3), 299–301

Lehnert-Schroth, C. (2007). Three-dimensional Treatment for Scoliosis: A Physiotherapeutic Method for Deformities of the Spine. Translated by C. Mohr, A. Reeves, D.A. Smith. Palo Alto: The Martindale Press

Martínez-Llorens, J., Ramírez, M., Colomina, M.J. et al. (2010). Muscle dysfunction and exercise limitation in adolescent idiopathic scoliosis. European Journal of Respiration, 36(2), 393–400

Negrini, A., Parzini, S., Negrini, M.G. et al. (2008). Adult scoliosis can be reduced through specific SEAS exercises: a case report. Scoliosis, 3: 20. doi:10.1186/1748-7161-3-20

Page, P., Frank, C.C., Lardner, R. (2011). Assessment and Treatment of Muscle Imbalance: The Janda Approach. Champain, IL: Human Kinetics

Sperandio, E.F., Alexandre, A.S., Yi, L.C. et al. (2014). Functional aerobic exercise capacity limitation in adolescent idiopathic scoliosis. The Spine Journal, 14(10), 2366–2372

Sweigard, L.E. (1974). Human Movement Potential: Its Ideokinetic Facilitation. New York: Harper and Row

Todd, M.E. (1937). The Thinking Body. Brooklyn: Dance Horizons

van Loon, P.J.M. (2012). Scoliosis idiopathic? The etiologic factors in scoliosis will affect preventive and conservative therapeutic strategies. In: Grivas, T. (ed.) Recent Advances in Scoliosis. InTech, pp. 211–234. Retrieved August 13, 2018, from: http://www.intechopen.com/books/recent-advances-inscoliosis/changes-in-conservative-treatment-of-spinal-deformities-based-on-increased-knowledge-on-etiology

Williams, D.M. (2011). Review of: Assessment and Treatment of Muscle Imbalance: The Janda Approach. Journal of Orthopedic and Sports Physical Therapy, 41(10), 799–800. Retrieved August 20, 2018, from: http://www.jandacrossedsyndromes.com/wp-content/uploads/2011/10/JOSPT2011JandaReview.pdf

Breaking up the pattern: motion is lotion

The goal of breaking up the fascial pattern works within two major aspects, the musculoskeletal aspect of fascial reshaping and the neuromuscular aspect of reprogramming the motor system. Reduce asymmetrical pulls within the body by positional release, individual pattern activation and restructuring with props. Create myofascial extensibility to concavities and compensatory fascial adhesions. The neuromuscular aspect involves repetitive motion in lateral shifting and rotary movements to move away from ingrained patterns due to preference and side dominance. Motion becomes lotion to create heat, lubricating joints, promoting fascial glide and encouraging fascial recoil activity.

Degree guidelines for severity of the Cobb angle

A = 0–10° Normal expected degree of spinal asymmetry

B = 10–20° Mild

C = 21–40° Moderate

D = >40° Severe

E = >70° Severe with possible medical breathing issues.

Use extra precaution with any operative clients that either have or do not have spinal or other hardware due to joint replacements.

☑ indicates the exercise is appropriate for either those with spinal fixation or for those who have not had any surgery.

⚠ indicates the exercise is not appropriate for those with spinal fixation.

Passive de-rotation positions

Passive de-rotation positions are a release technique where gravity assists fascial or passive muscular stretch. By positioning deeper into the asymmetrical shaper, muscle holding, called facilitations, begins to let go.

Connective tissue then experiences the creep phenomenon of soft tissue stretching due to the viscoelastic property of biologic tissues, changing shape as a load is placed over time, even after a relatively short time, such as 10 seconds. In terms of the asymmetrical spine, this technique also decompresses the vertebral transitional points where the spinal segments above and below the curves transition into a more normal vertebral alignment (Dunn & Silver, 1983; Nordin & Frankel, 2012; Jones et al., 1995).

Positional release with props

☑ *Constructive rest position (90/90) (Figure 9.1)*

The basic 90/90 position is more powerful than it appears. Originally a release for the psoas muscle in dancers, gravity aligns the pelvis into neutral. It aids hip dissociation, stretching deep and superficial fascial back lines along with gluteal fascia, and helps balance large hip musculature. The crossed arm position helps open the distance between the shoulder blades, softening the ribs and allowing gravitational effects to open the posterior girdle area, releasing the neck. A small towel roll underneath the curve of the neck is useful in relieving neck pain. *Note:* This is not a position for any client with recent disc herniation issues. A long box or the seat of a chair works. For disc or low back discomfort, place a small folded towel under the arch of the low back. For tenderness underneath the sacrum, place a small pad underneath the pelvis.

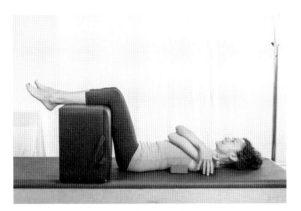

Figure 9.1

⚠ Baby Arc fascial stretching: A–D

Balance the entire trunk systematically with this series of stretches. Think of the trunk as divided into nine segments in a grid pattern similar to a Rubik's Cube. The Arc stretches serve to open each area in a safe, supported way.

Beginning a session with these stretches gives instant feedback as to how tight or uncomfortable a certain body area is that day. The set adapts as a home program on a home Arc, Therapy Ball or bolster.

Do not use tactile aid here to imitate full body work or physiotherapy. A soft grasp facilitates

Exercise

- Place the tongue behind the top teeth. The normal rest position of the tongue is on the soft palate.

- Place the wedge prop perpendicularly, parallel to shoulders, under the greatest part of the thoracic convexity, the heaviest part of the ribcage upon the mat, with the widest part of the wedge at the side of the body.

- Place a wedge under the pelvic side that the client reports is heaviest into the mat. Place a small towel roll underneath the neck and gently slide the head away from the feet until the nose appears to be in a central line with the spine line. Do not contort the body into an unnatural position. Move the thin side of the wedges closer toward the spine until the client feels a sense of relief and greater comfort.

- Cue gentle deep breathing for 8 counts in, 8 counts out, imagining the internal ribcage and pelvis expanding in width, seeing the bubbles from the gills of the posterior ribcage floating toward the ceiling. Vary the direction of the breath first in the widening direction, then in the spinal elongation from the top of the spinal chain at the crown of the head pulling away from the soles of the feet, then the trunk, expanding simultaneously toward the ceiling and the floor.

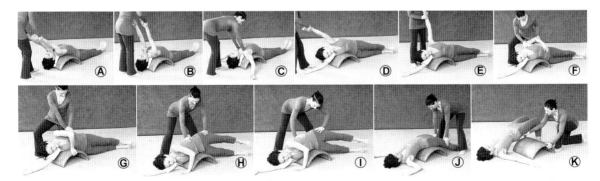

Figure 9.2

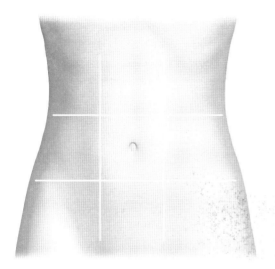

Figure 9.3
The Baby Arc fascial stretching aids the Visceral Core uniting the Upper Core and the Pelvic Core and housing the Inner Envelope.

fascial stretching. Focus first on making contact with the skin:

- Press gently into the skin to access the fascial body stocking underneath the superficial body fat layer. Engage the skin, then let your soft, flat fingers or palms tack down onto the fascial layer.

- Then move gently in the direction of pull for tensional release. Do not clasp the bones or pull them apart. Think of fascial biomechanical slings, instead of trying to massage or mobilize a joint. As a home program, the client moves through the various positions, using imagery and reach to gain the stretch.

The value of the tactile aid is that the client gains the sensory awareness to repeat the sensation of stretch during the home program. Those experiencing acute ribcage, spine or low back pain are not suitable for these series of stretches. When in doubt, refer out.

Exercise

Upper back: two supine stretches (Figure 9.2A–C)

Stretch 1

- Position the sternum facing upwards at the height of the Arc.
- Place a small rolled towel or pillow underneath the neck as needed. Gently clasp the forearm skin, not the wrists. Do not tug on the arms.
- The client exhales 3–5 times. Gently release. Use good body mechanics.

Stretch 2

- Position the arms to the side in a position of comfort. Open the arms sideways more than downwards toward the hands.
- The client breathes for 3–4 breath cycles. Gently release.

Sidelying upper ribcage: three stretches (Figure 9.2D–F)

Stretch 1: arm elevation

- Help the client change to the side position so that the chest is at the height of the Arc. The legs are stacked one upon the other. Line the pelvis up with the ribcage. A towel or pillow underneath the head or waist helps to prevent neck and back strain if there is any discomfort.
- Cue a gentle lie of tension from the client's arm to waist. Breathe for 3–4 breath cycles if no discomfort.
- Perform all the stretches on the same side before helping the client to reposition to the other side of the body.

Continued

One-lung Breathing on Baby Arc

Also a stand-alone exercise (see Figure 9.2G), the addition of this exercise restores rib mobility on the convex rib areas as well as providing the concave areas with the opportunity to increase volume. *Note:* it is not appropriate for those with osteoporosis or hypermobility.

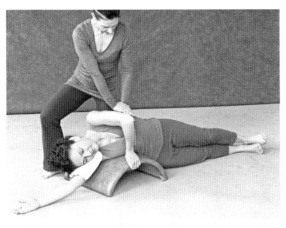

Figure 9.4

Since the client is already positioned sidelying with the chest at the height of the Arc, the PMME gently stacks two flat hands upon the client's ribs approximately lined up with the height of the Arc (Figure 9.4). Avoid placing the hands upon the floating ribs (bottom-most ribs) or making contact with the breasts. Cue the client to inhale for 4 counts, and with a 4-count exhalation. Perform this action about 4 times. The Activ-Wedge® prop increases effectiveness for home use.

Watch the video for the One-lung Baby Arc technique (Code 9.1).

Activ-Wedge® de-rotation mobilizations

The client consciously performs the work for voluntary, not automatic engagement with the wedge.

Supine pelvis: two stretches (Figure 9.2J and K)

Help the client to place the posterior pelvis at the height of the Arc in the following manner:

- Have the client sit a distance in front of the Arc, lean the ribs backwards to feel the Arc on the ribcage. Then use the feet to slide up to the top of the Arc.
- Avoid having the client sit at the height of the Arc and then attempt to lie backwards. If necessary, place a pillow upon the Arc, or underneath the client's ribcage to make the Arc height less steep.

Stretch 1: Psoas stretch

Do not use force down upon the client's thighs. Use only gentle arm weight and avoid over-pressure, a concerted force, toward the floor. Expect the client's low back to feel arched, yet do not stay in this position more than 2 breath cycles.

Stretch 2: Bridge stretch to remove Arc

A successful technique to remove the Arc is to perform a bridging position. Even if the client cannot elevate the pelvis very high, the Arc can usually be removed more easily and without much strain to the client. Inability to elevate the pelvis indicates psoas tightness.

Code 9.1 (free code)
One-lung breathing exercise

⚡ Imprinting compressions for the individual scoliosis pattern: A–D

'Imprinting' and 'compressions' are used interchangeably here to mean pressing the body down into the mat as if pressing pearls into sand. With isometric exercise, muscles tense, contracting, without full skeletal movement such as posterior rotation of the pelvis or large spinal flexion. It is listed here again, in addition to Chapter 7, to illustrate how to progress the exercise for the individual scoliosis pattern.

Activation of the musculature across the neck, the torso and the head opens concave areas promoting lengthening toward lighter areas of the body by pressing body weight into the mat. The props guide how to feel de-rotation out of the asymmetrical pattern creating more volume in the torso. Targeted isometric contractions create a counterforce against the client's usual scoliosis pattern. The lighter areas need stimulation to become

assertive against the scoliosis pattern. The concave areas need volume. Settling the shoulder girdle counters its spiral capacity to spin on top of the ribcage.

Add asymmetrical cues to the imprinting from the initial coordination exercise in Chapter 8. Refer to the profile for the client for eye and tongue cues. Compare your standing profile findings with the client now in the supine position. Activ-Wedge® checklist:

- Which shoulder side is higher off the mat?
- Which area of the ribcage is not touching the mat?
- Is one side of the waist more concave than the other?
- Is one side of the pelvis higher toward the ceiling?
- Is the back of one thigh closer to the mat than the other?
- Does one leg feel lighter against the mat?
- Is one leg turned out more than the other?
  - Or are both feet falling outwards? One?
  - Or are the feet straight up toward the ceiling?

Supine prop use and placement

Place the arm of the shoulder that is higher toward the ceiling in an easy open position with the hand touching the shoulder if able. Place one wedge under the more elevated ribcage area, a concavity between the body and floor. Place another wedge under the side of the pelvis that is lighter into the mat and higher toward the ceiling. Place both legs in easy neutral position with knees upwards toward the ceiling and hips in non-rotation, with the feet pointing upwards.

Watch the video to better understand the sequence (Code 9.2).

Code 9.2 (free code)
Supine Activ-Wedge® use

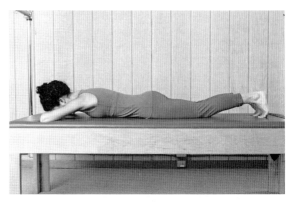

Figure 9.5

used with the wedge prop. It decompresses the facets of the vertebrae and creates volume in the concavities of the scoliosis pattern.

Clients who are either sway-backed or with hyperflexible lumbar spines benefit from strengthening of the natural lordotic curve of the lumbar spine.

⚡ *Balloon with pelvic bridge: A–D*

A child's balloon makes this pelvic bridge quite effective in opening the concavity of the ribcage and waist area, achieving greater volume.

⚡ *Prone ice cube exercise with wedge: A–D*

Progressing from Prone exercises in Chapter 8 (Figure 9.5), this exercise engages deep spine musculature of the multifidi and balances hip extension, reducing pelvic rotations. It promotes muscular counterforce to the asymmetrical spinal pattern when

Exercise

⚡ *Supine: A–D*

Part 1

- Inhale. Begin to exhale.
- Starting at the bottom of the body, sequentially imprint the wedge underneath the pelvis on the perceived lighter side: the wedge underneath the more concave area of the ribcage, the shoulder blade on the side of the elevated arm, the back of the head. Imagine the body is being ironed out as if ironing a tablecloth.
- Hold for 4 counts after the sequence. Repeat several times.

Part 2

- Add the eye and tongue use. Close the dominant eye. Place the tongue up behind the top teeth away from the side that dropped down in the Vertical Compression Test from the Client Profile.
- Repeat in the same manner as previously. Imprint the wedge underneath the pelvis on the perceived lighter side, the wedge underneath the more concave area of the ribcage, the shoulder blade on the side of the elevated arm, then the tongue and eye hold.
- Hold for 4 counts after the sequence. Repeat several times.

Exercise

- Place the prop perpendicularly underneath the ribcage area that protrudes to the front. The client attempts to move away from this wedge. Place another prop underneath the side of the pelvis that is lighter on the mat.

- Observe the client's pants' smile line. The prop goes on the pelvic side with the less developed smile line, indicating less hip extension on that side. Another prop underneath the concave waist area is appropriate for those with large lordotic curves. Use observation skills to determine the best placement. Avoid confusion. At times, both the rib area prop and the pelvic prop are on the same side.

- Watch the video to better understand the wedge with the Prone position (Code 9.3).

Code 9.3 (free code)
Prone Activ-Wedge® use

- Place the hands underneath the forehead, with the knees bent and ankles dorsiflexed with the toes extended. Cue the client to inhale and on the exhalation, press the elbows down into the mat, gently elevate the sternum, and lift the area of the ribs underneath the protruding ribs away from the wedge.

- Next, retract the navel away from an imaginary ice cube. Stay in this position. Then inhale, exhale and begin to extend the hips by straightening the knees, pressing firmly into the pelvic wedge of the lighter side, and also pulling the coccyx toward the feet. Stay and breathe, intensifying the areas of hold and then lower the knees. Repeat several times.

An important, often undeveloped, breathing muscle area called the serratus posterior consists of chevron-shaped breathing muscles above and below, yet underneath, the rhomboid area. They are important connectors for the deep shoulder and arm fascial lines, a missing rib link for those with ribcage asymmetry. An added bonus is the pelvic floor musculature effect, which receives extra challenge through changes in the internal pressure by blowing up the balloon. Increase in intrathoracic pressure optimizes the ZOA, and the challenge to the pelvic floor stimulates eccentric control while coordinating with inner unit musculature.

Laterality

Laterality, or directional bias of task limb preference, seems to be exaggerated for individuals with scoliosis until it is brought to the individual's attention. A major management goal is to identify these biases and preferences in directions of motion.

Sometimes one-sidedness is developed and promoted as a professional strength, for example in such fields as music and tennis. The goal of these exercises is not to change one's strategic outcome for optimal performance, but to open new possibilities for choices of direction.

Repetitive motion in the favored directions creates overuse problems. We all benefit from training into non-favored directions to counterbalance our everyday use tendencies. It is recommended to use lateral rolling and side-bending instead of classic Pilates Method sagittal rolling until the client is more advanced in order to avoid injury to the spinal curve transition points.

☑ *Sidelying handedness correctives: A–E*

Refer to Chapter 8 to review correctives for right or left-handedness under Functional group correctives. Perform the correctives periodically to keep handedness ramifications in check.

Exercise

Note: not for those with acute disc bulging or herniation. Those with osteoporosis are not advised to perform flexion exercises with exertional force of breath.

- Lie on a mat with the knees bent at approximately hip-width apart and the soles of the feet upon the mat. Stretch the balloon beforehand so that it is easy to blow up. Hold the balloon in the non-dominant hand. Inhale to prepare, exhale to begin slowly engaging the gluteals and elevating the pelvis from the tailbone, vertebra by vertebra toward the ceiling to the shoulder blades. Inhale, exhale and blow into the balloon for 6 counts.

- Keep the pelvis elevated. Check pelvic elevation balance and gluteal muscle activation. Lower and perform 4 more cycles.

- Check that the elevation of the bones of the pelvis appear to be equal heights and that both sides of the gluteals and hamstrings remain engaged. Lower the pelvis, beginning with lowering the breastbone, then the waist, the navel, below the navel and then bringing finally the tailbone down to the mat. Also, see Figure 8.7 in the pelvic bridge exercise from Chapter 8.

⚡ Baby Rolls: A–D

A seemingly simple exercise, it exerts a large impact upon breaking up side-to-side patterning. The main purpose is the fascial gliding. This exercise is not appropriate for those with osteoporosis, spondylolisthesis, and recent disc herniation. Refer to the SSPOT-2 in Chapter 7 (p. 109) for the exercise instruction.

⚡ X-rolls: A–D

This exercise is also part of the SSPOT-2, and benefits youth and non-symptomatic adults. Judicious sequential rotation of the spine combined with sequential imprinting of the torso promotes a flowing diagonal fourth dimensional path from the upper or lower limb, through the torso to the ipsilateral upper or lower limb. Refer to the SSPOT-2 in Chapter 7 for the exercise instruction.

⚡ Seated Core Pillow: A–D

Excellent for the daily regime and beneficial for desk workers, this exercise breaks up the pattern of sitting on one side of the pelvis. As a whole-body exercise, it accesses deep pelvic postural muscles along with the quadratus lumborum, often a sore area for those with scoliosis.

Any pillow or sitting therapy ball works if the core pillow is not available (Figure 9.6). Sitting with the feet free allows for more torso work:

- Move the pelvis from side to side, front to back, in circles each way, in diagonals (right front/left back, left front/right back).

- Perform about 5 repetitions of all the motion variations above. Emphasize smooth motion. Avoid initiating the motion from the legs.

⚡ Shift mobilization: A–D

Another daily routine mainstay, it mobilizes multiple facets and intervertebral joints. Similar to a McKenzie shift mobilization, it aids in breaking up the pattern of singular leg weight-bearing stance. Muscles recruited include the quadratus lumborum, gluteus medius, hip abductors and adductors, focusing on the pectineus. Glide and recoil occur through the lateral and spiral fascial lines:

- Press into the 'direction of ease' from the lateral sway test for the first side. Cross the arms into the 'genie' position, with the hands touching the elbows and the forearms not touching the torso. Standing close to the wall, place the pad of the ring at the greater trochanter (Figure 9.7). Point the feet forward, with the legs in 1st parallel. Step in toward the wall to hold the ring firmly into the wall. Gently and rhythmically press the ring into the wall in a smooth repetitive way. Strive to isolate the pelvis from the ribcage.

- Press in with an exhalation for 2 counts, return out of the position for 2 counts. Repeat 10 times. Then repeat to the opposite direction.

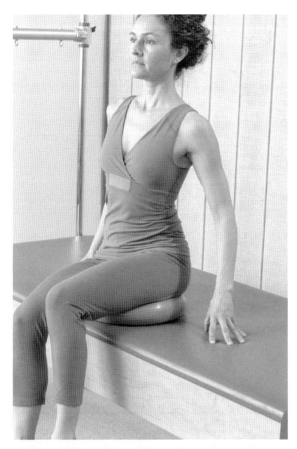

Figure 9.6

✔ Figure of eight with Magic Circle: A–E

Moving the ring in a figure of eight accesses unused musculature and creates heat to optimize fascial gliding.

- Stand in 1st parallel. Use the standing pull-up cues. Press gently yet firmly against the hand grips of the ring.

- Begin a figure-of-eight pattern moving from shoulder height to thigh level 6 times in each direction (Figure 9.8).

⚠ Standing disc rotations: A–D

It is easy to underestimate the ability of simple rhythmic rotation on fascial play and recoil. This is a safe, useful way to develop fascial extensibility:

- Place each foot in the middle of rotating discs and reach the hands up at head height onto the Trapeze Table uprights (Figure 9.9). Slowly, yet rhythmically rotate to one direction, then the other 6 times.

- Next, place both feet upon one disc, focus on the upright and rotate 6 times.

- Repeat on the other rotator disc, focusing on the upright.

Scolio-moves

Diagonal torso and rotary mat movements promote spinal, hip and shoulder action while adding to the recoil ability of the pelvis, ribs and spine. Watch the video (Code 9.4) to see how the use of the Z-sit, lateral rippling through the spine, and using the arm motions tracing an icosahedron shape are additions for movement development in stool and mat use.

✔ Diagonal Balloon Breathing: A–D

Vary the Balloon Breathing exercise from Chapter 8 by accentuating the diagonal movement through the torso. Inhale and breathe up toward the right shoulder and ear, expanding that area. Then exhale, send the breath to the left internal pelvis, gently distending the lower left abdomen. Attempt to keep most of the torso in contact with the mat. Perform about 6 repetitions and repeat to the other side.

✔ Icosahedron moves: A–D

- Sit toward the front edge of a chair.

- Curve the right arm from the right to the left, horizontally enveloping the space. Hold it there.

- Take the left hand and thread the hand through the right arm curve toward the right upper back diagonally. Then open both hands simultaneously, moving from a coronal plane to a diagonal where the left hand is up and back, and the right hand is low on the right. Feel the diagonal connection.

- Then dive the left hand from the upper left back area to the lower right area.

- Perform this 4 times and repeat to the other side. Follow the video (Code 9.4).

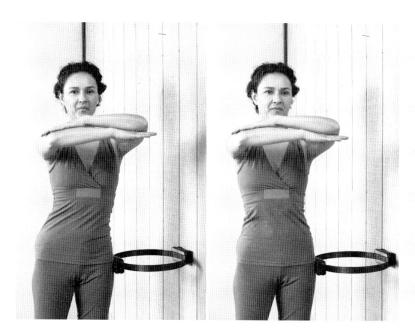

Figure 9.7

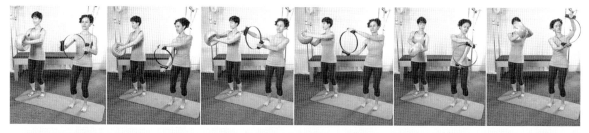

Figure 9.8

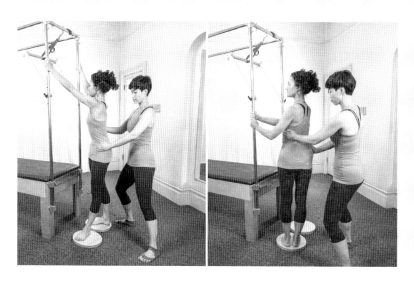

Figure 9.9

Code 9.4 (free code)
Four scolio-moves

⚡ *Rotational Z-sit progressions: A–C*

- First sit on the mat leaning back on both hands with flexed hips. Gently rock from side to side, lowering one inner leg then the other.

- Next, sit in the Z-sit to rotate toward the preferable direction first. In this example, sit with the left leg in front. Begin by gently rocking the right pelvis forward and back, using the abdominal and hip muscles to make the action.

- Begin spiraling the spine beginning with the pelvis, waist, shoulders and head to look toward the side. Then de-rotate back to the front again starting from the pelvis, waist, shoulders and head.

- After comfort is achieved, place the left hand in front of the body, the right to the side, both with softly curved horizontally held arms. Move the right hand toward the mid-line with the sideways rotation. Then on the de-rotation return the left hand in front of the chest.

- After several repetitions, let the left fingers pull an imaginary thread up toward the ceiling with the side rotation, then allow the right hand to pull up the thread on the de-rotation.

Watch the video (Code 9.4).

⚡ *Seaweed: A–C*

- Sit toward the front edge of a chair. Sway the body in a sequential manner as if a tree is softly blowing in the wind.

- Ripple up from the pelvis through the side of the ribs and shoulders up toward the ear. Then begin the ripple to the other side. Do not force any motion that does not feel good.

Watch the video (Code 9.4).

Bibliography

Dunn, M.G., Silver, F. H. (1983). Viscoelastic behavior of human connective tissues: relative contribution of viscous and elastic components. Connect Tissue Resident, 12(1), 59–70

Jones, L.H., Kusonose, R., Goering, E. (1995). Strain–CounterStrain. Boise: Jones Strain–Counterstrain

Nordin, M., Frankel, V.H. (2012). Basic Biomechanics of the Musculoskeletal System, 4th edn. Philadelphia: Lippincott Williams and Wilkins

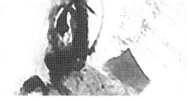

Redirect the pattern

Redirecting the pattern goes beyond remediation into acquisition of the skill of the Method; however, not all the exercises shown are suitable for every client. As an indispensable second pair of eyes and guide, the PMME begins to coordinate the entire body in its quest for altering the available changeable aspect of the asymmetry through fascial and muscular connections, critical in learning the basis of musculoskeletal and neuromuscular de-rotation. Functional solutions list detailed, practical and workable scenarios for the PMME. It is beyond the scope of this book to detail over 400 known Pilates exercises; however, a number of exercises are included in the list that are helpful for functional solutions along with insights relating to progressive acquisition of the Method for this population.

Note

A word of caution for those with spinal fixation

This chapter moves into larger spatial orientations. There is a special code for each exercise:

    ☑ indicates the exercise is permitted for those with spinal fixation

    ⚡ indicates the exercise is a contraindicated movement for those with fixation.

There are fewer exercise options in general than for a client who has not had surgery. A PMME must coordinate with the attending medical provider to ensure readiness and safety. Bone fixation, spinal surgery where the bones are re-shaped, is a severe trauma to the body, similar to mending multiple fractured bones. Heightened tissue sensitivity could last from around eight months to a year. It takes about eight weeks for the basic bone to knit, usually approximately three months to begin a program. Many types of fixation surgeries exist. Clients with older surgeries still need precaution. Be conservative. Never venture into areas of pain.

Functional solutions for the spine

Note

Words of advice and caution for all clients

- Start neutral before expanding into orientation planes. Use the wedge to individualize the spinal cues while remaining neutral in orientation.

- Delay any sagittal rolling or full flexion exercises until the client acclimates after several sessions. Save Short Spine and Mermaid for later advancement. I recommend omitting Pretzel altogether.

- Any corkscrew or criss-cross movements must remain within the frame of the body. Spiraling out of the frame is advanced. When beginning, keep the legs at least at a 45° angle to the horizon when supine. Place the wedges underneath both sides of the lower ribs in supine to facilitate more control when the legs lowering toward the floor cause more sway back and back extension past neutral as in typical leg circles.

- The cervical spine and neck are fragile. Use the cues to access head and neck, although suggestions in thoracic solutions in supine are most conservative. The eye cues relate to C1. The tongue cues relate to C3 as well as to the deep frontal fascial line.

Degree guidelines for severity of the Cobb angle

A = 0–10° Normal expected degree of spinal asymmetry

B = 10–20° Mild

C = 21–40° Moderate

D = >40° Severe

E = >70° Severe with possible medical breathing issues.

Unweighting; finding the spine

Taking the spine out of gravitational load and onto the mat aids the discovery of the internal spine length.

Fascial unwinding for functional movement

Safe de-rotation begins with this simple movement: see ⚠ Standing disc rotations in Chapter 9 (See Figure 9.9, page 160).

Exercise

⚠ *Mat 'C': A–D*

Lie supine on the mat. Grasp the hands together. Lengthen the feet away from the hands. Slide the hands and feet to the right, keeping the shoulders and pelvis flat upon the mat. Then lengthen and slide over to the left. Repeat 5 times.

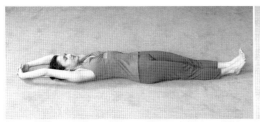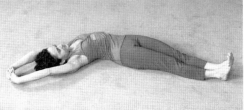

Figure 10.1

☑ *Sidelying hip flexion: A–E*

Lie on the concave side. Make 'O' arms and press off the side of the bottom upper arm to elevate the high ribs. Elongate. Flex the hips to 90° while maintaining neutral spine. Elongate and fully extend the hips to neutral, emphasizing smile lines of the pelvis. Repeat 5 times.

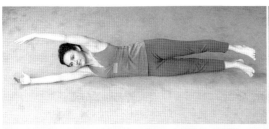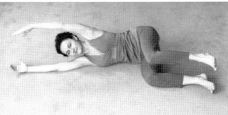

Figure 10.2

Stability training in the asymmetry cues

Exercise

☑ *Reformer foot work with wedges: A–D*

Watch the video for pointers with wedge use (Code 10.1).

Code 10.1 (free code)
Activ-Wedge® use on the Reformer

☑ *Reformer – No-springs abdominals: A–D*

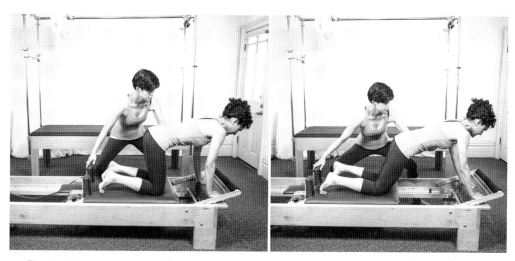

Figure 10.3

Use extra caution in spotting the client. Remove all springs from the spring hooks to heighten core use. Hold the carriage for safety. Cue the client to kneel onto the mat of the Reformer. Curl the fingers around the edge of the base for security. Hold the shoulder rest with one hand to block the carriage from sliding out. Gently hold the client underneath the protruding ribs to cue the concavity up toward the ceiling, evening out the thoracic rotation as much as possible. Cue the quadruped 'bull-dog' cues of bent elbows. Slowly allow the client's shoulders to move the carriage to slide back about 4 in (10 cm). Then allow the thighs to extend about 30°. Cue the pelvis to lift to flex the hip joints. Then allow the shoulders to return the carriage to the base. The motion sequence is: Shoulders move, then thighs move, lift the pelvis, thighs under hips and glide back to the base. Control the client in this fashion 5 times.

⚠ *Half-barrel or Arc Prone Swimming: A–D*

This typical Pilates exercise takes on a new level of complexity while attempting to balance prone on the Arc. This one is a favorite with youth. Check with the tolerance for those with fixation. If in doubt, leave it out.

Continued

☑ *Chair – Psoas Pumps: A–E*

Code 10.2 (free code)
Psoas trainer exercise on split-pedal chair

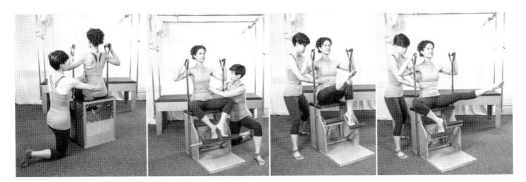

Figure 10.4

Set an appropriate weight of springs on the chair. Place a wedge underneath the heavier pelvic side diagonally between the IT and the coccyx. Lock the pedals. Pull down on the arm grips, lining up the sides of the ribcage and waist. Bring the head over the center of gravity and equalize the shoulder heights. Place the feet in the Pilates 'V'. Perform a rhythmic accent up-pump, repeatedly elevating the knees for 20 repetitions. Flex the hip above 90° to favor psoas flexion use over quadriceps dominance. Add one-legged variations after removing the dowel. Perform 10–20 pump repetitions. Watch the video (Code 10.2).

☑ *Traditional safe Pilates repertoire for spinal stability (4 parts): A–D*

These exercises are safe for those requiring the maintenance of neutral spine. Place the wedges in prone as advised in Chapter 8, with one wedge underneath the protruding rib area and the other underneath the lighter pelvic side. Slide it perpendicularly at the anterior superior iliac spine (ASIS) area and cue to press down onto it, engaging the posterior pelvic floor between the IT and the coccyx toward the head. For the elevated positions of Long Stretch and Jackrabbit, stand by the client and cue the anterior ribs and non-engaged pelvic side.

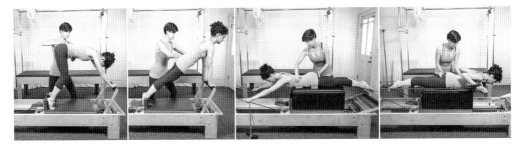

Figure 10.5
Part 1. Long Stretch, Part 2. Jackrabbit, Part 3. Long Box: pulling ropes, Part 4. Modified Swan: pushing ropes.

Traditional Pilates Chair for advanced clients

⚡ *Chair – Sidelying hand pedal presses: A–D*

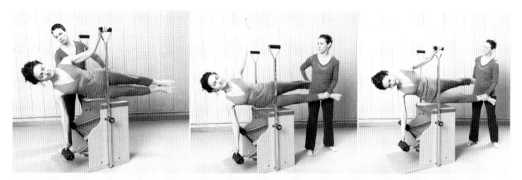

Figure 10.6

Use an appropriate amount of spring weight. Place the pelvis of the concave side on the seat. Place one hand on the hand grip, the other on the front pedal, using a 'duck' hand grip. Inhale lean over, exhale return by lengthening the body. Remain horizontal at the return. Perform 4 repetitions. Repeat on the convex side. Take this exercise to another level. Stand between the legs with the top leg to the back. Lean slightly back to cue leg tension combined with elongation. Cue dorsiflexion in the ankles. Monitor that the pelvis remains upright. Cue the client to grip the PMME's thighs throughout the exercise.

Elongation: holding against gravity

☑ *Trapeze Table Horse: A–D*

The Horse benefits awareness of the ribcage over the pelvis and strength of the waist. Cue the client onto the long box with the Arc on top, or an improvised version. The legs are in parallel with the ankles dorsiflexed. The hands go through the fuzzy loops and grasp the webbing. Exhale. Pull down on the loops. Elevate the torso and grasp the Arc with the hip adductors. Line up the seams of the mid-ribcage with the seams of the pants in a vertical line. Stay. Breathe 3 times. Relax down. Repeat twice more. On the third time, spot the client. Set up the position and release the arms reaching them sideways to see if the waist holds the position. Check the adductor pectineus lengths by spotting the client to sit equally on both sides of the pelvis, not off to one side. Cue the smile line engagement and control the anterior protruding ribs (see Figure 10.7).

Continued

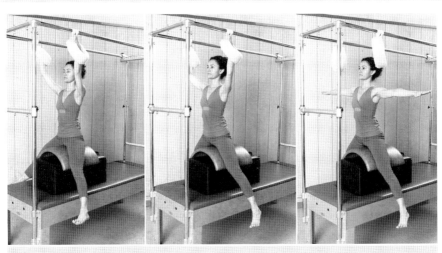

Figure 10.7

✓ 4-D de-rotation on Tower or Trapeze Table: A-D

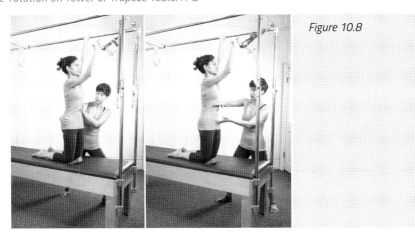

Figure 10.8

Kneeling on the Trapeze Table, or alternatively on a Tower Unit or even next to a wall are effective substitute locations. To access the fascial fourth dimension (4-D), place a wedge one-eighth of its length underneath the front of the lighter knee. Reach the arms up with the concave side, the side with the elevated hand lower in the assessments either higher on a wall or more in front of the other hand if on the table. These cues correct z-axis side-bend and help y-axis pelvic transverse rotation. Cue the anterior rib protrusion to gently contract, another y-axis cue. Cue the smile lines evenly, emphasizing the lift of the posterior pelvic floor. Cue the xiphoid to pubis to flex but elongate to cue the x-axis.

Add the eye closure and tongue position. Cue the client to breathe in, get tall, exhale, get taller with a SSHH-ing breath for 4 counts. Repeat 5 times and relax.

⚡ Balancing 'O' mat exercise

See SSPOT-2, Chapter 7 (Figure 7.31, page 113).

Articulation

Exercise

⚡ *Roll-down/Roll-up on Trapeze Table: A–D*

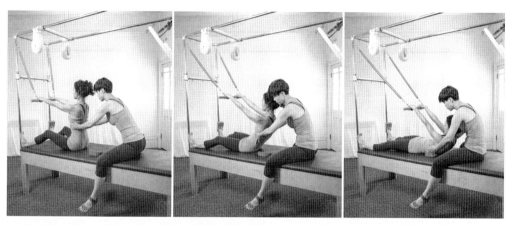

Figure 10.9

Place a wedge under the forefoot of the shorter leg against the upright pole. Sit behind the client and aid weighting the lighter pelvis side on the mat. Elongate the ribcage, guiding the concave area to lie as flat and lined up with the pelvis as possible down against the mat. On the return up, once again elongate and open the concave rib area by gently pulling back on it. Elongate the client onto the lighter pelvis. Cue the client to think of the coccyx reaching away from the head and creating the flexion. Cue the pull-up of the pelvic slings toward the head before rolling back. Chapter 12 offers more information on cueing pelvic lift, which is needed in cases of both hypermobility and prolapse.

⚡ *Sling Hip Circles: A–D*

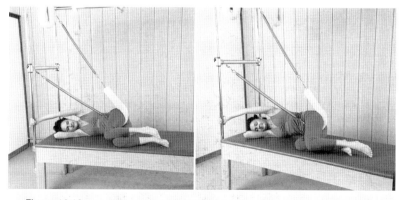

Figure 10.10

Continued

Use two moderately heavy leg springs, one placed lower than the other on the Trapeze Table. Cover a foot strap with a fuzzy loop to make a sling. Lie upon the convex side. Pull the sling around the top leg close to the pelvis within comfort level. Be sure the client braces the arms. Imagine an axis going through the greater trochanter of the top pelvis into the bottom. Guide a hip circle. Hike the top pelvis toward the ribcage, then back toward the back wall, then reach the sit bone toward the opposite end of the table. Complete the circle by reaching the top knee forward past the bottom knee. Try to make the circle with the pelvis and not just the legs. Repeat 5 more circles and move to the other side to repeat the whole exercise (Figure 10.10).

⚡ *Twisty Cat: A–D*

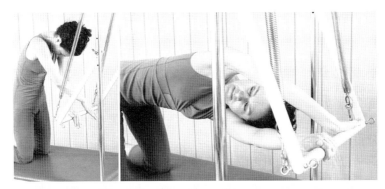

Figure 10.11

Use two moderate leg springs for support. Start in the direction of the easier way to twist. If you twist more easily to the left, then I place the right arm underneath the left. Palms face onto the bar. Go onto the knees in the 1st Parallel. Inhale. Hollow the waist and elongate to push the bar down. Lengthen the spine, keep the arms with the elbows bent and press down onto it. Lift the left elbow and look underneath it. Then de-rotate/cue the concave ribs to lift. Let the bar push the client back to roll up to the original position. Keeping the elbows bent on the return prevents the shoulder girdle from elevating. Perform 5 repetitions each way. A modification on the Reformer is in Chapter 12.

⚡ *Spinal spiral: A–C*

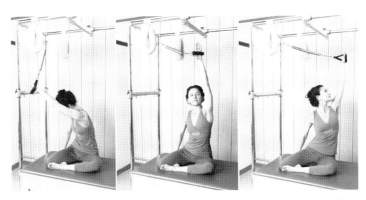

Figure 10.12

Start in the easier direction to rotate. Use one moderately heavy short spring clipped high upon the upright behind the client. Cue the Z-sit with the front tibia parallel with the table. Touch the internally rotated back thigh to the sole of the front foot. It is not necessary for the IT on that side to touch the mat. Cup the internally rotated calf. Hold the hand grip with the other hand. Inhale. Exhale and begin to rock the pelvis forward from the internally rotated hip toward the front thigh. Continue rotating the spine from the pelvis, waist, and shoulders. Turn the hand and reach it away from the bottom hand in a diagonal line. Lengthen/inhale and exhale, resist with the top hand, striving to keep the hand in the same spot. Return from the pelvis, waist, ribcage, shoulders, and curve to look at the hand cupping the calf. Do 5 repetitions on each side.

Functional solutions for the ribcage

Note

Words of advice and caution

Recall that the ribs are longer on the convex side and that actual bone shape changes will limit the ability of the ribs to rotate. Do not force rotation. Use the wedge, ball and Rooster hand positions for safe ribcage interventions before branching out to more difficult movements. Delay Mermaid exercises until the client has more ribcage articulation. Starting with the mat mobility exercises begins the process.

Mobility

Exercise

Mat: Arc/One-lung Breathing

See Chapter 9.

⚠ *Thoracic Mobilizer: A–C*

| *Code 10.3* (free code) |
| Thoracic mobilizer |

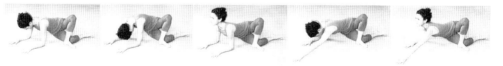

Figure 10.13

Lie on the side that is easier to rotate toward. Tip sideways to cross one leg over the other on the mat with the sole of the foot on the floor. Place the forearms parallel to one another in an angle more forward than straight to the side. Do not force the front forearm to touch the floor. Flex the spine, leading from the pelvis. Look at the navel. Then reverse the action. Anteriorly rotate the pelvis, extend the spine and look underneath an imaginary table. Watch the video demonstration (Code 10.3).

Fascial unwinding for functional movement

Exercise

☑ *Ribcage interventions = Rooster hands and ball: A–E*

Use a blue and red spring on the Reformer as appropriate. Bring the legs into the 1st Parallel. Form Rooster hands by bringing the thumbs and index fingers together. Lightly pinch the bridge of the nose with the thumbs and place the index fingers upon the forehead. Start to rhythmically rotate the legs in unison. Rotate the knees to one side in a flexed position as if describing the inside of an upside-down bowl. Then slightly push away from the foot bar. Stay there and flex the knees, make the semi-circle arc with the knees and change to the other side. The leg rhythm goes: bend, semi-circle, push. Bend again and stay there. Bend, semi-circle, push, bend again. Repeat this action rhythmically 4 times. Vary the position of the head by rotating it to one side while the legs continue for a while, then switch to the other side. Another variation is to hold a weighted ball, moving it in opposition to the knee directions.

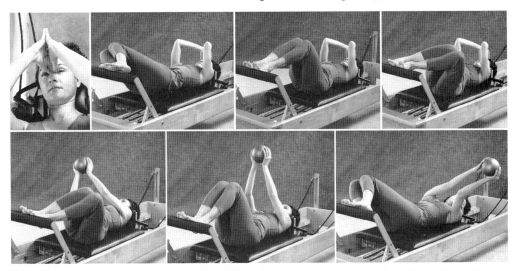

Figure 10.14

⚠ *Spine Corrector: fall and release with dowel or Mini Bar: A–C*

Reserved for youth, this exercise promotes sitting strength through range. Start with the convex side toward the height of the Corrector. Sit into the lip as in a Z-sit. Flex the front knee over the front edge. Elongate the arms with a dowel overhead. Slowly begin to make contact with the dome of the Corrector with the ribcage and lean over it toward the mat. Keep the muscles engaged. Then reverse the action, lean away from the mat in an elongated side-bend and sit up. Repeat this action 4 times. Then repeat 4 more times with a weighted Mini Bar as an option. Do the exercise on the other side. Never do only one side.

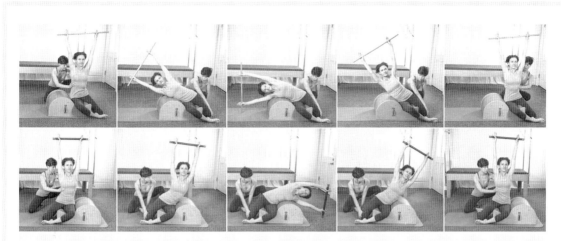

Figure 10.15

Stability training

Exercise

☑ *Reverse abdominals: A–D*

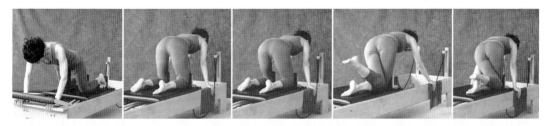

Figure 10.16

Use one blue spring. Go onto the Reformer in the quadruped position. Reach forward onto the sides and pull the whole shape toward the pulleys until the head is past the line of the hands. The arms press diagonally backwards. Hold the position. Isolate the hip flexion moving the hips from 90° to 120° to accentuate psoas use. Cue the asymmetry cues of the anterior ribcage hold and correct any hip hike. Place a wedge underneath the lighter knee as an option. Flex the hips 10 times, return to the base and repeat.

Elongation

Exercise

⚡ *Sidelying bar fall and release on Trapeze Table: A–C*

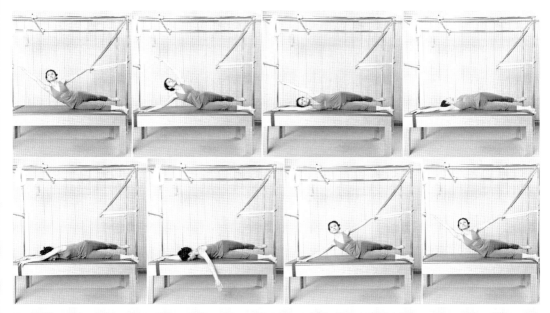

Figure 10.17

Go onto the side with the top leg to the back upright and the bottom leg to the front upright. Hug the uprights with the arches of the feet. Hang from the push-through bar . Place the free hand down upon the mat and begin to slide out, elongating and lifting the bottom waist. The top arm then reaches back easily, then reaches forward onto the edge of the table, elongating the fascial Spiral Line. Use momentum to then sweep the hand toward the floor, reach up with the ribcage and catch the bar. End in the bottom arm arc pose. Do 4 repetitions each side.

Articulation

Exercise

⚡ *Cleopatra variation: A–C*

Use one blue spring. Lie on one side. Start toward the direction that is easier to rotate. Place the bottom forearm on the end of the carriage mat. Cup the other palm with a duck hand on the foot bar at a comfortable height. Flex the legs and stack the tibias one on top of the other, close to the shoulder rests. Exhale. Extend the top arm. Rotate and look down into the well. Inhale. Return the carriage and look over the shoulder in a profile like Cleopatra on the barge. Repeat 4 times.

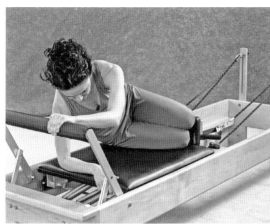
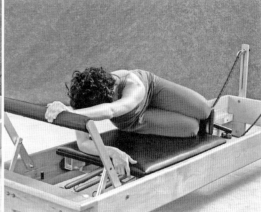

Figure 10.18

⚡ *Pigeon: A–C*

Figure 10.19

Becoming advanced as it progresses into deeper spinal rotation in three different arm holds, use one blue or red spring. Go onto the favored side and place the forearm on the dropped head rest. Cup the other hand on the front shoulder rest. Flex the hips to 90°. Place one parallel metatarsal head upon the foot bar toward the front. Rhythmically begin to gently flex and extend the leg in the same motion as the previous Rooster arms exercise. Rotate the top knee internally in a flexed position as if describing the inside of an upside-down bowl. Then slightly push away from the foot bar. Stay there and flex the knee, make a semi-circle arc with the knee and move to externally rotate the hip. The rhythm goes: bend, rotate, push. Bend again and stay there. Think of the bowl and the semi-circle. Bend, semi-circle, push, bend again. Repeat this action rhythmically 4 times. Next, advance to change the top hand to the opposite shoulder, rotating the upper body to look at the head rest. Repeat the leg activity 4–8 times. Lastly, move to the most challenging rotation by placing the palms on the shoulder rests. Repeat the same rhythmic leg activity.

Elongation: holding against gravity

 Sidelying bar fall and release on Trapeze Table

See previous section.

Functional solutions for the pelvis

[QR code]	*Code 10.4* (free code) Functional pelvis explanation

Note

Words of advice and caution

Solutions here include leg use, especially hip dissociation of the legs and development of hip extension strength. Prone work is an opportunity to use eye and tongue cues where change in antigravitational and vestibular muscle balancing has a direct effect upon underused muscle slings and systems.

Focus also on the dissociation mobility of the three bones of the pelvis. Watch the video to see how the pelvis operates in daily walking through the mobility of the separate bones (Code 10.4).

Dissociation mobility of legs from pelvis

Exercise

☑ *Trapeze Table triangle elongation/Reformer Elephant version: A–D*

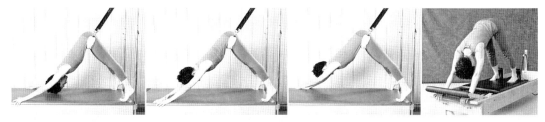

Figure 10.20

The elongation stretches help the concept of dissociation as well as addressing the length of the Superficial Back Fascial Line. The Trapeze Table set-up uses two long D-ring foot Reformer straps with a fuzzy loop sling made from a medium-length Reformer foot strap. Guide the client to place the fuzzy loop around the front of the pelvis close to the hip crease. Then walk the hands down to the table. Next, walk the feet back to the uprights. Spot the feet to prevent slippage. Do not stay in this stretch for an extended period, over 2 minutes. The Reformer modified Elephant version emphasizes the extended spine. Observe from the back which pelvic height is lower. Place a kneeling pad and/or a wedge underneath the forefoot of the lower pelvis. Watch the video demonstration (Code 10.5).

	Code 10.5 (free code) Activ-Wedge® use in plantigrade on the Reformer

☑ Quadruped sling: A–E

A common exercise that often promotes poor form and reinforces compensations, yet when done with a sling and precision, it reveals faulty strategies that are correctable.

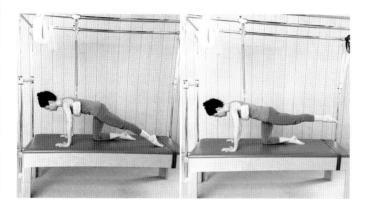

Figure 10.21

Use two moderately heavy leg springs with a fuzzy-loop sling on the overhead rail or a similar version on the Tower. Place the sling around the lower ribs. Guide the client into the quadruped. Start on the side that does not shift laterally the most. Exhale. Lengthen one leg, press the top of the foot to the mat. Breathe. Then extend the hip, attempting to control no lateral shift and/or drop of the ribcage, especially the anterior protruding ribs. Breathe 3 times, lower, return the leg. Alternate to the other side. Perform several sets.

⚡ Bilateral leg lift: A–C

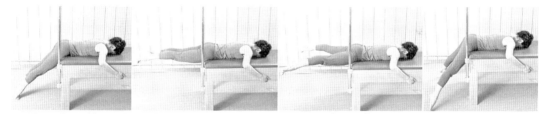

Figure 10.22

Lie prone on the end of the Trapeze Table with the legs on the floor. Feel the imaginary ice cube underneath the waist and the pelvic parachute toward the head. Exhale, elevate the lengthened legs. Open them past shoulder width. Lower them with control. Exhale, elevate the legs. Close the legs and lower with control. Be sure to fully extend the hips yet keep the legs below the horizon. Perform 10 repetitions.

Fascial unwinding for functional movement = connective tissue resiliency and recoil

Exercise

☑ *Reformer Half-kneel with Magic Circle: A–E*

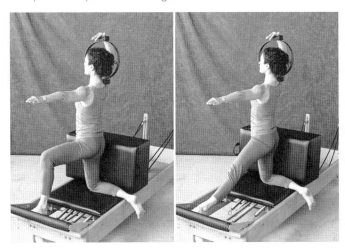

Figure 10.23

This movement supports pelvic obliquity balance, equalizing pectineal lengths and IT control. Experiment to find which leg does not promote the hip hike when kneeling on it and use that support leg first. Use one red spring. Place the knee in neutral rotation against the back-shoulder rest. Place the metatarsals of the other foot in the Pilates 'V' on the Reformer base. Use padding. Place the Magic Circle on the shoulder on the same side as the kneeling leg. Exhale. Extend the knee slowly, concentrating on the external rotation and vastus medialis control. Inhale, flex. Exhale, extend. Expect a small motion. Concentrate on the pelvic and asymmetry cues. Do approximately 6 repetitions on each side.

⚡ *Reformer Semi-circle: A–C*

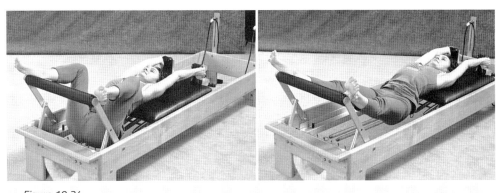

Figure 10.24

This is the traditional Semi-circle exercise. Use it for advanced work once the client has more spinal control and is deemed safe.

☑ *Dreaded Frog circles and scissors: A–D*

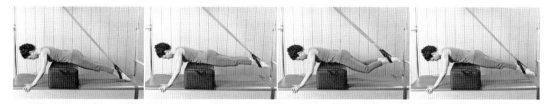

Figure 10.25

Use a Short Box set up with two yellow springs from the overhead bar. Cue the client to place the hip creases at the edge of the box, lie over it and brace the arms by pushing them. Place the foot loops on the soles of the feet, not the ankles. Spot the motion of the legs and prevent slippage of the loops. Use all the prone and asymmetry cues. There are three parts. The first two warm up the hip joints. Start with easy leg circles, eventually giving the client control. Next, guide scissor motion for a number of sets. The last part is the Dreaded Frog. Perform a Frog motion attempting to keep the heels in a horizontal line with the coccyx, opening the knees toward the ceiling. Inhale, flex the hips. Exhale, lengthen. Cue the non-engaging inner thigh and smile line to engage. Perform 6 repetitions as able.

Stability training

Exercise

⚡ *Half-kneel spine rotations: A–D*

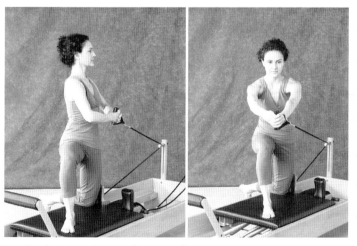

Figure 10.26

Use the direction of ease of rotation for the first rotation. Place one knee in neutral rotation against the back-shoulder rest. Place the other foot upon the front corner in relation to the supporting knee. Cue the pelvic asymmetry cues for IT control, hip hike, anterior rib protrusion, and head over center of gravity. Fold the hands into the

Continued

foot loops or hand grip. Experiment with which hand is placed on top of the other. Inhale, prepare. Exhale, rotate just within the frame of the body. Do not over-rotate. Next, extend the elbows, reach the hands out past the knee and lean, promoting balance and functional reach. Then bend the elbows with control toward the waist. Be sure to spot the client at this moment as balance is often lost here. Then rotate back to the original position. The motion goes: Rotate, reach, retract the elbows and un-rotate back. Perform around 8 repetitions on each side (see Figure 10.26).

☑ *Chair Sideways Mountain Climber: A–D*

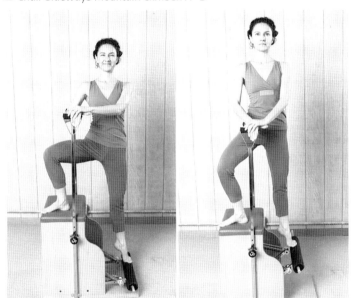

Figure 10.27

Start on the side that has less hip hike in the half-kneel position. Use the appropriate weight of springs. Spot the client closely for security of the foot on the pedal. Stand with one foot in the high half-toe (elevated heel) in the Pilates 'V' on the metatarsals if possible on the back pedal. Place the other foot fully onto the seat of the chair. Hold the arm grips with both hands on the front grip. Line up the leg with the middle of the side of the pelvis and the middle of the side of the ribcage. Imagine elevating the center of gravity using the adductors and pelvic slings. Levitate and gently pulse up and down in a mid-range off from the chair base for 10 pulses, accenting an upwards lift. Repeat to the other side. Never do only one side.

☑ *Weighted ball: A–D*

This exercise has three parts and is excellent for straightening out the legs and aiding inner thigh muscular balance:

- *Part 1.* Lie on the mat. Imprint the spine and use the asymmetry cues. Place a weighted ball between the ankles. Make sure to start the client in the 90/90 supine chair position. Then place the ball between the ankles to determine if the core strength is sufficient to handle the load. If not, place a pillow underneath the pelvis. Keep the legs in 1st Parallel. Align the knees with the second toes. Exhale. Elevate the ball. Inhale, return to the parallel tibia-to-the-floor position. Be sure the client's knees are more toward the face rather than listing away from the hip joint line to avoid lumbar strain. Repeat elevating and lowering 10 times.

- *Part 2.* Place the soles of the feet down on the mat with the ball between the ankles. Exhale. Flex the hips. Elevate the ball to the ceiling. Return through the parallel tibia-to-the-floor position and place the ball down. Repeat this action 6 times.

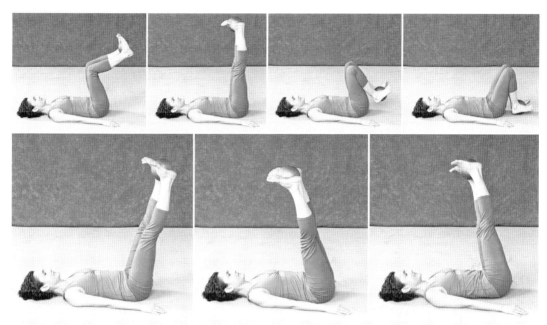

Figure 10.28

- *Part 3.* Keep the elevated ball up after softly extending the knees after the last repetition of Part 2. Now make an infinity sign, a sideways figure eight with the ball. Do around 10 repetitions each way. Attempt to make the motion form the pelvis instead of the feet.

⚠ *Confounded balance: A–D*

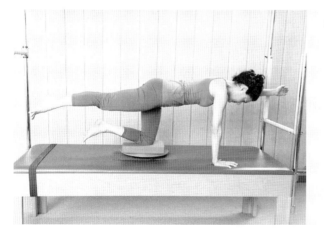

Figure 10.29

Place a wobble board on the Trapeze Table. Place a sitting pad on the wobble board. Start with the stronger leg first as found from the Quadruped Sling exercise. Guide the client to align the knee with the apex of the fulcrum of the

Continued

wobble board. Form a quadruped with the free leg extended behind as in the Quadruped Sling exercise. Exhale and levitate the free leg. Reach the opposite arm out in front. Attempt to keep the rim areas of the wobble board the same height off the mat. Breathe 5 times and lower. Repeat on the other side. Challenge the client by adding the asymmetric eye and tongue cues.

Elongation = strength and stability

Exercise
⚡ *Side-bend on Short Box with Mini Bar A–C*

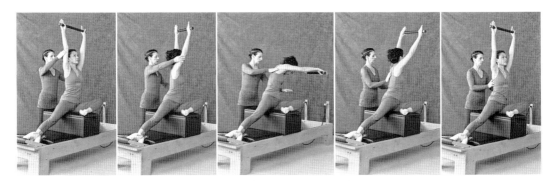

Figure 10.30

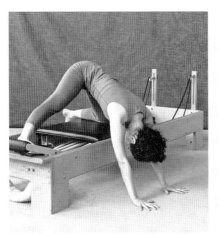

Figure 10.31

This side-bend series is different than the traditional Pilates exercise (Figure 10.30). The client sits on the Short Box with the hips in parallel (not the Pilates externally-rotated 'V' to balance pectineal length). Start on the concave side toward the pulleys for the first side. Use the eye cue. The PMME guides the client to hold the pole in a gentle grasp with mostly the fingers. Elongate the pole or Mini Bar into a side-bend. Then the PMME holds a forearm underneath the client's ribs for the client to rotate over. Attempt to get the shoulders even with the horizon. The client then changes hand grip on the pole so that the skin of the gently flexed fingers curls over the pole with the thumbs on the same side as the fingers. Next exhale and roll up the spine, allowing the weight of the pole or bar to stretch the fascia of the superficial back and spiral lines. Rotate back to the beginning pose. Repeat 4 times each side.

⚠ *Inverted abductions: A–D*

This exercise looks dramatic, yet most people can do it (Figure 10.31). Use the side with the less pelvic hip hike to begin. Place a sitting-box sideways against the shoulder rests. Use one blue spring and one red spring. Guide the client to place the hands and walk the knees onto the carriage and then down to the floor beside the Reformer. The client places one foot toward the front of the Reformer base on an angle across the edge of the base to hold the leg steady. The legs are in neutral rotation. Use the asymmetry cues as the client exhales and moves the carriage, abducting the hip repeatedly. Repeat about 10 times and perform the exercise on the other side.

Articulation

Exercise

⚠ *Dreaded Frog = open chain*

✅ *Wobble Board foot-to-core sequencing: A–E*

This series has four parts. It greatly benefits lining up a vertical stance between the legs and the torso, promoting foot-to-core sequencing. Use a wobble board with a flatter rather than rounded fulcrum on the bottom for safety (Figure 10.32).

- *Part 1.* Open the legs in parallel rotation. Stand on the edges of the board. Perform 3 motions. Rock side to side. Tilt the board front to back attempting to elevate the body with the heel lifts. Then trace the rim of the board in a circular motion, allowing the knees to bend spontaneously.

- *Part 2.* Place one foot in the middle of the apex of the fulcrum on the bottom. Bend the other leg. Do straight leg heel rises, tipping the board front to back yet emphasizing the elevation of the torso. Do about 15 repetitions.

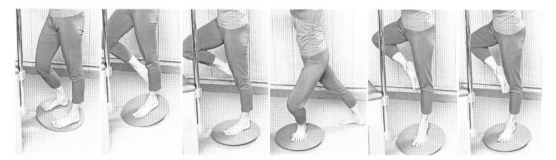

Figure 10.32

- *Part 3.* While standing on the same leg, rotate both hips, touching the little toe of the bent leg in front of the support knee. Next, rotate to parallel and touch the inside of the elevated foot on the inside of the support knee. Rotate out and in 10 times.

Continued

- *Part 4*. Remaining on the same leg, rotate to the Pilates 'V'. Step back with the elevated foot, placing on the floor behind the board. Then reverse the action and return the little toe in front of the support knee again. Do about 10 repetitions. Repeat the whole series, Parts 1–4, to the other side. Watch the video demonstration (Code 10.6).

Code 10.6 (free code)
Wobble board demonstration

Scolio-moves

Include some of these specific pelvic moves from Chapter 9. Watch them on the video (see Code 9.4).

- ☑ Diagonal Balloon Breathing
- ⚡ Rotational Z-sit progressions
- ⚡ Seaweed
- ☑ Icosahedron moves.

Stability of the pelvis with arm motion

☑ *Figure of eight with Magic Circle (Figure 10.33)*

Refer to Chapter 9 for the exercise instruction.

⚡ *Elongated Side Reaches*

⚡ *Elongated Rotations*

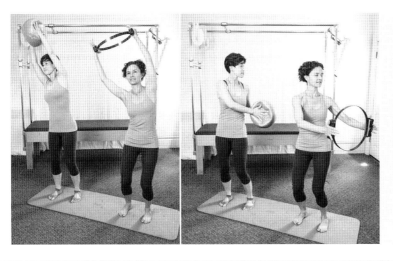

Figure 10.33

Correct the pattern: 3 Es into everyday life

"Practice means to perform, over and over again in the face of all obstacles, some act of vision, of faith, of desire. Practice is a means of inviting the perfection desired."

Martha Graham

Correcting the pattern is a dedication of love. The 3 Es of ergonomics, exercise and emotion along with Body Skills bring sensible spinal asymmetry management into everyday life. One joke is that while it is possible for an elephant to ride a unicycle, it definitely is a balancing act! Troubleshoot with the client by offering daily tools encouraging better back health habits that affect everyone, not just those with spinal asymmetry. Although training new habits seems artificial at first, requiring trial and error when faced with individual asymmetry and changes over time, the major benefit is taking control of one's comfort level in order to simply enjoy life.

Ergonomics

Ergonomics involves sitting, standing, walking, sleeping, and all the activities that revolve around those basic functions.

Sitting

Sitting is one of the most difficult activities for those with spinal asymmetry. It is critical to find individual strategies for work and leisure. The exercises strengthen and develop body awareness, yet fatigue onset naturally increases through the day. Try some of the strategies below.

Put it into practice

The use of a sitting orthotic, such as the Activ-Wedge®, helps to balance out the spine for more comfort. Place it underneath the heavier pelvic side on a diagonal between the IT and the coccyx. If the client has spinal fixation hardware, use trial and error because perhaps bolstering up the lighter pelvic side provides more relief.

Place a micro-bead thoracic pillow lengthwise behind the ribcage in the space between the shoulder blades toward the waist. Place a wedge underneath the forefoot of shorter leg (in line with the foot) while using an electronic device.

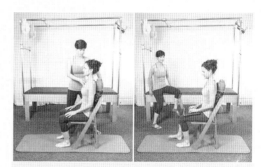

Figure 11.1

The use of a higher foot rest aiming to have the knees higher than the hips relieves swayback. A chair seat that is too high for the lengths of the legs also increases swayback. When a chair seat is too high, sit forward in the chair, bending forward from the hips, and consciously hold an erect spine. When fatigue sets in, change positions with the legs, use the Straw exercise as a Body Skill (see Figure 8.21).

Adjust an automobile seat in order to sit close to the pedals. Use a back rest in the low back area, usually placed horizontally across the lumbar spine. Place the head back against the headrest several times during the trip. Sitting with the seat too far from the pedals either increases dowager hump or over-emphasizes the lumbar curve.

TV slump leads to a dowager's hump and strains the neck and shoulders. A slumped, strained reading position in a head thrust position strains muscles of the head and neck.

Students need leg room underneath the desk top. Avoid sitting for long periods at lab tables where the legs are rotated in a direction not in line with the shoulders. When not typing or taking notes, sit with the pelvis back into the chair and bring the head over the pelvis to rest.

Standing

Good posture is not a simple matter of standing tall. It takes attention and practice. People with asymmetry perhaps do not understand that a good percentage of upright posture is a matter of choice. Several strategies help the navigation of standing. Image an optimal erect posture line dropped from the ear through the tip of the shoulder, middle of the pelvis, back of the kneecap (not the knee), and in front of the ankle. For asymmetrical individuals, a simple way to find this posture is with the ZOA and Inner Envelope maneuver from Chapter 8. The standing version of the Straw exercise, shown in sitting in Chapter 8, reinforces the ability to maintain the ZOA and Inner Envelope posture. These two skills are indispensable for standing comfort.

> ### Put it into practice
>
> Allow reasonable rest periods to prevent strain and pain in everyday activities. Compression and fatigue increases as the day increases. Lying down for even a quick 10-minute rest at midday or mid-afternoon refreshes both body and mind.
>
> Practice and reinforce both the Standing Straw exercise and ZOA and Inner Envelope Posture.
>
> When performing chores at a counter or kitchen sink, open the cabinet below and place a foot upon

the raised cabinet floor, or use a small stool to place underneath the foot of the concave waist side.

When performing chores that must lean over the work, bend the knees and brace the legs against the table or cabinet if able. Lean upon the forearms, bend at the hips (dissociate the pelvis from the legs). Lift the sternum and maintain the lordosis of the spine while initiating pull-up of the pelvic and abdominal muscular slings.

When visiting museums, attending standing social events, initiate the Straw exercise several times during the event. Alternate sitting with standing. Wear padded shoes with good supportive insoles. Avoid locking the knees to stand. Keep re-initiating the Straw exercise and ZOA and Inner Envelope posture. Start with the feet. Imagine the number 7 at the bottom of each foot. Press the weight onto the outsides of the heels. Hold that firm. Then press the first metatarsal into the floor, then the little toe side into the floor. Moving from the lateral heel to the first toe then to the little toe inscribes two mirror image number 7s underneath the feet. Then reach up sequentially through the spine as in the Straw exercise. In addition, wearing a back brace or compressive garment to add support when standing for long durations is helpful.

When holding heavy items, keep them close to the body at waist height if possible.

When bending down to the floor to pick up a heavy item, first guestimate the weight of the item before full lifting. Determine if help is needed. If not, bend from the knees and hips, keep the spine straight. A little humor with the term 'butt-ski out-ski' position gives clients a buzzword to remember. Most people know the phrase, lift from the legs. Be sure to engage the inner unit, then lift the item close to the body to carry it. Heavier loads separated into lighter loads always makes good spine sense. Use the legs, not the spine.

Teach the Arc arch with spinal roll in Chapter 12. Although reserved for those without current spinal issues besides the basic asymmetry, such as most youth and young adults, it is so helpful in coaching how to engage the pull-up and inner bracing needed for balance while the head is in an inverted position.

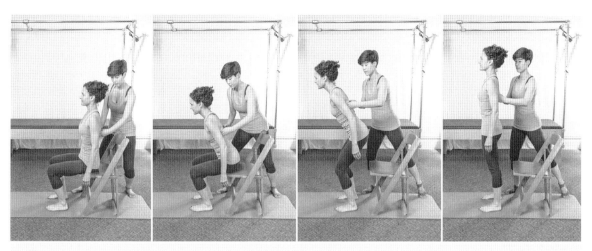

Figure 11.2

Transitioning sit to stand

Sit to stand is a movement everyone does naturally. However, those with spinal asymmetry need to
attend to good hip dissociation and spinal form along
with mixing up habits that often reinforce the internal twisting alien.

Put it into practice

Sit toward the edge of the chair. Lean forward in a
flat back, dissociating from the hips. Guide the client
from the ribcage to lift up on a diagonal with the nose
far forward of the knees in space. If there is a tendency to shift toward a certain leg, usually the longer
leg, guide the client toward a more middle position.
Encourage the ability to stand without using the
hands to push off from one side repetitively. Begin by
using the hands upon the thighs if the squat strength
is weak. Focus on the full extension of the hips at the
end of the stand phase to ensure that the pelvic stabilizers and Inner Envelope are active (Figure 11.2).

Stair stepping

Stair stepping is where pelvic obliquity is most apparent. The tensor fascia lata (TFL) balancing exercises
are helpful along with these strategies.

Put it into practice

Going up and down stairs is similar to the sit-to-
stand motion. Reinforce the ability to use the legs
and the pull-up of the core, jokingly referred to as
rump lifting. The paradox of stair climbing is that
the hamstrings and posterior fascial chain ideally
press downwards as the torso elevates upwards.
Keeping the chest lifted and using the legs and
trunk pull-up is the key. Think of the coccyx relating to the heel of the foot as the foot fully places
upon each step. Avoid toe-stepping where the foot
barely makes contact with the step. Engage the
pelvic stabilizers with the imagery of the magnets
between the sit bone connection and also each
sit bone relating to the coccyx to avoid hip hiking
on one particular side, usually the side with the
waist concavity.

General walking

Walking is the most fundamental of functional activities, but is complex in analysis. While full attention to
gait training is beyond the scope of this book, a quick
synopsis and tips for those with asymmetry help to
understand the basics.

Put it into practice

Slightly bend both knees with the shoulders upright. Place the heel of one foot ahead of the other. Activate the longitudinal posterior sling which includes the peronei, biceps femoris, sacrotuberous ligament, thoracodorsal fascia, and erector spinae, by everting the foot and dorsiflexing the ankle. Pointing the little toe to the sky, press the heel down into the floor and pull the heel in a backwards direction, keeping contact with the floor. This force elongates the upper torso and stabilizes the sacroiliac joint, engaging the inner thigh and hamstrings. Posterior sling strength is essential for acceleration, deceleration and speed necessary in most athletic activities. This motion brings the knee forward in line with the second toe, and activates the lateral sling (adductors, gluteus medius). The lateral sling gives stability in standing on one leg. Soften the foot. Stand on all four corners of the foot. This creates the tripod of the ankle/foot complex. Activating the adductors and the lateral sling also activates the anterior oblique sling of the hip adductors internal and external rotators along with abdominal fascia, allowing the free leg to swing forward. People with asymmetry need attention in this transfer, minimizing lateral shift of weight, helping to keep the body weight more centered. When both anterior oblique and lateral slings are activated, the hamstrings pull the pelvis into neutral from below while the abdominals pull the pelvis into neutral from above, creating a transfer of weight balance point. A visible 'scoop' of the lower abdominals, the hollow, occurs as the lower abdominals and pelvic stabilizers coordinate to allow the psoas to stabilize the trunk with momentum and/or forceful leg motion. Activating the gluteus medius (lateral sling) causes the gluteus maximus to also activate the posterior sling of the opposite gluteus maximus and contralateral latissimus dorsi. Contracting the posterior sling brings the shoulders back and also brings the pelvis back into neutral, and the cycle begins again (Gough, 2017; Lee, 1999).

Highlights for those with asymmetry include the engagement of the posterior sling, attention to the minimization of transfer of weight as one leg swings forward, and minimization of hip hike, the increase in pelvic obliquity when the longer leg strikes the ground.

Sleeping

Sleep habits, positions and bedding often confound those with spinal asymmetry due to the compromise between the need for a good night's sleep while attempting to not exacerbate the asymmetry. A little extra attention here goes a long way as many hours are spent in bed.

Put it into practice

Form good sleep habits. Winding down and getting proper rest is important for those with asymmetry due to the fatigue element. Even if young, reasonable rest is important.

Think of reading in bed to help to wind down and create the atmosphere needed for deep sleep. Lying supine on an angle with a pillow arrangement including a neck roll and low back support, and perhaps underneath the knees support, helps to keep the spine elongated in a semi-reclined position. Avoid sitting upright and hunching over the device or book.

Most people cannot sleep in one position throughout the night. However, train by beginning sleep in the supine position. Elevate the pelvis, wipe the low back from the ribs along the back of the pelvis to the legs and then lower the pelvis to find an elongated spine. It is advised to use one long pillow instead of many; however, having a variety of different small rolls can help during the night. The general rule of thumb is to always find the elongation while preserving the lumbar lordosis. Using the Balloon Breath, breathing for a minute or two before going off to sleep, settles the spine and promotes parasympathetic calmness.

When rolling to the side, bend the knees and move the shoulders at the same time with the pelvis to avoid twisting. Train to sleep mostly on the concave side of the waist. Place a pillow between the knees and flex the hips slightly to take pressure off the low back.

There is also the three-quarter pose option. From the side, roll back and place a long pillow behind the shoulders and pelvis to take pressure off the side, allowing relief for the back from too long of a duration upon the back.

Avoid habitual sleeping on the stomach. Use this position for a brief relief position. Lie prone, then perform the Ice Cube exercise, tightening the abdominals and gluteals. Elongate the body and then change to another position. If prone is indicated due to a sacral issue or disc herniation, wedge the whole torso with double bed pillows underneath the trunk and let the legs fall below the horizon level of the trunk. Place the hands underneath the forehead or use a rolled towel underneath the forehead and breathe in this position and try to sleep for a while.

Bedding makes a huge difference. A topper on a medium to heavy mattress is preferred over foam mattresses since falling into the foam perhaps increases the spinal twist.

Staying in bed too long also takes a toll. Asymmetric spines do better with motion. Remaining sedentary more than three days is not advised during painful episodes. Walking is *the* spinal health exercise. Get enough aerobic activity to ensure enough fatigue in order to sleep through the night.

Waking up through the night is common with spinal asymmetry. Use long duration breathing, the Balloon Breathing exercise, to calm down and return to sleep. Long exhalations of 15 counts with the tongue placed on the upper soft palate relaxes the mind. Feel the bedclothes with the fingers and the toes and literally think, this feels good, to pull the mind away from the pain side of the pain–pleasure continuum toward the pleasure end.

Exercise

The third part of this book is devoted to the framework of the basic spinal asymmetry and scoliosis program. One element of a program is how to implement it. Daily maintenance of breaking up pattern is similar to brushing the teeth, a daily habit that greatly aids general health. The PMME begins the training of these habits with the initial education and adds on for daily homework as the client progresses in understanding. Habit formation takes a dedicated input in the initial phases yet becomes more efficient as time goes on and skill level improves. A daily maintenance format combined with corrective exercises formulated from the GPOA and SPPOT, the use of Body Skills, selections from the neurodevelopmental

sequence along with additions to address comorbidities and conditions comprise an individualized program. Chapter 12 gives more detail on programming for the individual.

Daily basic maintenance

Several basics are critical to daily maintenance:

- Use of the scoliosis cues: dominant eye closed and tongue position for all or part of any exercise
- Core Pillow pelvic motions from Chapter 9
- Side hip shifts from Chapter 9
- Ring overhead lengthen daily (see Figure 10.33)
- Wobble board use from Chapter 10 (see Figure 10.32 and Code 10.6)
- Daily stretch for opening the Deep Frontal Facial Line
- Stand in a doorframe, facing away from a Trapeze Table or from a ballet barre. Lean forward and breathe. Watch the video for this exercise which starts my mat class (Code 11.1).
- Mat 'C' exercise from Spinal Solutions in Chapter 10
- Sidelying knee bends from Spinal Solutions in Chapter 10.

Code 11.1 (free code)
Wobble board demonstration

Baker's Dozen Body Skills

Body Skills are essential skills not only for training with the client but also in daily management of asymmetry. Watch the video for ideas on how to coach Body Skills with clients (Code 11.2).

Code 11.2 (free code)
Body skills explanation

Put it into practice

Relieving techniques. Outlined in the ergonomics section, bracing with pillows, compressive garments, breathing and positioning, such as constructive rest from Chapter 8, help along with a dedicated health-care team.

Breath. Concentration on development of functional breathing and potentiating the concave areas of the ribcage are primary as in Chapters 7, 8 and 9.

Acquiring strength and coordination of the the Inner Unit. Aligning the best vertical spinal alignment: optimize ZOA posture, organize the four diaphragms, and reduce gravitational stress upon asymmetric structures, as in Chapter 8.

Re-training stance through behavior modification in order to automatically assume the *1st Position Parallel* with legs about 2.5 inches (5 cm apart) and toes facing for

Unlocking laterality and preferences. Changing daily habits includes breaking up fascial patterns and directional biases. Scolio-moves, such as describing a figure of eight in space with a Magic Circle, cross the body's mid-line, an important element in breaking up rotational favoritism. Scolio-move demonstrations appear in Chapters 9, 10, and 12.

Stimulating the vertical spinal reflexes two ways. Balance point exercises in seated position on the ischial tuberosities, as in Chapters 7 and 10, increase segmental multifidi engagement. The Straw exercise from Chapter 8 establishes sitting and standing postural muscle reactivation when fatigued.

Bringing the head over the center of pelvic gravity. Coordinate the postural muscular slings of the Deep Frontal Line along with the Posterior Slings to oppose the exacerbating dominance of the spinal erectors, because those with spinal asymmetry perhaps are unable to fully straighten the spine. Finding the head over the pelvic center of gravity is a good second option. Multifidi training brings the head over the center of gravity as well as using the ZOA postural cues to connect the xiphoid to the sacrum.

Dissociation of the pelvis from the legs. This skill interrupts the compensatory leg patterns reinforcing the spinal curvature. Learning to squat is an essential element to protective spinal body mechanics. Functional solutions for the spine and pelvis in Chapter 10 offer many opportunities to train this skill. Implementing the concept daily prevents spinal exacerbations.

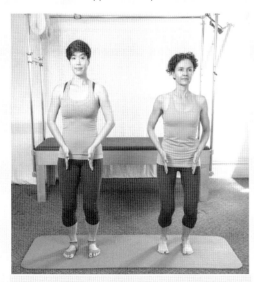

Figure 11.4

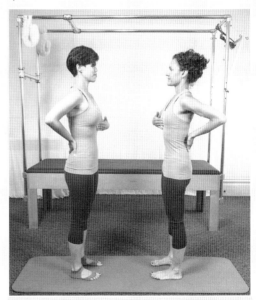

Figure 11.3

Coordinating the ankle/foot complex with pelvic movement. Foot-to-core sequencing begins with finding the pelvic stabilizers in the Core Pillow exercises and continues with wobble board reinforcement in Chapter 10.

Striving toward the equalization of transfer of weight in gait. Minimizing in particular one-sided preference in stance and walking lessens strain on hip, knees, ankles, and feet. Pelvic solutions along with attention to gait pattern in the previous Ergonomics section address these issues.

Adding asymmetry cues and neurological aids. Although not mandatory for every exercise or continual use, done periodically these break up vestibular and compensatory dominance. Combining the use of the wedge in various positions along with the eye and tongue placement complete the whole-body experience for a whole-body condition. Training with the client then empowers the client for independent use in stance. For instance, the y-axis cues help both to lengthen the shorter leg as well as control anterior rib protrusion. The z-axis attention lengthens the concave waist and extends the quadratus lumborum at the waist, correcting the anterior hemi-pelvic hip joint. The x-axis optimally connects with the ZOA posture of connecting the sacral base with the xiphoid area. Ease comes with practice.

Use of the body orientations of the neurodevelopmental sequence. Begin the initial foundation found in Chapter 8 and continue through Chapter 10. Although it is not necessary to employ each position in each session, the three-dimensional aspect of spinal asymmetry warrants not only a three-dimensional but also the fourth-dimension fascial engagement approach.

Adapting mat exercises such as the Side Kicks for the spinal asymmetry population is one example of how to use the neurodevelopmental concept with traditional Pilates Method mat exercises (Figure 11.5). Propping on the forearm elongates the spine. Watch the video (Code 11.3).

Code 11.3 (free code)
Adapted mat Side Kicks

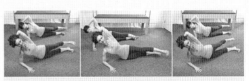

Figure 11.5

Emotion

Everyone experiences emotions. The PMME influences both physical and emotional development of clients. Spinal asymmetry influences each person in a different way, some more than others. Four areas where PMMEs help include breathing exercises, the choice of exercise body positions, vocalization and interoception, the recognition of how one feels in relation to a body experience. Deliver the suggestions in a detached yet compassionate matter-of-fact way. Over-focus on a particular element of distress is not always in the best interest of the client. Have a licensed psychology counselor in your referral list to steer appropriate clients toward the emotional help needed to realize their physical goals. Here are some tips on how to address the four main emotional areas.

Put it into practice

Breathing exercises

Breathing guidance is a part of all Pilates Method exercises. The very act of conscious breathing, particularly attention to the number of breaths per minute and style, begins a pull toward the parasympathetic nervous system, as opposed to the sympathetic fight or flight pathway. However, match the breath to the motion – a running theme throughout all the exercises.

Choice of body positions and qualitative motion

Certain movements align with four common emotions of anger, fear, happiness and sadness. Insight relating to clientele body language is helpful along with how to re-direct a client in a positive way.

- *Anger* movements are strong, sudden, direct and advancing, meaning coming closer into personal space. Notice cues of dislike of space invasion. Keep cue guidance and demonstrations slow and smooth. Encourage smooth motion in the mid-range. The three salient characteristics to upend anger are slow, controlled and mid-range. Help a client at times of disappointment during injury or discovering limitations that often sets off anger.

- *Fear* is a cousin of anxiety, a prevalent emotion in society. People usually seek out the Pilates Method (PM) because of concern. Fear movements are retreating backwards, shrinking, binding, and enclosing. Certain PM repertoires involve leaning backwards and flexing the spine, and require stability, a sort of binding. For this reason, be sure to re-frame the Pilates repertoire to highlight its expansive nature. For instance, emphasize the leaning backwards in the Reformer Rowing Series as an elongating motion by focusing on the sternal lift in the tilt. For spinal flexion, emphasize the elongation of a Trapeze Bar Roll-down by helping the client feel the traction of the action. Emulate the traction upon the return curl-up. Always strive to create the most elongated flexion. The Twisty Cat modification on the Reformer teaches the deepening of the anterior body as the thighs remain attached to the foot bar upon the return of the Reformer carriage after the spinal extension. When giving stability exercise, focus on the term engagement rather than contract. Emphasize the lengthening anti-gravitational nature of the muscles rather than the shortening nature of muscle pull.

- *Happiness* is an elusive mood state associated with rhythmicity, verticality, upwards motion, jumps and ease of motion. The rhythmic motion of the Standing Disc Rotations, Core Pillow rocks, the Magic Circle hip shifts, leg motions of the Wobble Board and Footwork all contribute to an increased sense of contentment and lightness. Any glide on the Reformer serves this purpose. Training verticality with the Chair Psoas Pumps, the Balancing 'O' or the simple Straw exercise empower the client to move up and out of the vortex of the spinal asymmetry. Following the protocol of beginning one-sided exercises into the direction of ease makes the more challenging side just a little bit more doable.

- *Sadness* is both warranted during periods of grief and loss and perhaps is an unwelcome, unwarranted emotion when grappling with an irregular body. Signs of sadness are passivity, sinking, head lowering and arm hugging. Emphasizing the proactive nature of lifestyle management rather than the crisis aspect of asymmetry care empowers the individual. Everyone improves, and everyone close to the individual benefits. Integrate multiple aspects of wellness involving school, play or work into the client's personal goals, inspiring variety and consistency over a duration of time. Most clients begin with hope, but faith in the process requires fostering. Give the client an anchor by repeating the mantra of imagine, think, and feel as a strategy of movement acquisition. Repeat the mantra at each time of challenge. Be sure to include the happiness movements in both the studio and home use. This is why particularly simple motions, such as the Core Pillow and Magic Circle exercises, performed regularly renew the quest against the gravitational pull of the internal alien (Shafir et al., 2016).

An added element to emotional stability is vagal nerve stimulation. Humming, vocalizing, and use of the eyes in an upwards direction all encourage parasympathetic activity. Incorporate this concept simply by directing the eyes up during selected exercises such as Twisty Cat or even Chair with Pike. Encourage humming as a lung or breathing exercise (Porges et al., 1994).

Although emotions are not shaped and trained like muscles, learning to recognize and acknowledge our emotions helps us to understand the physiological responses to them, and not become overwhelmed by them.

Bibliography

Gough, M. (2018). Functional training for the posterior chain. Retrieved August 22, 2018, from: http://trainingdimensions. net/tdArticles/Functional%20Training%20for%20the%20 Posterior%20Chain.pdf

Lee, D. (1999). The Pelvic Girdle : An Approach to the Examination and Treatment of the Lumbo-Pelvic-Hip Region. London: Churchill Livingstone

Porges, S.W., Doussard-Roosevelt, J.A., Maiti. A. K. (1994). Vagal tone and the physiological regulation of emotion. Monographs of the Society for Research in Child Development, 59(2–3), 167. Retrieved August 14, 2018, from ResearchGate: https://www.researchgate. net/publication/15215400_Vagal_Tone_and_the_ Physiological_Regulation_of_Emotion

Shafir, T, Tsachor, R., Welch, K. (2016). Emotion regulation through movement: unique sets of movement characteristics are associated with and enhance basic emotions. Frontiers in Psychology, 6(2030), 9–11

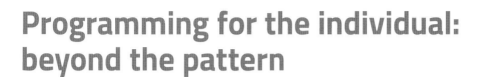

Programming for the individual: beyond the pattern

It is not necessary to have an encyclopedic knowledge of every condition to be a safe and effective PMME. In addition to the actual spinal aberration of the scoliosis, both youth and adults present with a wide variety of confounding and overlapping conditions, illnesses and diseases beyond the scoliosis itself. Referred to as comorbidities, PMMEs aid or support these simultaneously occurring situations. Due to the number and complexity of possible scenarios, several are listed here with possible programming suggestions and formats.

PMMEs can rest assured that comorbidities benefiting from the Method include juvenile rheumatoid arthritis (Svantesson et al., 1981), fibromyalgia (Altan et al., 2009), multiple sclerosis (van der Linden, 2014), Parkinson's disease (Which Pilates exercises are good for someone with Parkinson's disease?, 2017) and osteoporosis (Betz, 2005).

There are also conditions that coexist with and are linked to scoliosis such as abnormalities in chest development. A common one is pectus excavatum, where the sternum is sunken inside the medial ribs, indicating tight pectoral muscles as well as impacting the deep and superficial fascial arm lines. These clients must be followed by cardiologists and pulmonologists due to the pressure being exerted on the heart and lungs (Jaroszweski et al., 2010).

Another condition is Straight Spine Syndrome, where the sagittal curves either do not develop fully or the curves alter and lessen due to prior surgery and/or emerging spinal bone pathology (Virginia Spine Institute, 2017).

Individualized programs fluctuate between general applications for asymmetry training and the needs of specific comorbidities and conditions requiring urgent attention.

Do not focus upon the asymmetry when other comorbid issues take priority, including those with post-operative spinal fixation. Reserve asymmetry training for later when the client is more able to focus upon the asymmetry. A whole Medical Team is indispensable at certain times.

General applications of asymmetry training include creation of the individual asymmetry profile and cues from the assessments. Next, proceed to individual correctives and initial education with and without the use of wedges. Then include exercises in neurodevelopmental positions as well as standing and gait promotion.

Follow the mantra: identify the curves, break up the curves, re-direct the curves, correct the curves, and go beyond the curves. Going beyond the curves implies prioritization of either addressing impending factors first that interfere with asymmetry training as well as detailing more aspects involved with body type, time of life issues, surgical history and other comorbidities such as frailty, osteoporosis, spinal pathology, osteoarthritis, or other conditions such as autoimmune and neurologic conditions.

Creating cues from the assessments

The asymmetry cues, starting from the top to the bottom, include eye dominance, tongue position, head over center of gravity, concave waist elongation, anterior rib protrusion, hip-hike/sit-bone control, 1st position parallel leg position, weight into shorter leg/ pelvic stabilizer use and tripod of the feet. The use of the yoga strap with the Inner Unit exercise and initial line of the spine supine compressions are two great ways to ingrain the multiple cues. Start with a few and add on from there.

Precautions

Observe ☑, indicating the exercise is permitted for those with spinal fixation. The symbol ⚠ indicates the exercise is a contraindicated movement for those with fixation. Follow the degree guidelines listed with the exercises.

> *Degree guidelines for severity of the Cobb angle*
>
> **A** = 0–10° Normal expected degree of spinal asymmetry
>
> **B** = 10–20° Mild
>
> **C** = 21–40° Moderate
>
> **D** = >40° Severe
>
> **E** = >70° Severe with possible medical breathing issues.

Some clients who have not had spinal surgery are skeletally stiff due to the shapes of the convexities and abnormal bone growth along with body general body type or operative fixation devices. Adults in general stiffen with age. For this reason, avoid movements within the repertoire that are particularly difficult for scoliosis and abnormal spines.

An abnormal spine is any that is not aligned with the usual central vertical spinal line with typical gravitational curves. Start with neutral and expand from there. The Arc stretches in Chapter 9 aid in acquiring pliability within reason over time to advance past neutral posture strength toward larger orientation movements.

The following is a repertoire known for its difficulty with this population, along with some replacements. Start with the substitution options until the client shows more proficiency in understanding how to maneuver the spine and ribcage.

> *Arc stretches from Chapter 8.* The Arc stretches are contraindicated for operative clients. Substitute Trapeze Table Roll-down/Roll-up for stiff non-operative clients.

> *Mermaid on the Reformer or Chair.* Substitute selections include Mat Thoracic Mobilizers, standing disc rotations, Twisty Cat on the Trapeze Table from Chapter 10 or the modification on the long box on the Reformer listed under the Hip and knee replacement section in this chapter. Begin Mermaid after working on these exercises for at least a month.

> *Short spine/long spine.* Navigating the transition points presents challenges until the client achieves controlled flexion, therefore substitute the Roll-down on the Trap Table with the wedges from Chapter 10. Begin to attempt these flexions after the client navigates the Roll-down and the Twisty Cat repertoire with control.

> *The Twist on the Reformer.* The pretzel shape with the hands and feet fixed and the carriage glides into full body spinal rotation should be avoided in general, even if the client is an advanced mover.

> *Rolling like a ball/Seal.* Replace these with the lateral rolling from Chapter 9 until the client accomplishes controlled flexion.

Pain

When pain is present, perform relieving somatic exercise. Be sure to consult with the Medical Team as necessary.

- Positional release with props in Chapter 9
- Balloon Breathing in Chapter 8
- Imprinting Compressions from Chapter 9.

Sacral instability

Postnatal clients often experience sacral instability. Be sure to consult with the Medical Team as necessary:

- Prone sacral stabilizers from Chapter 8
- Constructive rest from Chapter 8
- Inner Unit performed independently from Chapter 8.

Youth, hypermobility, females and athletics

Youth

⚡ *SSPOT-2: A–D*

The SSPOT-2 assessments from Chapter 7 provide a template on how to proceed with youth. Use the foundational Initial Education from Chapter 8 to train the correct form for the SSPOT-2. The Pelvic imbalance solutions from the SSPOT-1 are more appropriate for adults.

A typical beginning-to-intermediate program for non-operated, without spinal fixation, youth is as follows.

Exercise

All the exercises include the asymmetric cues:

- Arc stretching with One-lung Breathing from Chapter 9
- SSPOT-2 selected exercises starting with Planks three ways, using the concepts of initial education from Chapters 7 and 8
- Mat: wedge compressions from Chapter 8
- Balloon with pelvic bridge from Chapter 9
- Arc Prone Swimming from Chapter 10
- SSPOT-2: X-rolls from Chapter 7
- Spine Corrector – fall and release with dowel or Mini Bar from Chapter 10
- Chair Psoas Pumps from Chapter 10
- Reformer reverse abdominals from Chapter 10
- Figure of eight with Magic Circle for crossing mid-line development from Chapter 9
- Dreaded Frog circles and scissors from Chapter 10
- ⚡ Sidelying Hang with Pull-up: A–C. For detail see below.

⚡ *Sidelying Hang with Pull-up: A–C*

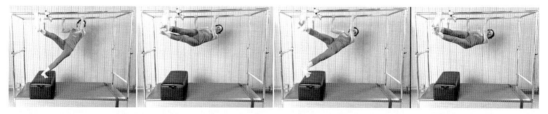

Figure 12.1

Challenge the youth with this exercise, combining strength with elongation. It is an advanced version of the SSPOT-2 Sidelying Shooting Star Hip Lift. The PMME must guarantee enough strength to spot the youth appropriately. Follow these stages to prepare the youth for the ultimate exercise:

Continued

- First, test the grip strength. Wipe the hands and place gripping liner on the overhead rails. Cue the youth to stand in the middle, gripping the overhead rails with one hand on each rail at the sides.

- Keep the elbows bent, bend the knees and test how the hands hold the body weight.

- Cue some pull-ups.

- Place the Short Box on the table. Cue the client to face the Box, stand upon the Box and perform pull-ups again with both feet on the Box.

- The last stage tests pull-up strength with one foot in the loop and the other remaining on the Box.

Once this action of using both hands (one on either side of the table) feels secure, try the one-sided hang.

Start with the hands in place and the feet in the middle of the table. Spot the client and cue moving the hands onto the outside of the overhead rail. Both hands hook onto the overhead rail behind the foot in the loop.

Important: be sure to use the stronger arm first as the arm farthest away from the feet. Keeping the elbows very bent is critical for safety since this keeps the biceps brachii in the best mechanical advantage for strength. The farthest hand is curled *underneath* the rail. The hand closest to the feet grips *over* the rail.

Walk up the Box, turn sideways toward the table, and place the top leg into the *front* loop. Be sure to dorsiflex the ankle strongly to keep it in the loop. Next, prepare to spot the client by climbing up onto the table bed. Support the client's pelvis. Cue the bottom leg to lift. Support the leg. Cue the client to perform pull-ups. As the client gets stronger, cue the client to open and close the legs while the arms perform the pull-ups. Perform 4 repetitions on each side.

☑ *Reformer Feet in Straps Leg Circles, Bow and Arrow, Frog: A–D**

*Since these Reformer exercises are typical Pilates repertoire, they are not described in detail.

⚡ Trapeze Table Arc arch with spinal roll

This incorporates the Squat and Roll-up from the SSPOT-2, described here (A–D).

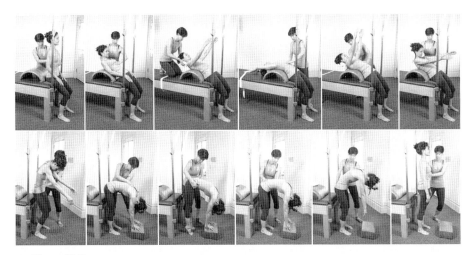

Figure 12.2

An excellent ending to a session, the Arc arch with spinal roll calms down the back after a workout as well as training proper stance. Place an Arc close to the end of the table. Guide the client to sit at the end.

Press the spine back onto the Arc. Slip the hands underneath the belly belt. Splay the hands. Control the inner pelvis with a pelvic parachute lift. Engage the solar plexus. Keep the shoulders away from the ears as much as possible but narrow the arms toward the head. Breathe 3 times.

On the next exhalation, release the hands. Reach the hands up to the ceiling. Cue the client to look down the expanse of the body. Reach the hands toward the wall in front of the feet. Peel off the Arc. Deepen the abdominals. Hollow and reach the hands to the floor or to a small box. Guide the pelvis upwards at the anterior superior iliac spine (ASIS). Cue the client to brace for balance with pelvis cues and weight into the fingers. Cue the client to elevate the heels; hold the hollow above the pubic bone. Then twist one elbow and hand up to the ceiling. Place it back down. Then twist the other way. Cue the tailbone to become heavy, the head is heavy. Then guide the tail to drop heavily with a coccyx to heel connection. And roll up. Repeat this sequence twice more.

For the hypermobile individual

Hypermobility is a poorly understood connective tissue condition. A hypermobile joint is one that moves beyond an expected flexibility range when observed with the eyes or measured with a goniometer. Although not a scoliosis or asymmetric-specific condition, scoliosis often accompanies joint hypermobility. It is more prevalent in single curve scoliosis. Controversy exists over whether increasing spinal mobility through exercise for those with scoliosis is appropriate. As previously referenced by Dr Martha Hawes, over-stretching for those with a spinal asymmetry is not advised. Especially for those with hypermobility, an already loose spinal segment could lead to actual joint instability causing pain, loss of true joint function and possibly the need for surgery.

Do not confuse the words instability and unstable! Spinal physicians use the term instability to indicate that a joint or a motion segment (three vertebrae in a row) is literally dismantling from coupled motion and falling apart to some degree. The term unstable means lack of stability, which in the world of the PMME and PT means unable to exert core and joint control.

Healthy hypermobile joints do exist. However, a person who does not understand their hypermobility runs the risk of injury. The wise PMME's job is to help the client function within their best mechanical zone, strengthening mid-range motions while avoiding an unsupported end joint range.

Coordination, motor control and special attention to all joint proper mechanics matters. Use the guide in Chapter 7 to gauge the hypermobility level (Knight et al., 2012). The Ehlers-Danlos society recently presented new classifications for hypermobility. PMMEs should familiarize themselves with this condition if working with this population (EDS International Classification, 2017; Czaprowski et al., 2012).

Exercise

A typical curriculum of exercises includes:

- Organize and stabilize the ankle/foot complex with the wobble board from Chapter 10.
- Organize and stabilize the wrists using the image of a claw hand (Figure 12.3). Place the cupped hand on the foot bar with the thumbs on the same side as the fingers, if possible, in Long Stretch, Jackrabbit, and similar exercises. Avoid sole contact with the heels of the hands with the wrists extended on the bar.

Continued

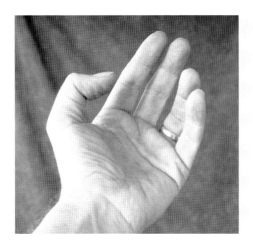

Figure 12.3
The claw hand posture aids a neutral wrist position.

- Sidelying bar fall and release on Trapeze Table from Chapter 10.
- Chair Psoas Pumps in Chapter 10.

Concentrate on stable isometric spine:

- Inner Unit from Chapter 8
- No-spring abs from Chapter 10
- Reformer carriage push out from base:
  - Start from the Inner Unit position facing the pulleys on the carriage. Use one red and one blue spring. Push out the carriage. Glide from a triangle position to a plank 3 times, then return the carriage to the base through the Inner Unit pose.

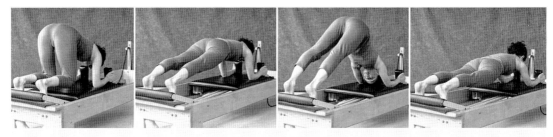

Figure 12.4

- Adductor balancing in stance: this exercise is beneficial for valgus knees. Simply place the ball as high in between the legs as possible. Stand in 1st Parallel. Perform a small squat. Then repeat elevating and lowering the heels with extended knees. Repeat both 6 times (see Figure 12.5).
- Weighted ball exercise from Chapter 10.
- Spine Corrector full side-bend with pole from the Youth section.

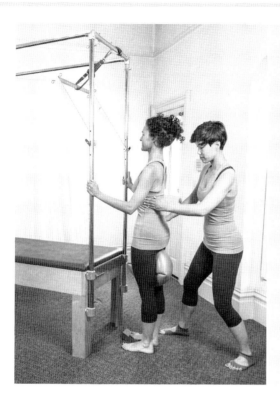

Figure 12.5

- Chair Psoas Pumps from the Youth section (see Figure 10.4).
- Arc arch with spinal roll from the Youth section (see Figure 12.2).

Fascial stretches

Several stretches are included here for youth and may be appropriate for others, especially those associated with the performing arts. Note that those with hypermobility also need fascial stretching in order to avoid tight muscles pulling and potentially dislocating joints. One general benefit of stretching the hips and legs is that often a person wishing to use or acquire the stretch needed for performance over-stretches the spine instead of the legs and hips. Attempt to keep a neutral spine through these stretches.

Youth benefit from stretching because of the opportunity to make significant changes before adulthood impact the lumbar spine. Learning foam roller, ball body-rolling and stick fascial self-release is invaluable in promoting beneficial stretch and circulation. It potentiates direct stretching, as demonstrated here.

The full scope of stretch acquisition is beyond the scope of this book. Refer to my other titles, such as *Stretching*, for more detailed programs. A complete stretch acquisition program for performance entails floor stretches, barre stretches and foot-in-hand standing stretches.

Stretches on the Trapeze Table to promote hip dissociation are demonstrated here.

Front stretches

Stand on the Trapeze Table. Keep the legs in neutral hip rotation in the 1st Parallel position (Figure 12.6).

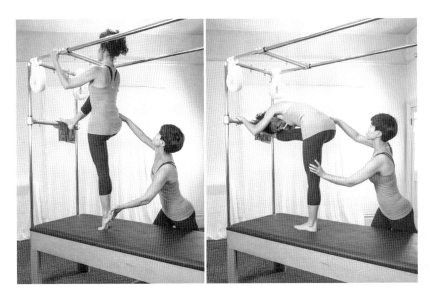

Figure 12.6

- Start with the easier side first. Place one foot on the sliding side bar. Lunge up, elevating the standing heel, flexing deeply into the front leg's hip. Attempt to keep the pelvis square, not shifting out to either side. Feel the stretch on the standing side's front of pelvis. Breathe for 5 breath cycles.

- Alternate by lowering the standing heel, straightening the top knee without locking it. Attempt to bow the head toward the top knee.

- Check the distance between the legs. Avoid swaying to one side. Breathe for 5 breath cycles. Repeat twice more and change to the other side.

Side stretches

For the side, place one foot upon the side bar and hold onto the overhead bars (Figure 12.7). Be sure the stance leg is behind the level of the foot upon the bar, otherwise the hip will hike. Guide the support knee in line with the second toe of the foot. The legs are in the Pilates 'V' shape, not parallel. Bend both legs and breathe for 6 breath cycles. Straighten up and repeat once more.

Leg stretches to the back

- The Trapeze Table makes this stretch possible (Figure 12.8). Place the top of one foot upon the sliding side bar. Padding helps here. Then turn away from the foot, hold onto the overhead rails.

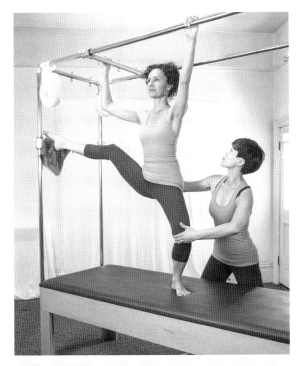

Figure 12.7

- Walk the hands and hop the foot more away from the back foot to achieve the full line. The legs are in the Pilates 'V'. Bend and straighten

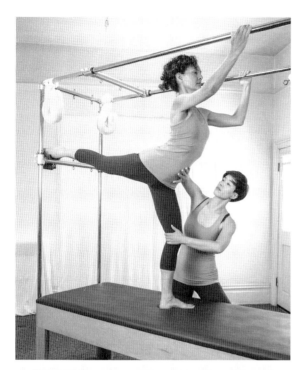

Figure 12.8

the bottom knee. Cue the lift from the anterior pelvis up through the respiratory diaphragm and support the body weight with the arms to keep the spine from compression.

- Recall the presentation by Dr Peter Lewton-Brain (see Ch. 3, p. 35) of the intent for this movement.

Programming for the athlete

Youth or adults engaging in athleticism need extra conditioning and balancing in the legs with these exercises:

- Weighted ball from Functional solutions for the pelvis in Chapter 10

- Wobble Board series from Functional solutions for the pelvis in Chapter 10.

Scoliosis: the female experience

Scoliosis and pelvic pain

Scoliosis is associated with female pelvic pain. The PMMEs usually receive education in the support for prenatal and postnatal clients, and often breast cancer support. This is a situation where the PMME definitely needs a Team. However, the following gives the PMME insight as to a number of conditions associated with spinal asymmetry.

Pelvic pain often arises from increased or decreased tone in internal or external hip rotators, hip flexor shortness and myofascial abnormalities.

Symptom areas of pelvic floor pain include the suprapubic, perineal, pelvic floor, or deep rectal regions.

Evidence suggests the rate of pelvic pain is higher for those with scoliosis than without. Pelvic pain and low back pain are often interrelated due their proximity. Scoliosis can influence pelvic joint alignment, tone of pelvic muscles and the relationship of nerves to surrounding tissue (Tate, 2015).

Scoliosis and pregnancy

The PMME should be aware of the multiple risks that increase during pregnancy for those with scoliosis. Breathing may be impacted and require ventilatory support due to difficulty adapting to the natural upward displacement of the diaphragm which may reduce vital capacity and residual volume of the lungs.

Know that a PMME needs to take extra steps with not only pregnancy and scoliosis, but even more so with those with the hypermobility of EDS. These clients are at high risk for uterine hemorrhages or rupture, miscarriage, and premature deliveries due to cervical incompetence.

At delivery time, those with a severe scoliosis may not be able to have spinal anesthesia. The PMME helps by encouraging the use of, and coordinating with, the midwife, doula, or other providers to prepare the client for a safe birth.

The PMME's role is to concentrate on educating the client on center of gravity shifts as well as focusing on joint comfort during sessions as well as in home and work life (McNaughton et al., 2008).

Scoliosis and pelvic organ prolapse

Women with scoliosis, and especially so if they also exhibit hypermobility, are at risk for pelvic organ prolapse (POP). This is where the connective tissue ligaments become too weak or unbalanced due to the alteration of loads from an unbalanced spinal column. As a result, the bladder, vagina, urethral or rectal areas literally 'fall out of place,' as the Latin term prolapse suggests.

Urinary incontinence is a common symptom of this condition. Evidence suggests that typical Kegels do not help these conditions. Where singular Kegel exercises may not completely address the stretched fascial slings, a sophisticated PMME has the potential to give comprehensive attention to full pelvic core health (Women's International Pharmacy, 2013).

For clients with any prolapse (uterus, vagina, bladder or rectum), it is critical to avoid spinal rolling where the client's body weight bears down upon a moving pelvis, such as in Roll-downs, until pelvic pull-up control is closely achieved.

Use the image of attempting to lift a raisin up inside the pelvic floor to begin. Explain the four bony points at the bottom of the pelvis, the two sit bones, the pubis and the tail. In sitting, bring the pubis to the tail (puborectalis) and one sit bone to the other (ischio-coccygeus/coccygeus/quadratus femoris).

Then imagine lifting the soft tissue between the sit bone to the tail (ischiococcygeus) toward the head (posterior pelvic floor), as if bungee cords were attached to the raisin, and elevate it toward the head.

Another simpler version is to imagine the front, urinal area and the back rectal areas floating like a parachute toward the head. Working in supine with a neutral spine and exercises from the preceding section with emphasis on neutral spine priority all work for this population.

Sidelying exercises are especially beneficial to keep internal organ pressure out of gravitational load. Focus also on single leg standing exercise using the bungee cord pull-up image and the left of the posterior pelvic floor.

Clients with prolapse may need to use a pessary device, a removable medical device similar to the outer ring of a diaphragm, to control the condition. Be sure you know what device is being used and are aware of any recommendations from the Medical Team.

Scoliosis, osteoporosis and athleticism

Osteoporosis is certainly correlated with aging, especially in post-menopausal women, but with men as well. In fact, men catch up with women in their risk at the age of 70 (Osteoporosis in men, 2017).

For women, scoliosis tends to be associated with osteoporosis due to its association with a low BMI. In addition, osteoporosis is associated with athleticism in females. The American College of Sports Medicine in 1998 produced a position paper on this issue, identifying three possible interrelated risks for females participating in sports: amenorrhea (disruption or loss of menstrual periods), eating disorders, and osteoporosis (The Female Athlete Triad, 2011). Scoliosis is also potentially associated with abnormalities in bone-cell-binding enzymes such as calmodulin (Rowe, 2004).

A young woman in her 30s is still in a bone-building life stage and requires a different approach than a 50- or 60-year-old with osteoporosis, who is perhaps more fragile.

At a meeting of FORE (Foundation for Osteoporosis and Research), an endocrinologist opined that when bone-thinning begins, in its first decade the wrist is most at risk for fracture. In the second decade of bone-thinning, it is the thoracic spine, and in the third decade, it is the hip. For this reason, concentrate on mat arm-weight-bearing exercises such as the rotisserie planks of the SSPOT-2. Be sure to include a number of prone exercises and the prone pelvic functional exercises from Chapter 10.

Younger women (adolescence and girlhood)

Younger women are at risk for the consequences of low bone density due to the problems of the Athlete Triad, discussed above, in combination with the issues of adolescent idiopathic scoliosis (low BMI, stress fractures and stress reactions, or a less-than-fracture bone injury) (The Female Athlete Triad, 2011; Burwell, et al., 2009).

Furthermore, in younger women with scoliosis, identification of osteopenia (thinning of the bones) or osteoporosis is difficult since traditional screening begins at post-menopause.

For young women and girls, preventive conditioning and functional training, using the Pilates Method as a gateway to larger exercise, combines to avoid joint injury as well as limit accidents that could lead to fracture (Borghuis et al., 2008).

General adult practice and modifications

Begin with assessments from Chapter 7 to provide a template on how to proceed. Establish the asymmetry cues and begin with the pelvic imbalance correctives appropriate to the client, which dovetail with the initial education positions from Chapter 8.

Adults tend to lose the ability to lift their center of gravity in the pelvis, a useful skill for balance and a

necessary skill to be able to stand up from the floor. They also have more compensations due to typical life injuries such as ankle sprains and childbirth trauma.

Be conservative with expanding the range of the spine since osteoarthritis is common with aging. Use discretion with the Arc stretches from Chapter 8. Substitute the disc rotations from Chapter 10 to safely open fascial lines instead if stiffness is present. Use the wedges in a variety of the neurodevelopmental positions from Chapters 8 and 10 to allow time for a learning curve in body awareness to use the asymmetry cues appropriately.

Expect slower progress. Focus on spinal elongation and de-compression. A typical beginning program for an adult in general without focus on a present issue is:

Exercise

- Roll-down on Trapeze Table from Chapter 10

- Disc rotations from Chapter 10

- Inner Unit from Chapter 8

- Pelvic Floor exercise from Chapter 8

- Reformer: Compressions and Footwork with Activ-Wedge® under the concave ribcage/lighter area on the mat and another wedge placed perpendicularly underneath the lighter pelvic side. Use the familiar Footwork series.

- Partial Side hip lift from SSPOT-2 in Chapter 7

- 4-D de-rotation on Tower or Trapeze Table from Chapter 10

- Chair Psoas Pumps with wedge from Chapter 10

- Reformer leg circles with wedges

- Use the traditional leg circle series

- Elephant on Reformer with wedge from Chapter 10

- Wobble Board: 2-feet and 1-foot balance from Chapter 10.

The aging individual

Case example

One client of mine, who suffered from long-term Type 2 diabetes, finally developed spinal infections from the treatments and was severely kyphotic and side-bent due to his condition. I lovingly cared for him as a fragile elder rather than attempting

to correct such a situation. I managed to bolster and support him through gentle arm and rocking motions on the Trapeze Table. Although in a state near death, he appreciated the human contact and connection with his own body. It allowed him to relax to the other side.

The aging adult with scoliosis and asymmetry is particularly vulnerable, especially females. Women are more likely to reach old age and are more likely to have scoliosis and to be recipients of both knee and hip replacements (Kirkwood, 2010).

Joint replacement necessity often occurs as a comorbidity due to bodily compensations, resulting in osteoarthritis (Levine et al., 2009). Onset of arthritis is common in people with asymmetries.

Spinal arthritis correlates with spinal asymmetry. Scoliosis which developed in adolescence or manifested in adulthood tends to progress with age, sometimes rapidly as age increases, to become adult degenerative scoliosis.

Many question the concern over spinal asymmetry when there is no apparent problem. Reasons to address spinal asymmetry, even when there is no pain, are numerous.

Natural history of long-term progression of those with treated and untreated spinal asymmetry is incomplete in research. However, existing evidence shows that spontaneous improvement without some sort of attention appears not to be a practical approach.

A Saint Justine Cohort Study of 1476 subjects with adolescent idiopathic scoliosis suggests that back pain interfering with walking, socializing, lifting, and managing the pain is responsible for a considerable amount of disability and handicap in later life (Mayo et al., 1994).

Degenerative joint disease

Degenerative joint disease (DJD), also known as disc disease, is arthritis of the spine causing stiffness and stenosis, mostly narrowing of the areas between the vertebrae where the nerves exit. It needs decompression through flexion and traction.

However, if osteoporosis is present, use only neutral spinal positioning and substitute breathing exercises, particularly in the prone position.

Fostering lumbopelvic rhythm through flexion exercises promotes traction between the vertebrae as well. Include this beneficial list in your work (see below). Always cue the decompression of the concave areas whenever possible.

Table 12.1
Incidence of curvature progression in scoliosis: adults

Study	No. of cases	Beginning Cobb angle (range)	Incidence of progression
Ascani et al., 1986	187	<20 – >60°	100%
Bjerkrein & Hassan 1982	70	10 – 154°	60%
Collis & Ponseti 1969	134	<50 – >100°	69%
Korovessis et al., 1994	91	>10°	67%
Weinstein & Ponseti 1983	102	15 – 135°	68%

Reproduced from Hawes, M.C. (2010). Scoliosis and the Human Spine. Willowship Press, p. 25. Reproduced with permission from Martha C. Hawes.

Exercise

- Rotator discs with hand elevation from Chapter 10

- Roll-down/Roll-up on Trapeze Table with wedge from Chapter 10

- Twisty Cat (see Figure 12.13)

- Elephant with wedge from Chapter 10

- Chair with pike.

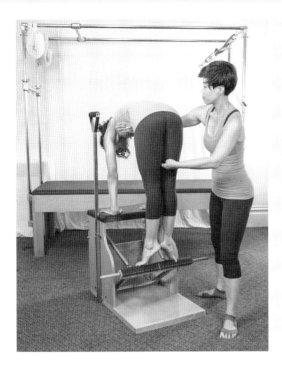

Figure 12.9

This traditional Chair exercise helps those who need spinal decompression. Use the asymmetry cues to open the concave ribs and waist through deeper flexion. Cue the adductors to meet to balance pelvic shift.

Spondylolisthesis

Spondylolisthesis is where one vertebra is slipped forward of another, creating a disruption in the normally smooth sagittal 'S' curve of the spine. It is a logical occurrence at the transition points between the curves.

Most people with an asymmetrical spine probably experience this effect to some degree whether youth or adult. However, some people are in specific danger from this condition. They usually know who they are, due to having received a medical diagnosis.

Controlled flexion and breathing exercises are best in general to help the condition. Neutral spine needs monitoring to ensure sway back and low back compression do not occur. Avoid spinal rotation and extension, especially when the arms or legs are extended out away from the body (Richardson et al., 2004).

Do not use the rotator discs with these people. Try the following exercises. Be sure to work in a pain-free zone. The use of rotator discs is contraindicated.

Exercise

- Trapeze Table bar Roll-down/Roll-up with wedge from Chapter 10
- Chair with pike with asymmetry and pelvic adductor cues
- ⚠ Stomach massage variations with small box support: A–D.

Continued

Part A. Use one red and one blue spring for the Stomach Massage Variation

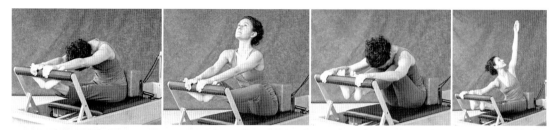

Figure 12.10

Place the small box against the shoulder rests. Place the metatarsals upon the foot bar in 1st Parallel. Grasp the foot bar with the palms of the hands. Inhale, exhale and extend the legs, pulling backwards by hollowing the abdominals. Gently cue the concave side of the ribs from the front to expand. Breathe 3 times. Inhale, reverse the action, flexing the hips and extending the spine.

Depress the convexity of the ribcage by gently encouraging the ribs down toward the waist. If the convexity is larger in the lumbar spine, use the same technique in this location. Repeat 4 more times.

Part B

Place the feet in the Pilates 'V' upon the foot bar. Grasp the foot bar with the palms on the inside of the 'V' on the foot bar. Inhale, exhale.

Lengthen the legs. Simultaneously reach the arm up and rainbow the arm on a diagonal angle away from shoulders. The body leans at an angle creating a thoracic rotation. Reverse the action by exhaling, elongating the hand, painting the ceiling and returning back to the foot bar as the hips simultaneously flex and the spine flexes. Repeat 4 more times alternating sides.

Disc herniation

Disc herniation is a serious condition that needs prioritization for healing. Avoid flexion of any kind including prolonged supine positions. Place a small folded towel underneath the lumbar spine for any supine or bedtime activities. Avoid any supine leg work below 45° to the horizon including leg circles. Prone work is beneficial. Lumbar spine stability is key.

- Inner Unit from Chapter 8
- Isometric Body Setting from Chapter 8
- Prone sacral stabilizer from Chapter 8
- Sidelying sacral stabilizer from Transverse Abdominals (TA) Correctives from Chapter 8
- All the neurodevelopmental positions from Chapter 8.

Hip and knee replacements

Both hip and knee replacements affect the anterior outer chain coordinating adductor to opposite oblique abdominals. Almost all fascial lines receive impact.

The Deep Frontal Line and, especially, the Lateral and Spiral Lines are disrupted due to scar tissue build-up. Rotary compensations into the legs both up and down the chains create more twist, pain, and discomfort.

Avoid the Arc stretches from Chapter 9. Observe all precautions from the Scoliosis Medical Team.

Concentrate on general strength in neutral spine. Avoid crossing the legs. Start with standing exercises or simple mat recommended from the PT to begin until full healing takes place about one year out.

Hip and knee replacement fascial stretches

These two stretches directly address multidirectional fascial stretch needed to allow the muscular links to re-coordinate. Do not stay in this stretch more than 5–10 minutes.

Exercise

☑ *Part A. Modified Magician Elongation: A–D*

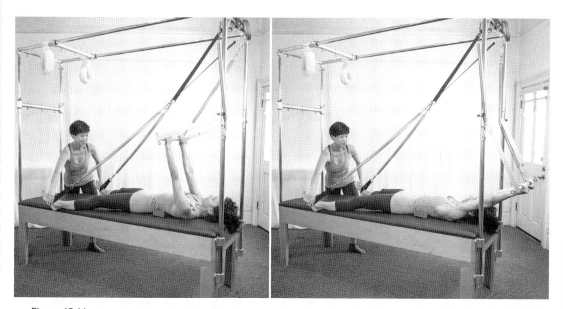

Figure 12.11

Attach a pair of yellow springs to D-ring medium length Reformer foot straps. Place the feet into foot loops. Lengthen the arms behind the head with the push-through bar. Use the asymmetry cues and wedges. Place one wedge under the lighter pelvis, and one under the ribcage that has less contact with the mat. Stay and breathe 5–10 minutes.

☑ *Part B. Leg Straightener: A–D*

This exercise benefits those with both knock knees as well as bow legs. Long-sit, in front of a mirror if possible. Place a strong stretchy band around the thighs, a rubber band around the great toes, and a ball between the knees. A wedge can also be placed underneath the heavier pelvic side between the IT and the coccyx, or underneath the lighter side for operative clients. Line up the second toe with the mid-patella and hip joint at mid-pant line. Note the girth of the lateral thighs. On the side where there is less girth, cue the thigh to slightly press away from the mid-line (abduction) Then take a weighted ball and hold it overhead.

Continued

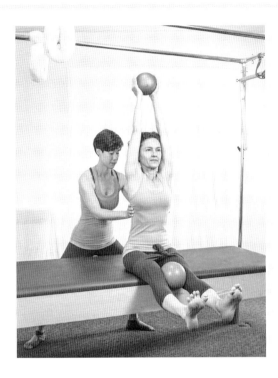

Figure 12.12

Cue the client in their specific asymmetry cues. Then 3 times, cue breathe in, grow tall, exhale, grow taller. Attempt to stay in the pose for 1–2 minutes.

Exercise

⚡ *Twisty Cat with hands on Long Box on Reformer: A–D*

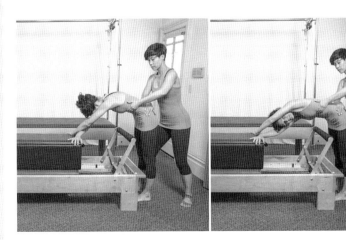

Figure 12.13

This exercise is a mainstay in my repertoire. Direct the reach from the shorter hand side from the vertical compression test. Cue the concave ribcage areas to open on the return after the push-out.

Use one blue spring. Start in the direction of the easier way to twist. If you twist more easily to the left, then place the right arm underneath the left. Leg position is 1st Parallel. Hollow the waist. Exhale. Move the legs to the foot bar, lean onto it. Cue the client so that the bar does not move. Lengthen the arms and spine. Lift the left elbow and look underneath it. Then de-rotate/cue the concave ribs to lift. Let the carriage push the client back to the original position. Perform 5 repetitions each way.

Additional beneficial exercises are:

- Chair Psoas Pumps from Chapter 10
- Elephant with wedges from Chapter 10
- Inverted hip abduction from Chapter 10.

Note that the inverted abduction exercise is for knee replacement clients only and not intended for those with hip replacements.

Spinal post-operative conditions and others requiring baseline extensions

Clients with spinal fixation, spinal bone spur pain and bone thinness due to osteoporosis need core strength too. Strengthening the engagement of deep spinal musculature in static positions with little or no spinal motion but with breathing and arm motion plus spring and carriage motion resistance greatly aids this group.

Quadruped, supported anterior waist prone and kneeling give additional support without compromising structures. Clients who are approximately one year post-operative should still start in standing, quadruped, sitting, kneeling and prone.

Exercise

☑ *Rib Shift control: A–E*

Figure 12.14

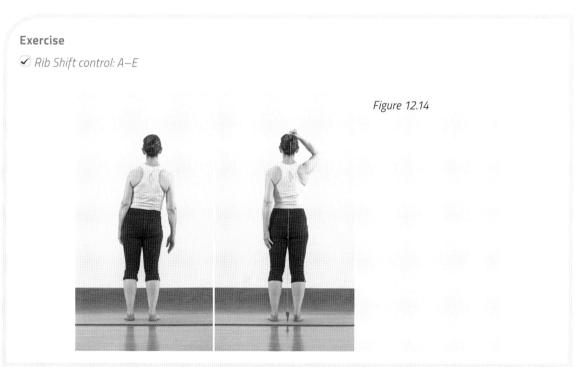

Continued

It is of utmost importance to acquire rib shift control post-operatively, but it is also an important skill for everyone.

The fixation of surgery does not hold the spine up against gravity. The body half from the waist up is very heavy. Some older clients with Harrington Rods have actually broken the rods.

The Straw exercise Body Skill from Chapter 8 teaches non-operative clients to elongate and attempt to balance the horizontal lines of the shoulders and pelvis. Rib Shift Control is a Body Skill for operative clients to learn to stand up inside the fixation by elongating and keeps the ribcage inside the frame of the vertical pelvis.

☑ *Isometric Proprioceptive Neuromuscular Facilitation (PNF): A–E*

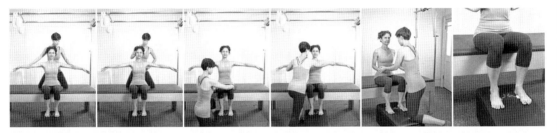

Figure 12.15

PNF concepts help post-operatively. The client sits upon the Trapeze Table with the legs in 1st Parallel. Place two 'feet mice' (lamb's wool or unrolled cotton from tampons) underneath the soles of the feet.

- Cue the client in a Short Foot exercise. Feel as if the sole is lifting the cotton upwards, shortening the distance between the heel and the metatarsals. Avoid curling the toes.

- Cue the client to elongate the spine. Stand behind the client and place two flat hands on the space between the shoulder blades while the client breathes 3 times.

- Then systematically move the hands to the next locations starting at the shoulders and proceeding out along the arms around the elbows and forearms, maintaining easy, steady pressure for the breathing client.

- Next move to the front of the body. Place each hand on the outside of the thighs and press toward the mid-line as the client resists. Then alternate and place the hands on the inside of the knees and press outwards as the client attempts to preserve the 1st Parallel. Perform only one set of breathing in each location.

Inner Unit

See Chapter 8.

4-D de-rotation on Tower or Trapeze Table

See Chapter 10.

☑ *Kneeling Reformer series: A–D. Four parts*

Be sure to cue the asymmetry cues of the anterior rib protrusion hold, weighting the lighter knee, engaging the sit bone to tail equally, along with other appropriate cues. All use one blue or red spring:

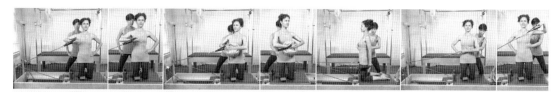

Figure 12.16

Part 1. Horizontal adduction of the arms

- Kneel in the middle of the carriage with the knees in 1st Parallel with a wedge underneath the lighter knee.
- Place one hand in the front loop (direction being faced) or hand grip with the forearm parallel to the floor below the chest height. Place the other hand rounded on the side of the pelvis and press toward the pulleys as the top hand slices across the chest in a horizontal motion. Repeat 5–9 times more.

Part 2. Ball rotation

Place a soft ball between the abdomen and the clasped hands. Hold the headlights of the pelvis forward as the spine rotates within the frame of the body away from the pulleys. Do not exceed a normal, comfortable range. Use the eye dominance cue to help rotation to the more difficult direction. Repeat 5–9 times more.

Part 3. Chest expansion

- Place one wedge underneath the lighter knee. Place the knees farther away from the shoulder rests to use the wedge. Splay the fingers and place the thumbs into the smile lines. Increase the pressure into the legs as able. Exhale as the hands move backwards.
- Stay and exhale as the chin deliberately turns to one side and tilts slightly toward that shoulder while, elongating the clavicle on the opposite side. Repeat 5–9 times more.

Part 4. Pull sword

Face toward the side again. Place the legs in 1st Parallel. Hold the pelvis with the hand by the pulleys. Pull the loop from the pelvis to the chest and up toward the shoulder and return back down to the hip. Start with low resistance. Repeat 5–9 times more.

☑ *Dynamic Plantigrade: Moving Quadruped: A–D. Two parts*

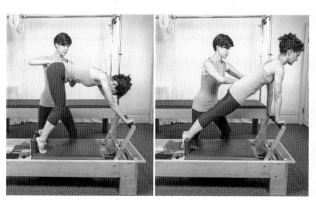

Figure 12.17

Continued

Dynamic plantigrade exercise safely engages whole body core without compromising the post-operative spine. Perform these typical Pilates exercises from Chapter 10:

- Part 1. Jackrabbit.
- Part 2. Long stretch.
- ☑ Prone Long Box Reformer Pulling and Pushing Ropes (modified Swan): A–D. Two parts:
  - Part 1. Prone Long Box pull ropes without thoracic extension: facing pulleys with either one blue or one red spring.
  - Part 2. Prone push ropes; modified Swan without thoracic extension; facing the base using one blue spring.

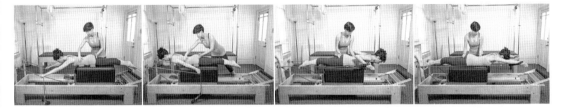

Figure 12.18

☑ *Standing arm work: A–C*

Standing arm work with springs from the Trapeze Table or Ped-o-Pull is excellent for this group. Face the Table. Dog paddle the hands.

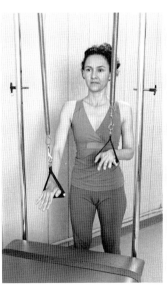

Figure 12.19

☑ *Wobble Board sequence from Chapter 10 (Figure 10.32):*

Emphasize single leg use. Start with the stronger leg and repeat with the weaker leg.

Bibliography

Abei, M. (2005). The adult scoliosis. European Spine Journal, 14(10), 925–938. doi:10.1007/s00586-005-1053-9

Altan, L., Korkmaz, N., Bingol, U., Gunay, B. (2009). Effect of Pilates training on people with fibromyalgia: a pilot study. Archives of Physical Medicine and Rehabilitation, 90, 1983–1988. Retrieved January 26, 2017, from: http://myalgia.com/PDF%20files/Pilates%20for%20Fibromyalgia%202010.pdf

Alves de Araújo, M.E., Bezerra da Silva, E., Bragade Mello, D. et al. (2012). The effectiveness of the Pilates method: reducing the degree of non-structural scoliosis, and improving flexibility and pain in female college students. Journal of Bodywork and Movement Therapies, 16(2), 191–198. doi:10.1016/j.jbmt.2011.04.002

Ascani, E., Bartolozzi, P., Logroscino, C.A. et al. (1986). Natural history of untreated idiopathic scoliosis after skeletal maturity. Spine (Phila Pa 1976), 11(8), 784–789

Asher, M.A., Burton, D.C. (2006). Adolescent idiopathic scoliosis: natural history and long term treatment effects. Scoliosis, 1: 2. doi: 10.1186/1748-7161-1-2

Balanced Body. (2014). Selected bibliography of recent research articles on Pilates. Retrieved August 26, 2018, from: www.pilates.com: https://www.pilates.com/BBAPP/V/pilates/library/bibliography.html

Balsamo, S., Willardson, J.M., Frederico, S. de S. et al. (2013). Effectiveness of exercise on cognitive impairment and Alzheimer's disease. International Journal of General Medicine, 6, 387–391. Retrieved February 5, 2017, from: http://europepmc.org/articles/PMC3668090

Betz, S.R. (2005). Modifying Pilates for clients with osteoporosis. IDEA Fitness Journal, 46–55. Retrieved January 29, 2017, from: http://www.ideafit.com/fitness-library/pilates-osteoporosis

Białek, M., Pawlak, P., Kotwicki, T. (2009). Foot loading asymmetry in patients with scoliosis. Scoliosis, 4 (Suppl. 1): 019. doi: 10.1186/1748-7161-4-S1-O19

Bjerkrein, I., Hassan, I. (1982). Progression in untreated idiopathic scoliosis after end of growth. Acta Orthopaedica Scandinavica, 53(6), 897–900

Blom, M.-J. (2012). Pilates and fascia: the art of 'working in'. In: Schleip, R., Findley, T.W., Chaitow, L., Huijing, P.A. eds. Fascia: The Tensional Network of the Human Body. New York: Churchill Livingstone Elsevier, pp. 449–456

Borghuis, J, Hof, A.L., Lemmink, K.A. (2008). The importance of sensory-motor control in providing core stability: implications for measurement and training. Sports Medicine, 38(11), 893–916

Burwell, R.G., Ranjit K Aujla, R. K., Grevitt, M. P. et al. (2009). Pathogenesis of adolescent idiopathic scoliosis in girls – a double neuro-osseous theory involving disharmony between two nervous systems, somatic and autonomic expressed in the spine and trunk: possible dependency on sympathetic nervous system and hormones. Scoliosis and Spinal Disorders, 4: 24. doi: 10.1186/1748-7161-4-24

Chaitow, L. (2012). Breathing pattern Disorders. Retrieved August 26, 2018, from: http://leonchaitow.com/2012/01/23/breathing-pattern-disorders-and-lumbopelvic-pain-and-dysfunction-an-update/

Collis, D.K., Ponseti, I.V. (1969). Long-term follow-up patients with idiopathic scoliosis not treated surgically. Journal of Bone and Joint Surgery, 51(3), 425–444.

Core Dynamics and Pilates. (2007). All about Eve. Santa Fe,New Mexico, USA

Czaprowski, D, Kotwicki, T., Pawlowska, P. Stolinksi, L. (2012). Joint hypermobility syndrome in children with idiopathic scoliosis. Scoliosis, 7(Suppl. 1): 069. doi:10.1186/1748-7161-7-S1-O69

EDS International Classification. (2017). Retrieved September 1, 2017, from The Ehlers–Danlos Society: https://www.ehlers-danlos.com/2017-eds-international-classification/

Eisen, P. F. (1981). The Pilates Method, Vol. 1. New York: Warner Books

The Female Athlete Triad. (2011). Retrieved September 1, 2017, from www.acsm.org: http://www.femaleathletetriad.org/wp-content/uploads/2010/03/FATC_Slideshow_2011.pdf

Hawes, M.C. (2003). The use of exercises in the treatment of scoliosis: an evidence-based critical review of the literature. Pediatric Rehabilitation, 6(3–4), 171–182

Henneman, E., Somjen, G., Carpenter, D.O. (1965). Functional significance of cell size in spinal motoneurons. Journal of Neurophysiology, 28(3), 560–580

Jaroszweski, D, Notricia, D., McMahon, L., et al. (2010). Current management of pectus excavatum: a review and update of therapy and treatment recommendations. Journal of American Board of Family Medicine, 23(2), 230–239

Kaya, D.O., Duzgun, I., Baltaci, G. et al. (2012). Effects of calisthenics and Pilates exercises on coordination and proprioception in adult women: a randomized controlled trial. Journal of Sport Rehabilitation, 21(3), 235–243. Retrieved September 1, 2017, from: http://www.academia.edu/1123285/Effects_of_Calisthenics_and_Pilates_Exercises_on_Coordination_and_Proprioception_in_Adult_Women_Randomized_Controlled_Trial

Kendall, F.P., McCreary, E.K., Provance, P. G., eds. Muscles: Testing and Function, 4th edn. Baltimore: Williams and Wilkins

Kirkwood, T. (2010). Why women live longer. Scientific American, pp. 34–36. Retrieved February 5, 2017, from: https://www.scientificamerican.com/article/why-women-live-longer/

Knight, I., MacCormick, M., Bird, H. (2012). Managing Joint Hypermobility – A guide for Dance Teachers. London: South West Music School

Korovessis, P., Piperos, G., Sidiropoulos, P., Dimas, A. (1994). Adult idiopathic lumbar scoliosis. A formula for prediction of progression and review of the literature. Spine, 19, 1926–1932

Larsson, M. (2013). All about Eve. Retrieved August 13, 2018, from: http://coredynamicspilates.com/wp-content/uploads/2014/10/AllAboutEve-SantaFe-NM.pdf.

Levine B., Kaplanek, B., Jaffe, W.L. (2009). Pilates training for use in rehabilitation after total hip and knee arthroplasty.

Clinical Orthopaedics and Related Research, 467(6), 1465–1475

Lewton-Brain, P.A. (2008). Back-bend or spinal extension? Biomechanics and multi-sliced computed tomography and movement intention. Centre Hospitale de Princesse Grace. Monaco: Centre Hospitale de Princesse Grace

Lin, J.J., Chen, W.H., Chen, P.Q., Tsauo, J.Y. (2010). Alteration in shoulder kinematics and associated muscle activity in people with idiopathic scoliosis. Spine, 35(11), 1151– 1157

Lowe, T.G., Burwell, R.G., Dangerfield, P.H. (2004). Platelet calmodulin levels in adolescent idiopathic scoliosis (AIS): can they predict curve progression and severity? European Spine Journal, 13(3), 257–265

Mayo, N.E., Goldberg, M.S., Scott, S., Hanley, J. (1994). The Ste-Justine Adolescent Idiopathic Scoliosis Cohort Study. Part III: Back pain. Spine (Phila Pa 1976), 19(14), 1573– 1581

McNaughton, S., Farley, D., Staggs, R., et al. (2008). Pregnancy, fertility, and contraception risk in the context of chronic disease: scoliosis. Journal for Nurse Practitioners, 4(5), 370–376

Mueller, M.G., Lewicky-Gaupp, C., Collins, S.A. et al. (2017) Activity restriction recommendations and outcomes after reconstructive pelvic surgery, a randomized controlled study. Obstetrics and Gynecology, 129(4), 608–614

Myers, T.W. (2014). Anatomy Trains: Myofascial Meridians for Manual and Movement Therapists, 3rd edn. Edinburgh: Churchill Livingstone

National Center for Chronic Disease Prevention. (2013). The State of aging and health in America 2013. Retrieved February 5, 2017, from Center for Disease Control: https://www.cdc.gov/aging/pdf/state-aging-health-in-america-2013.pdf

Negrini, A., Parzini, S., Negrini, M.G. et al. (2008). Adult scoliosis can be reduced through specific SEAS exercises: a case report. Scoliosis and Spinal Disorders, 3: 20. doi:10.1186/1748-7161-3-20

Osteoporosis in men. (2017). Retrieved August 26, 2018, from National Institutes of Health: https://www.bones.nih.gov/health-info/bone/osteoporosis/men

Phrompaet S., Paungmali, A., Pirunsan, U., Sitilertpisan, P. (2011). Effects of Pilates training on lumbo-pelvic stability and flexibility. Asian Journal of Sports Medicine, 2(1), 16–22

Pilates, J.H. (1945) [2010]. Return to Life Through Contrology. Miami, Florida: Pilates Method Alliance

Pilates Method Alliance. (2017). The 2016 Pilates in America Study. Retrieved August 28, 2018, from: https://www.pilatesmethodalliance.org/i4a/pages/index.cfm?pageID=3821

Rabago, D., Slattengren, A., Zgierska, A. (2010). Prolotherapy in primary care practice. Primary Care, 37(1), 65–80

Rapoport, I. C. (2016). A Day with Joseph Pilates. Retrieved January 27, 2017, from: http://icrapoport.com/category/onassignment/sports-illustrated/

Richardson, C., Hodges, P.W., Hides, J. (2004). Therapeutic Exercise for Spinal Segmental Stabilization in Low Back Pain: Scientific Basis and Clinical Approach, 2nd edn. Edinburgh: Churchill Livingstone

Rock, J.A., Roberts, C.P., Jones, H.W., Jr. (2010). Congenital anomalies of the uterine cervix: lessons from 30 cases managed clinically by a common protocol. Fertility and Sterility, 94(5), 1858–1863

Saccuci, M., Tettamanti, L., Mummolo, S. et al. (2011). Scoliosis and dental occlusion: a review of the literature. Scoliosis, 6: 15. doi:10.1186/1748-7161-6-15

Schoeneman, S. (2007–2008). Implementing Pilates into my practice. Retrieved August 28, 2018, from Balanced Body: http://www.pilates.com/BBAPP/V/pilates/library/articles/implementing-pilates-into-my-practice.html

Silva, F.E., Lenke, L.G. (2010). Adult degenerative scoliosis: evaluation and management. Neurosurgery Focus, 28(3), E1. Retrieved February 2, 2017, from http://thejns.org/doi/pdf/10.3171/2010.1.FOCUS09271

Svantesson, H., Marhaug, G., Haeffner, F. (1981). Scoliosis in children with juvenile rheumatoid arthritis. Scandinavian Journal of Rheumatology, 10(2), 65–68

Tate, L. (2015). Prevalence of scoliosis in a Pelvic Pain Cohort. Journal of Women's Health Physical Therapy, 39(1), 3–9

Thompson, B. (2016). Case of 2 female elderly cadaver donors with scoliosis. Interview with Bonnie Thompson, Institute for Anatomical Research (http://www.anatomicalresearch.org/) (S. Martin, Interviewer).

van der Linden, M.L., Bulley, C., Geneen, L.J. et al. (2014). Pilates for people with multiple sclerosis who use a wheelchair: feasibility, efficacy and participant experiences. Disability and Rehabilitation, 36(11), 932–939.

Virginia Spine Institute. (2017). Spinal Curvatures. Retrieved February 4, 2017, from Spine MD: http://www.spinemd.com/symptoms-conditions/flat-back-syndrome

Watson, J. (2012). Sarcopenia in older adults. Current Opinions in Rheumatology, 24(6), 623–627

Weinstein, S.L., Dolan, L.A., Spratt, K.F. (2003). Health and function of patients with untreated idiopathic scoliosis: a 50-year natural history study. JAMA, 289(5), 559–567

Weinstein, S.L., Ponseti, I.V. (1983). Curve progression in idiopathic scoliosis. Journal of Bone & Joint Surgery, 65(4), 447–455

What is Lifestyle Medicine? (2015, January 1). Retrieved January 26, 2017, from American College of Lifestyle Medicine: https://www.lifestylemedicine.org/What-is-Lifestyle-Medicine/

Which Pilates exercises are good for someone with Parkinson's disease? (2017). Retrieved January 29, 2017, from MedicineNet.com: http://www.medicinenet.com/script/main/art.asp?articlekey=78165

Women's International Pharmacy. (2013). Pelvic organ prolapse: what can be done to prevent it? Retrieved February 5, 2017, from Connections: An Educational Resource of Women's International Pharmacy: http://womensinternational.com/connections/prolapse.html

Summary and final words

Embrace the complexity and uniqueness of each client. Use the summary as a guide. Cookbook-style exercise instruction is best avoided. One way to avoid becoming overwhelmed with the sheer enormity of the material is to read through it and implement it in stages, not all at once. Give time for some unconscious thought for both you and the client. Often clarity arrives later, after a time of being away from the client's personality. Intuitive solutions often occur when the conscious mind is not straining for a solution.

Start systematically. That is the purpose of the GPOA and SSPOT. They begin the conversation.

Educate everyone with the 3 Es. Always infuse art with the science. Dive deeper within exercises, mixing the somatic element with larger exercises or layer the depth of an exercise from session to session as the movement becomes more familiar. Imagine. Think. Feel. Monitor the form points of the exercise. Then cue the layers of imagery, anatomy, alignment, and match up the physicality to the emotion, which is optimally a pleasant experience, even if challenging. Strive for a whole-body experience, using the four diaphragm images to connect the body.

Degree guidelines for severity of the Cobb angle

A = 0–10° Normal expected degree of spinal asymmetry

B = 10–20° Mild

C = 21–40° Moderate

D = >40° Severe

E = >70° Severe with possible medical breathing issues.

Use extra precaution with any operative clients that either have spinal hardware or other hardware due to joint and bone repairs or replacements.

PMME goals

Understand the profound influence of the PMME. A leader impacts other people, sets a direction, sets a standard, and is a role model. To become a great role model, stick to the important tasks of educating the client, prioritizing your sessions, and staying on point. Focus on helping others achieve their goals and dreams. Be systematic. The overriding goal of the PMME is to organize and to build a functional body, centralizing the vertical body as much as possible. Perform frequent Scoliometer® readings to screen for curve progression. Clients with measures above 35 degrees mandate a team approach. The PMME operates as an anti-seismic function, bolstering the structure against earthquake activity.

Goals for youth

- Educate that good general posture is mandatory for clients with asymmetry

- Educate youth appropriate to age comprehension ability

- Educate and support parents/guardians and Team members

- Stabilize the progression of a deformity

- Support brace use (usually for 20° and higher)

- Support post-brace physical development

- Promote strength physical development delivery in a palatable way to promote compliance and consistency – make it fun

- Support post-operative lifestyle physical adaptations.

Goals for adults

- Educate for lifestyle factors for nutrition, work life, home life according to time of life
- Prioritize for co-conditions and co-morbidities, including post-surgical spinal interventions
- Promote spinal extension – emphasize waist elongation
- Improve gait and balance
- Promote postural exercise to avoid osteoarthritis
- Promote larger muscle group exercise to lessen the effects of sarcopenia and osteoporosis for aging adults
- Promote consistent use of Body Skills
- Encourage complementary physical pursuits such as travel, child care, gardening, sports, social life that align with physical development.

3 Es

- Ergonomics
- Exercise
- Emotion.

3 phases of exercise

- Somatic
- Corrective
- Conditioning.

Table 13.1
Goals for times of life

Time of life	Educate	Encourage	Manage
Children	Use SSPOT to start	Play for adherence Enroll parental participation in exercise	Study postures, book bag postures
Adolescence	Use graduated education, giving information in stages Start with SSPOT	Body Skill development Coping skills Group participation and support	Study postures Consistency – forming a habit of Body Skills and SSPOT skills
Child-bearing years	Prenatal core, leg and spine care Positioning for breast feeding Staged restoration of post-natal time Both sexes need help in how to handle unwieldy weight of small children	Staged return to exercise post-natally Positive sleep habits Ergonomic aides for infant care and childcare	Prenatal and postnatal laxity Sleep deprivation for men and women Occupational prolonged sitting and standing Foot issues
Mid-life	Need for rib mobility, lumbar stability, gait balancing	Prophylactic attention to potential waist collapse, beginning of muscle diminishment	Waist collapse Leg imbalances Balance and fall prevention
Menopause	Importance of weight-bearing exercise, pelvic exercises	Prophylactic attention to pelvic weakness Continuation of cardio exercise	Pelvic and leg weakness Single leg balance Equal gait
70+	Need for bone health Need for nutrition Need to attend to muscle tone and girth	Staying the course for a functional life Goals of participation in travel, childcare, leisure activities, sports	Community program accessibility Exercise inclusion into all activity areas

Dual influences for spinal asymmetry care

Neuromuscular (neurological influences on the muscular system)

- Balance
- Laterality in tasks – handedness and leg use
- Eye dominance
- Innate asymmetries
- Learned skills.

Musculoskeletal (fascia–muscle–tendon–bone–ligaments)

- Innate asymmetries in cranial region, respiratory diaphragm, pelvis
- Developed asymmetries in head bones, vertebrae, rib lengths, arm lengths, leg lengths
- Physical developed asymmetries due to strategies.

Common areas of typical difficulty in spinal asymmetry

- Eye vision imbalance
- Head balance over center of gravity (COG) (implications for inner ear use)
- Protruding anterior costal cartilage (usually in the region of the false ribs 8–10, which attach to the 7th rib by cartilage only)
- Rib rotation dysfunction
- Ribs on the convex side are stiff and more elevated
- Ribs on the concave side are depressed likely with tighter internal fascia
- Winging shoulder (serratus anterior imbalance)
- Serratus posterior imbalance (breathing imbalance)
- Hip hike (quadratus lumborum and tensor fascia lata dominance)
- Collapsing waist (inner unit core weakness)

- Pelvic obliquity (imbalance in pelvic floor, large hip musculature, and pelvic rotator cuff)
- Stride and foot strike imbalance (spine, pelvic and leg joint wear and tear).

Follow the order

- Identify the pattern
- Break up the pattern
- Re-direct the pattern
- Correct the pattern
- Beyond the pattern.

Identify the pattern

- GPOA-1 and GPOA-2
- SSPOT-1 and SSPOT-2.

Lay the foundation

Attend to the codes: ☑ indicates whether it is also indicated for those with spinal fixation, ⚡ indicates the exercise is contraindicated for those with fixation. If in doubt, leave it out.

Start with breath, posture, introduce the ND positions and correctives from the SSPOTs.

Optimizing the ZOA and spinal asymmetry

- ☑ Standing ZOA cues
- ⚡ The Pelvic Spool
- ⚡ Breath of Fire
- ☑ Counting to 15 during exhalation.

Neurodevelopmental positions

- Supine
- Prone
- Sidelying
- Sitting
- Quadruped

- Kneeling
- Half-kneeling
- Plantigrade (Down Dog)
- Standing – one leg.

Initial body coordination

- ☑ Imprinting compressions
- ☑ Isometric Body Setting
- ☑ Prone sacral stabilizer
- ☑ Lower body toner
- ☑ Pelvic Floor exercise
- ☑ Straw exercise
- ☑ Inner Unit exercise
- Pelvic imbalance solutions (from the SSPOT in Ch. 7), Part 1
- Three functional core muscle group test correctives from the Straight Leg Raise tests.

Transverse abdominals (TA) correctives

- ☑ Sacral stabilizer
- ⚠ Articulating bridging.

Multifidi (MF) correctives

- ☑ Multifidi training
- ☑ Inner Unit exercise.

Pelvic Floor (PF) correctives

- ☑ Lower body toner
- ☑ PF exercise
- ☑ Prone sacral stabilizer
- Functional group correctives (from the SSPOT in Ch. 7), Part 2
- Tensor fascia lata (TFL) dominance correctives:
  - ☑ Lower body toner
  - ☑ Psoas trainers and Toe Touches
  - ☑ Half- kneeling cueing.

- Functional group correctives (from the SSPOT-1 in Ch. 7), Part 3

Sidelying handedness correctives

- ☑ Sidelying hip rotation and adduction

Breaking up the pattern

Incorporate some type of fascial motion. Youth work well with the Arc, rolling, and Activ-Wedges®. Adults work well with wedge products used for passive stretching as well as Activ-Wedges®, rotator discs, and rings. Select a few.

Be sure to attend to the codes since many of the exercises in this section are not intended for post-fixation use: ☑ indicates whether it is also indicated for those with spinal fixation, ⚠ indicates the exercise is contraindicated for those with fixation. If in doubt, leave it out. Many exercises in this section are not intended for those with spinal fixation.

Positional release with props

- ☑ Constructive rest position (90/90)
- ⚠ Baby Arc fascial stretching
- ⚠ One-lung Breathing on Baby Arc.

Activ-Wedge® De-rotation mobilizations

> **Wedge use: quick check**
>
> - ☑ *Supine:* which shoulder is off the mat? Which pelvic side is higher or lighter off the mat?
> - ☑ *Prone:* which rib area is falling into the mat? Which pelvic side is lighter off the mat?
> - ☑ *Sidelying:* which side has more light under it?
> - ☑ *Sitting:* which pelvic side seems heavier into the mat?
> - ☑ *Kneeling:* which knee not as heavy into the floor?
> - ☑ *Half-kneeling:* which knee is less vertical and which forefoot needs more weight?
> - ☑ *Inversion:* which heel is higher off the mat; which side of the pelvis is lower from the ceiling?
> - ☑ *Standing:* which side of the pelvis has more lateral sway?

- ⚡ Supine prop use and placement
- ☑ Prone Ice Cube exercise with (see Figure 8.12)
- ⚡ Balloon with pelvic bridge.

Laterality

- ☑ Sidelying handedness correctives
- ⚡ Baby Rolls
- ⚡ X-rolls
- ⚡ Seated Core Pillow
- ⚡ Shift mobilization
- ☑ Figure of eight with Magic Circle
- ⚡ Standing disc rotations
- ⚡ Scolio-moves.

Re-direct the pattern

Incorporate elements of the spinal, ribcage and pelvic solutions as the client advances in familiarity, skill and tolerance of the system. Attend to the codes: ☑ indicates whether it is also indicated for those with spinal fixation; ⚡ indicates the exercise is contraindicated for those with fixation. If in doubt, leave it out.

Functional solutions for the spine

Unweighting

- ⚡ Mat 'C' exercise
- ☑ Sidelying hip flexion.

Fascial unwinding

⚡ Disc rotations from Chapter 9.

Stability training in the asymmetry cues

- ☑ Reformer footwork with wedges
- ☑ Reformer: No-springs abdominals
- ☑ or ⚡ Half-barrel or Arc Prone Swimming
- ☑ Chair Psoas Pumps
- ☑ Traditional safe Pilates repertoire for spinal stability:
  - Part A. Long Stretch

- Part B. Jackrabbit
- Part C. Long Box: pulling ropes
- Part D. Modified Swan: pushing ropes
- Traditional Pilates Chair for advanced clients
- ⚡ Chair Sidelying Hand Pedal Presses.

Elongation

- ☑ Trapeze Table Horse
- ☑ 4-D de-rotation on Tower or Trapeze Table
- ⚡ Balancing 'O' Mat Exercise from SSPOT-2, Chapter 7.

Articulation

- ⚡ Roll-down/Roll-up on Trapeze Table
- ☑ Sling Hip Circles
- ⚡ Twisty Cat
- ⚡ Spinal Spiral.

Functional solutions for the ribcage

Mobility

- ⚡ Mat; Arc/One-lung Breathing from Chapter 8
- ⚡ Thoracic Mobilizer.

Fascial unwinding for functional movement

- ☑ Ribcage interventions = Rooster hands and ball
- ⚡ Spine Corrector: fall and release with dowel or Mini Bar

Stability training

☑ Reverse abdominals

Articulation

- ⚡ Cleopatra
- ⚡ Pigeon.

Elongation

⚡ Sidelying Bar Slides on Trapeze Table.

Functional solutions for the pelvis

Dissociation mobility of legs from pelvis

- ☑ Trapeze Table triangle elongation/Reformer elephant version
- ☑ Quadruped sling
- ⚡ Bilateral leg lift.

Fascial unwinding

- ☑ Reformer Half-kneel with Magic Circle
- ⚡ Reformer Semi-circle
- ⚡ Dreaded Frog/circles and scissors.

Stability training

- ☑ Half- kneel spine rotations
- ☑ Chair sideways mountain climber
- ☑ Weighted ball
- ⚡ Confounded balance.

Elongation

⚡ Side-bend on Short Box with Mini Bar

☑ Inverted abductions.

Articulation

- ☑ Dreaded Frog
- ☑ Wobble Board
- ⚡ Scolio-moves.

Correct the pattern: 3 Es into everyday life

Keep reinforcing and discussing life skills. Select one or two each session.

Ergonomics

- Sitting
- Standing
- Transitioning sit to stand
- Stair stepping
- General walking
- Sleeping.

Exercise

- *Daily basic maintenance:* select exercises appropriate to either those without spinal fixation or those with fixation.
- ☑ Baker's Dozen Body Skills.

Emotion

Encourage stable emotions in the four areas where PMMEs help, which include breathing exercises, the choice of exercise body positions, vocalization and interoception.

Beyond the curves

- Create individualized cues from the assessments. Be sure to use the neurologic asymmetry correctives of handedness, eye and tongue use, at least intermittently. This strategy provides a safe back door to exercise skill acquisition, particularly if the client is unable to access large movements because of the need for precaution, especially after spinal fixation surgery.

- Acknowledge difficult moves within the Method along with addressing pain or sacral instability first. Employ judicious spinal flexion in those without fixation, making sure that the client is able or not able to bend in the sagittal directions, either due to lack of skill, lack of pliability, or due to contraindication for medical diagnoses. Work in neutral until safety is determined.

- Use programming appropriate to the times of life by differentiating between an approach for youth and an approach for adults.

- Follow the guidelines for hypermobile clients and athletic clients.

- Be mindful of the presence of female pelvic pain, and the special issues for women regarding pregnancy and prolapse.

- Note that osteoporosis not only occurs with aging but can also affect athletic women.

- Follow proper guidelines for spinal conditions such as herniation, degenerative disc disease and joint replacements. When in doubt, refer out.

- PMMEs hold a special place of influence for post-bracing and postoperative spinal asymmetry clients. Work with the Team.

Final words

A Method is a way or a path to accomplish something. Before you begin, go inside yourself. Ask yourself if you are a person who wants to make a difference. No Method is strong enough to replace discipline and passion. These characteristics do not come from a Method, they come from the soul. If you make those two things active in your practice, the Method will work for you.

Filling a gap in care as a client negotiates how to weave in, through, around and, possibly, out of a medical model is beyond monetary value. Every client is an opportunity to donate to the asymmetrical pool with wellness. Give the gift of life. Every action begins with thought. Imagine, think and feel. The client may not turn into what you thought the person was meant to be, yet the client will become who they are meant to be. I have faith in you.

INDEX

T